Rehabilitating Bodies

Rehabilitating Bodies

Health, History, and the
American Civil War

LISA A. LONG

PENN

University of Pennsylvania Press

Philadelphia

10 9 8 7 6 5 4 3 2 1

Published by
University of Pennsylvania Press
Philadelphia, Pennsylvania 19104-4011

Library of Congress Cataloging-in-Publication Data

Long, Lisa A.
  Rehabilitating bodies : health, history, and the American Civil War / Lisa A. Long.
    p.   cm.
  Includes bibliographical references and index.
  ISBN 0-8122-3748-X (cloth : alk. paper)
  1. United States—History—Civil War, 1861–1865—Historiography.   2. United
States—History—Civil War, 1861–1865—Health aspects.   3. United States—
History—Civil War, 1861–1865—Psychological aspects.   4. United States—History—
Civil War, 1861–1865—Literature and the war.   5. Ontology.   6. Ontology in
literature.   7. Knowledge, Theory of.   8. Knowledge, Theory of, in literature.
9. Body, Human (Philosophy)   10. Body, Human, in literature.   I. Title.

E468.5.L66   2004   2003060200
973.7—dc22

Contents

Introduction
Year That Trembled and Reel'd beneath Me

But in silence, in dreams' projections,
While the world of gain and appearance and mirth goes on,
So soon what is over forgotten, and waves wash the imprints off the sand,
With hinged knees returning I enter the doors (while for you up there,
Whoever you are, follow without noise and be of strong heart).

—Walt Whitman, "The Wound-Dresser"

On July 21, 1861, hundreds of Washington, D.C., residents packed picnic lunches and headed to a country hillside to watch the first large-scale battle of the Civil War. Able to see little but smoke, spectators soon panicked as the performance on the field threatened those in the audience; shells began to explode around them, and in the hazy stampede of equally frightened, inexperienced Union forces retreating to Washington, soldiers became indistinguishable from civilians. As one agitated *Harper's Weekly* observer later explained to shaken Northern readers:

It is impossible yet to tell the story of the day. The newspapers have teemed with differing accounts. Apparently there was victory at hand, if not in possession, when a sudden order to retreat dismayed the triumphant line. The soldiers, who from exhaustion or whatever cause had been sent to the rear, and the teamsters and civilians who hovered along the base of our active line, were struck with terror by a sudden dash of cavalry from the flank. They fled, panic-stricken, in a promiscuous crowd: while the soldiers who were really engaged fell back quietly and in good order. It was the crowd of disengaged soldiers, teamsters, and civilians in the rear who rushed, a panting rabble, to Washington, and who told the disheartening story that flashed over the country at noon on Monday.[1]

This relatively brief but telling account of the first battle of the Civil War reveals much about the war, though it conveys little information about the details of the military engagement—conventionally thought to be the stuff of Civil War narrative. Rather, the anonymous author introduces the concern that I argue compels subsequent rewritings of the

Civil War and that motivates this study: the violently aroused, disordered condition of those who both populate and attempt to tell the "story of the day." The *Harper's Weekly* correspondent (writing under the nom de plume "The Lounger") insists that it is "impossible" to determine what happened at Bull Run, even as he or she remarks upon the many stories carried in newspapers across the country. Thus, authoritative Civil War narratives are revealed as relative and elusive objects, both engendered and imperiled by the outbreak of hostilities. The qualifier "yet" implies that Civil War writers would eventually recover from the shock of battle and agree upon an accurate outline of the day's events. However, the journalistic community's initial inability to agree upon the facts and, then, the distant observer's difficulty in discerning the "real" story signal the narrative predicament realized in successive tellings of the Civil War. Walt Whitman would later reflect that this battle was lost by "a fiction, or series of fictions" rather than by cowardice or military weakness. It is Whitman's insistence on the crucial role of the imaginative in propagating Civil War histories, as well as his realization that "battles, and their results, are far more matters of accident than is generally thought," that makes the Civil War shockingly unreal, unpredictable, and ultimately untellable.[2]

As much a matter of concern to the *Harper's Weekly* observer as fellow journalists' inability to get their stories straight is the "panting rabble" of impassioned amateurs who scooped the professionals with their "disheartening" tales of the battle. The stories originating in such a throng would surely be as "promiscuous" as the population that produced them: indiscriminate, idiosyncratic, and confused. The proliferation of these personal and supposedly limited experiences of the war would serve only to fragment and muddle, not standardize, war narratives. "The Lounger" promotes the notion that these Civil War stories are unreliable by implying that the tellers clearly are not in their right minds: they are "panic-stricken" and "panting" with "terror" and excitement. This scene of war reveals not only soldiers "disengaged" from the battle at hand but also a whole array of elusive bodies cut loose from the strictures of social convention and good sense. It is no coincidence that, despite the article's focus on the panting rabble, the illustration accompanying this story, titled "Retreat of Our Troops from Bull Run by Moonlight, Colonel Blenker's Brigade Covering," depicts uniform rows of identical, faceless men stretching endlessly under a placid, moonlit sky (Fig. 1). In this way, the magazine rehabilitates the horrifying scene, reestablishing the good name of the Union forces on the seemingly firm foundation of disciplined bodies. Civil War writers increasingly relied on the realignment of promiscuous, fleeing bodies to straighten out their stories and to eradicate the "panic" that pro-

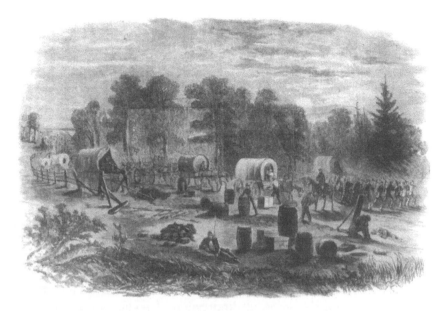

Figure 1. "Retreat of Our Troops from Bull Run by Moonlight, Colonel Blenker's Brigade Covering." *Harper's Weekly*, August 10, 1861. Courtesy of the Rare Book and Special Collections Library, University of Illinois at Urbana-Champaign.

pelled Civil War writers and their narratives beyond the bounds of propriety, beyond the limits of knowledge.

In order to dramatize the incoherence of individual and social bodies, Civil War writers turn again and again to the conflict's appalling carnage. In this way, Civil War texts keep readers continuously and painfully alert to the vexed nature of the corporeal knowledge so soon embodied in the trope of the war. In yet another version of the fallout from the First Battle of Bull Run, *Harper's Weekly* correspondent Henry J. Raymond encounters one retreating soldier, Quartermaster Stetson, a member "of the Fire Zouaves, who told [him], bursting into tears, that his regiment had been utterly cut to pieces, that the Colonel and Lieutenant-Colonel were both killed, and that our troops had actually been repulsed."[3] Although Stetson does not relate the details of the battle, he does bear witness to its aftermath, most notably the dismembered corps of his regimental body. The image of the butchered corps, like the promiscuous, fleeing rabble, allies the business of Civil War with an essential lack of corporeal integrity: both social bodies are volatile and discontinuous, always in the process of vanishing before the viewer's eyes. Significantly, Raymond turns his reader's attention toward Stetson's individual body, solidifying a connection between emotional and corporeal pain. The Zouave's surprising storm of tears is meant to register the incommunicable trauma of his corps' physical destruction. Yet Stetson's overpowering, wordless emotion does not make his or his fellows' pain communicable; rather, it makes the teller's body and his narrative as unreliable as the dead bodies his tears are meant to indicate.

Subsequent Civil War writers affirmed that physical and emotional explosions of the sort that overwhelmed this one soldier and galvanized the fleeing crowd of which he was a member produced aftershocks that reverberated through representations of the war. Much like these *Harper's Weekly* correspondents, many who wrote about the Civil War strove above all to understand and convey the material changes the war wrought in individual and national lives, to simply state "what happened." Indeed, Civil War writers repeatedly employ a meticulous and scientific accounting of those changes in efforts to make sense of the broken bodies and emotional outbursts that defy reason. In this way the Civil War has emerged as a powerful cultural hermeneutic that expresses not only altered social, political, and economic relationships but also an emergent self-consciousness, an impression of metaphysical distortion that lingers long after the war. Writers have attempted to convey the era's essence through complex and ultimately indeterminate investigations of the proximities and distances between disciplined troops and panting rabble, between the Zouave's butchered corps and his emotional outburst—between stolid corporeality and unnerving incorporeality.

The texts I have gathered in this project insist on the intimate relationship between the Civil War and a variety of invisible wounds, illnesses, and infirmities that beset modern Americans throughout the nineteenth century: nerve injury, neurasthenia, hysteria, hyperaesthesia, phantom limb pain, and degeneracy are just a few. Twentieth-century additions to this list would include post-traumatic stress disorder, depression, chronic fatigue syndrome, and stress. Such disorders strained, and continue to strain, the boundaries between organic and environmental illness, and physical and mental well-being. They are inextricable from the social diseases—malignant racism and sexism, for example—which, most scholars agree, constituted nineteenth-century medical discourse and infected the culture-at-large. Because whites and African Americans, both men and women, were situated in drastically different ways in biological, historical, and medical discourses of health before the war, their relationships to the already existing corporeal rifts the Civil War magnified were not the same. For example, although African American writers were as enmeshed in the discourses of health and history as their white counterparts, their texts rarely explore battlefield injuries in much depth. Instead, they focus on the war's power to both express and mitigate the racial "degeneracy" that supposedly made African Americans fractions of men and women. Yet in all cases the Civil War has been written as a cataclysmic event felt in, displayed by, and accounted for with mysteriously ailing bodies. As the *Harper's Weekly* articles exemplify, narrative anxiety stems from consistent unease with writers' and protagonists' bodies, demonstrating how neither the modern protocols of health nor history are able to capture the constantly moving and multiple dimensions of aberrant forms. To be human and hurting is, nominally, to be diseased in these texts. And diseased, unstable bodies— bodies traumatized not only by postwar injury, illness, and grief but also by newly racialized and gendered political and biological truisms— provided at best a shifting foundation for American history and identity.

In efforts to materialize and communicate the illusory and idiosyncratic nature of a reality founded on the perceptions of diseased human bodies, many writers analogized the war as a volcano or earthquake. As my subtitle from Walt Whitman's 1865 paean to the war, *Drum Taps*, implies, the Civil War was a time that "trembled and reel'd beneath" many Americans.[4] Whitman was not the only writer to employ tectonic imagery to convey the instability the war experience epitomized. In perhaps the nineteenth century's best-known Civil War novel, *Miss Ravenel's Conversion from Secession to Loyalty* (1867), John William De Forest writes, "No volcanic eruption rends a mountain without stirring the existence of the mountain's mice." Writing in 1904, Rebecca Harding Davis still noted that "to the easy-going millions, busied with their farms or shops, the onrushing disaster was as inexplicable as an earthquake."[5] Tectonic imagery was useful because volcanoes and earthquakes were foreign to most Americans' experiences during the war era.[6] At the same time, these representations made the cataclysm of the war a natural, enduring phenomenon. The trauma of war revealed the fault lines that *always* lay beneath the substratum of American culture and identity. Thus the quaking imagery usefully absolved individuals of responsibility for the slaughters of the Civil War, for such seismic events are beyond anyone's control. Most important, volcanoes and earthquakes kept readers ever mindful of the fully physical disorientation of the war. No one near the site of a quake or eruption is exempt from feeling its effects. Even those quite far off from the event feel the ground shake or find their view obscured by smoke and ash.

Yet volcanic eruptions do not merely shake the ground, but they also force fissures in Earth's crust. The Civil War is not only the trembling terra firma beneath our feet, but also the gap left behind; it is the silent space between health and disease, freedom and slavery, past and future, reality and perception. The long-standing belief that the "real" war remains untold, first penned by Whitman in 1882 and reiterated in Daniel Aaron's influential *The Unwritten War* (1973), reflects the fact that the regional conflict was *surreal* for so many.[7] Mountains made up of volcanic detritus may form over the site of such bewildering eruptions; indeed, this book argues that the asserted coherence of the Civil War and the mountain of scholarly and artistic attention it has elicited have made the war into a remarkably stable and powerful cultural trope. But I am also compelled by the bizarre chasms beneath the volcano, the hollow chambers that we have worked so hard to *habile*—to clothe, to cover over. These hollowed spaces have become hallowed ground, venerated and protected because of their supposedly sacred nature. And the timeless "abysms of New World humanity" beneath (to borrow Whitman's language) hold not only a calamitous past but also the promise of an equally earth-shattering future.[8] These past, present, and future moments exist beyond the temporal boundaries of the Civil War, but the attention the war elicits suggests that such corporeal traumas may best be expressed through the trope of the Civil War. Thus I posit a war-era and postbellum corporeal ideology that is not simply the effect of a material cause; for example, Civil War deaths and dismemberments caused cultural and individual instability. Rather, our continued processing of Civil War diseases and disabilities expresses an ontological and epistemological phenomenon that continues to lend unstable shape and meaning to the inner lives and social realities of many Americans. The war is not unwritten—nothing so finite—but, rather, it is rewritten and rewritten and rewritten. Like an inactive volcano, the Civil War seems to sleep, yet its rumble remains palpable; it will not let us rest easy.

Rehabilitating the Civil War

Unable to still the shaking ground or subsequently to reverse the damage done by the cataclysmic event, Civil War writers increasingly turned their attentions toward the unbalanced bodies that occupied this martial landscape. Indeed, upon closer inspection, tectonic imagery is disturbingly equivocal, for the difference between the foundational reformations of the war (evident in my study in evolving medical, historical, and psychological notions of selfhood and citizenship) and individual diseases became confused: Did the natural calamity of the Civil War produce diseased individuals, or did inherently diseased individuals produce the Civil War? Unwilling to address this chicken and egg conundrum—insisting in their volcanic imagery that the former was true, even as their texts subtly suggested that the latter was the case—writers and thinkers set their sights on the seemingly possible task of fixing bodies.

I use the term *rehabilitate* in this study because it suggests the many ways that Civil War writers attempt to fix the unnerving changes of the Civil War. In modern parlance, we use the term *rehabilitate* most often to connote a physical or psychological return to good health. Following the lead of medical writers, novelists, historians, journalists, and memoirists sought not only to stabilize a martial citizenry disturbingly out of kilter but also to sustain the revolutionary changes (i.e., emancipation) that filled the breach. *Rehabilitate* also means "to reestablish on a firm or solid basis." Thus Civil War writers and thinkers sought to secure bodies by making individuals and the events in which they participated predictable, unalterable, and static. As coverage of the First Battle of Bull Run postulated, fixed bodies could ensure definite stories, and rehabilitative Civil War texts offered the promise of the converse as well: fixed stories might produce definite bodies.

It is on this front that the disciplines of medicine and history—both emerging as discrete, scientific professions in the war-era and postbellum periods—colluded, as their practitioners developed strategies to narrate and organize radically particular bodily experiences. Disciplining the bodies and behaviors of both the professionals and the subjects of their study, history and medicine offered the possibility of Civil War rehabilitation. Let me clarify that although I invoke medicine and history here, I do not intend to chart their disciplinary developments per se. Rather, I contend that the basic questions of corporeality, narratability, and knowledge that generally troubled nineteenth-century representations of the Civil War simultaneously dictated the evolving disciplinary practices and narrative strategies of historians and doctors. Both history and medicine are premised on the existence of a corporeal and often critical reality that their practitioners cannot know fully. Yet the professional's disciplinary mission remains to access what he or she can and to contribute to totalizing, restorative narratives of human experience crafted from fragmentary knowledge of individual bodies and behaviors. History and medicine gained power in the war-era and postbellum periods precisely because they were compelled by the epistemological limits of unstable bodies.

War writers precede Michel Foucault in their keen awareness of the volcanic nature of the epistemes that serve to stabilize modern Western disciplinary culture.[9] At the heart of the scientific method crucial to both professions is a pose of stability and objectivity gained through adherence to regulated protocols of study. Both physical bodies and historical artifacts became objects to be scrutinized, tested, and then interpreted by the trained professional. Indeed, this project charts how physical bodies *became* historical artifacts for writers of the Civil War, making healing narratives contingent on stable, rehabilitated bodies and vice versa. However, investigations of the Civil War reveal not only how bodies are bound by disciplines such as medicine and history but also how the internal features and forces of bodies and psyches might be theorized.[10] Civil War texts so thoroughly enmeshed in the politics of these emerging disciplines assume that although knowledge of bodies, historical or not, cannot be comprehensive, those bodies are comprehensible.

The practice of professional historians in the postbellum era speaks to the correspondence between the two disciplines and their essential connection to matters of the Civil War. As one Gilded Age historian contended, historical seminars functioned like "laborator[ies] of scientific truth" where specimens were passed about to be examined. Another scholar of the era hoped that the scientific historian of the future would work "like the anatomist, who cuts through this sensual beauty to find beyond, in the secrets of its interior organization, beauty a thousand times superior."[11] Here the male historian believes in the existence of conventionally feminized, sublime knowledge; after all, the ultimate end of scientific pursuit is complete knowledge and, consequently, complete stability. It is not surprising that Civil War writers and thinkers would exploit this emerging scientific rhetoric in hopes of settling unsettled historical bodies. If one followed strict rules regarding the handling and interpretation of specimens (whether material remnants of people's lives or bodies themselves), these new scientists believed one would be able to reproduce results, and it is that reproducability that ensured accurate history, healed bodies, and secure self-knowledge.

Yet as I've begun to suggest, Civil War bodies seemed adamantly diseased, that is, unreceptive to disciplinary regimes of soma or text. Given that medical discourse revealed the pathologies of the bodies producing historical and medical narratives, Civil War texts concomitantly promote and undermine the scientific basis of such textual productions. Concern with fixing biological origins became the bailiwick of both professions, as identifying a more rational and dispassionate—in short, a healthier—race of historians and doctors seemed the most expedient means of ensuring the validity of both history and medicine. Just as scientific method galvanized the modern historical profession, history was crucial to the development of biological and medical sciences in that it provided a narrative template that chronologically organized human bodies, actions, and responses that were so spectacularly disordered.[12] In medical science, postbellum doctors transformed evolutionary history into genetic immutability: for example, white women were forever weak because of their wombs; African American men and women were perpetually childlike because of their small skulls and brains.[13] Scientific historians of the nineteenth century were similarly obsessed with national origins, a preoccupation that led to racist and nativist efforts to imagine the most eugenically fit American pedigree. It is widely accepted that white postbellum Civil War historians, Northern and Southern, predicated national reconciliation on the regions' shared acceptance of new evolutionary theories of racism.[14] Thus, for many, historical rehabilitation of the Civil War was founded on the unchanging degeneracy of African American bodies.[15]

Given the primacy of war-era and postbellum corporeal scientific praxis, it is no surprise that the discourse of bodies proves foundational in renderings of the Civil War. After all, bodies matter in that real people lived and died during the Civil War, and their bodies bore the wounds of the sectional conflict. As Elaine Scarry explains, "What matters (what signifies, what has standing, what counts) has substance: mattering is the impingement of a thing's substance on whatever surrounds it." [16] Though the trauma may be incommunicable, the matter of those bodies makes the war real on some basic level. This insistence on the legibility of bodily matters is at the core of Civil War rehabilitation. At the same time, Civil War writers insist that bodies *don't* matter, although such a claim may seem counterintuitive. After all, their texts are full of bodies: nervous bodies, hungry bodies, enslaved bodies, grief-riven bodies, mutilated bodies, dead bodies. The writers I treat here are obsessed with the matter of bodies, minutely detailing their physical afflictions and their emotional responses to the conflict. And yet they despair of ever being able to firmly fix how others or even they themselves feel or to determine what really happened during the war. Here, bodies are constantly in the process of falling apart, subject to perception-skewing attack or disease.

That specific diseases emerged in specific ways according to the gendered or racial identification of the sufferer is a basic premise of this book. We have become used to Civil War books that focus on a particular group through the lens of contemporary identity politics: we are familiar with the so-called woman's response to the war; slowly, we are getting works that treat the "African American response" to the war. The "white man's response" to the war is the invisible default, of course. Ultimately, however, I have found these configurations untenable for my purposes. Though gender and race are salient categories in this project—as they were for the writers I treat—my goal is to foreground the theoretical connection between corporeality and history as a field of discourse that many different writers entered in particular ways. All of the pliant Civil War bodies I examine exist outside of the mythical norms of health and history, for they are unable to feel right, unable to impress themselves upon the world, and, ultimately, unable to gauge what really matters.

Notably, in this latter case they are unable to legitimate invisible ills or to credibly narrate what happened.

I work under the assumption that bodies matter to the Civil War—they just matter differently from what is traditionally thought to be the case. As Judith Butler suggests in her exploration of the discursive limits of "sex," such "unsettling of 'matter' can be understood as initiating new possibilities, new ways for bodies to matter." As I will explain at length, the unsettling of bodily matters during the Civil War created a liberatory climate for many. However, to "problematize the matter of bodies may entail an initial loss of epistemological certainty."[17] And the rehabilitative disciplines of history and medicine emerged precisely to comfort in the face of such loss. The prefix *re* in *rehabilitation* presumes an originary state of bodily habiliment that marks the epistemological solidity of health and of history. That crucial *re* ensures a preceding authenticity, promising that we can get back to an essential wholeness. Thus the disciplines of health and history assume that the bodies/documents that mark the existence of a disordering event are incontrovertible, entities merely awaiting retrieval. As one recent defender of history against the encroachment of postmodern theory insists, historians have always known that they can "see the past only 'through a glass, darkly.'" However, such accessions do not challenge the basic notion of scientific discovery, which relies upon the belief that knowledge is preexisting, that historical bodies are "entirely independent of the historian," waiting for him or her to simply stumble upon them.[18] I find that those who write of the Civil War during the nineteenth century—indeed, those transcribing their reactions even as they stand in its midst and suffer its pains—find the Civil War just as elusive as those who still seek to know it now. These Civil War writers have no sure sense of the real that seemingly materializes before them or of the accuracy of the documents they produce while the war is raging. A history founded on the expressions of bodies is by some definitions an "ambulant form," for "the body is at best *like* something, but it never *is* that something."[19] Complete recoveries of health or history seem impossible in such Civil War texts—even to those who believe they are fully engaged in acts of recovery.

To illustrate, let me briefly turn to two rehabilitative texts: one historical, the other imaginative, but both intent upon the Civil War's fundamental relationship to invisible ills and dead bodies. Attempting to document regimental losses three decades after the cessation of hostilities in his military history, *Regimental Losses in the American Civil War* (1889), Civil War veteran William F. Fox writes, "The bloody laurels for which a regiment contends will always be awarded to the one with the longest role honor. Scars are the true evidence of wounds and the regimental scars can be seen only in the records of its casualties."[20] Here

Fox links the number of dead sustained in battle to the "bloody laurels" of victory. Thus, intangible characteristics such as "honor" are made perceptible through the list of dead bodies. But bodies are integral not only to the Civil War's accountability—its status as a verifiable event— but also to the war's basic knowability: the distinction between wounds and scars. In this passage, the "regimental scars" attest to the invisible wounds. As this book will demonstrate, Civil War doctors were stymied by the number and variety of invisible wounds suffered by their patients. Yet even if initially visible, physical wounds are a transitory phenomenon. With the passage of time they usually heal enough, or kill. It is significant that Fox is careful to differentiate scars from wounds, electing the former to stand in for the unrecoverable individual pains and historical reality of the Civil War. He enacts his own form of rehabilitation, as the scars cover over the wounds that persist metaphorically beneath the surface in many bodies and minds. In a well-known passage, Scarry writes of pain that it is "at once something that cannot be denied and something that cannot be confirmed . . . to have pain is to have *certainty*; to hear about pain is to have *doubt*."[21] Thus the "regimental scars," that is, the number of dead bodies, foreclose any efforts to revivify or authenticate the pain of individual wounds. Indeed, Fox insists that those scars are sufficient evidence for the sacrifices of the living and the dead and for the bloody laurels deserved by badly decimated regiments. But of course others' pain is always unknowable, though its effects cannot be ignored. Fox demonstrates that although postbellum Americans knew that bodies mattered, they also knew that their comrades' pain could not be resurrected, that surviving bodies didn't feel the same after the war, and that such feeling could not be conveyed. I contend contra Scarry that Civil War pain provided no certainty, even to those in its grips.

Fox's rhetorical strategies were typical in the postbellum period, and they shaped the parameters of subsequent study of the Civil War and of American history more generally. Fox asserts, for example, that it is only through accurately recovering the number of dead in each battle that scholars of the Civil War can know "where the points of contact really were; where the pressure was the greatest; where the scenes of valor and heroism occurred" (574). Here he uses terms such as *contact* and *pressure* to insist that the Civil War matters; his sensory language suggests that we must somehow feel its reality in our individual and national bodies. And yet those bodies are unreliable. He concludes his meticulous tally of the thousands killed during the war:

In a conversation with the late Col. Robert N. Scott, USA concerning [counting the dead and wounded] that officer remarked "We will do these things better in the next war." The question arises, will the "we" of the future do these things any better? In the turmoil and excitement will not "these things" be again over-looked?, and gallant regiments be again disbanded without leaving scarcely a trace to show how well they fought? Will not History be again neglected and despoiled? (574)

Interestingly, Fox and his contemporaries were not concerned with better war-making or with avoiding such deadly military engagements altogether. Rather, they were interested in better representational strategies. Without bodies, there is no proof of wartime activities and feelings. More important, Fox suggests that there is no history without bodies. History is personified and done a grave wrong by the military's inability to provide the statistics it needs to substantiate its raison d'être. Yet Fox's forceful and questioning tone suggests that he is aware that those bodies and the intangible states he argues they represent will continue to elude him. Without history, bodies leave "scarcely a trace." Just as Whitman darkly predicts, the Civil War will produce "no history ever—no poem sings, no music sounds, those bravest men of all" for their bodies "crumble[] in mother earth, unburied and unknown."[22] Bodies become universal signifiers, their mere existence needed to guarantee nineteenth-century Americans the possibility of knowledge. Thus the inability to (ac)count for bodies—and the subsequent dissolution of history—signal more than lack of knowledge about the Civil War. The impossibility of bodies means the impossibility of knowledge itself.

Whitman's poem "The Wound-Dresser" (1865), excerpted at the outset of this chapter, plumbs the depths of the instability Fox delineates. Whitman invokes the Civil War as the imaginative repository of inner life, a surreal yet bounded place whose "doors" writers will traverse again and again, bringing their readers with them. He abandons the notion that the Civil War is an accountable, verifiable event and asserts instead that war experiences are "dreams' projections," an iteration of the American subconscious writ large. In Whitman's poem, the Civil War is still a space filled with the mangled bodies produced by the self-destructive war of a diseased society. But it is also the home of the wound-dresser; though his actions are ultimately ineffective in healing those who perish around him, the wound-dresser is validated by the crucial work he has undertaken. Consequently, a defining characteristic of Civil War literature is that the war accrues therapeutic value. Though physical and mental health were so often ruined in the volcanic cataclysm, the war also became the metaphoric site of rehabilitation, where socially stigmatized Americans presumably were able to refashion themselves by assuming practically powerful roles. Like the wound-dresser, many postbellum writers were compelled to return to the Civil War in order to reclaim the promise of cultural authority and subjectivity that their contemporaneous culture of anomie, even antimodernism, vehemently denied.

But this lesson in history is achieved only when the wound-dresser imagines his body literally walking into the cataclysmic past. When asked by young men and maidens to "be witness again" to the Civil War, Whitman's aged wound-dresser must lead his listeners into the Civil War hospital (3, 9). "With hinged knees returning I enter the doors," he tells us, traversing the threshold of time to become a Civil War nurse once again (23). His sensual imagery evokes the physical dimensions of this psychic journey. The wound-dresser faces a pair of "appealing eyes," moves on to the next bed to dress a "crush'd head," examines "the neck of a cavalry-man with the bullet through and through" (31, 40, 41). The poem progresses through the fragmented body parts of different, anonymous men, moving down to the "stump of the arm, the amputated hand," "a wound in the side," and "the perforated shoulder, the foot with the bullet-wound" (45, 50, 53). In disregarding an individual soldier in favor of the many parts of many anonymous men, the wound-dresser depicts a national body and tells a national story. However, although his listeners clamor for him to "paint the mightiest armies of earth," to depict "hard-fought engagements or sieges tremendous," these silent bodies are the "deepest remains" of the war for him (9, 12, 11). I argue that the wound-dresser represents the Civil War doctor-historian as he attempts to re-member the national body through his ministrations. The wound-dresser's archive is the Civil War hospital, his documents the dismembered bodies of the patients.[23]

Even the undeniable, gut-wrenching force of infected, suffering, dying bodies cannot substantiate this history. Though his own body is unwounded, his memories remain mediated and surreal, "dreams' projections" suggesting his double distance from the events: this poem is not even a dream, but a projection of a dream. The anonymity of the dying soldiers who people the wound-dresser's memory distance him and us from the events. In looking into the eyes of a dying boy he claims, "I think I could not refuse this moment to die for you, if that would save you" (38). But of course he cannot die for the boy; and though he may be powerfully empathic, his clinical description of the soldiers' wounds do not provide access to how they feel. Interestingly, Whitman published "The Wound-Dresser" the year the war ended. Yet he already imagines the war through the distance of age and time and memory loss, as an "old man bending" toward the past that he imagines as obscured, as "imprints" in "sand" that the "waves" continually "wash . . . off" (1, 22). Whitman suggests that the war is an experience alien and transient even to those living through it.

The Rewritten Civil War

And yet the war experience continues to grip his psyche as Whitman's wound-dresser revisits the Civil War hospital again and again. It is not just Civil War writings themselves that interest me here, but also the dynamics of this incessant rewriting. Scholars have produced tens of thousands of books on the war, the vast majority concerned with "the quest to understand."[24] Dominated still by military and political history, this body of scholarship is largely interested in causes and effects: What caused the Civil War? Why did it take place when it did? Why did the North win and the South lose? What were the decisive military engagements of the conflict? Which men were heroes, and which were cowards? New social histories have expanded the set of questions and the narratives that answer, looking beyond the great men to examine how civilians in general, white women, African Americans, and others experienced the Civil War.[25] Although such work questions the presumed objectivity of historical praxis, it does not challenge the premise that historical experience is a verifiable, knowable place, though we may not be able to get to it.

In their assessment of Civil War historiography, James McPherson and William J. Cooper Jr. liken their profession's progress to "several blind men who tried to describe an elephant—each historian seems to have run his hands over a different part of the evidence . . . so each one has described a different animal."[26] This story (common in scientific circles) acknowledges the particularity of perspective; moreover, it suggests how one's proximity to the Civil War evokes bodily disability, or at least forces one to reconsider the nature of one's sensory relationship to the objects of study, to the bodies of the past. However, the story also relies on the material reality of the elephant—one could not choose a larger and more weighty body to stand in for the presumed coherence and undeniable knowability of the Civil War. It is not the elephant's fault that no one gets it right. Yet in endowing this historical project with life, McPherson and Cooper suggest that the past is not dead and insentient. Elephant bodies—just as human bodies—are mutable and mortal; perhaps each historian *has* described a different animal.

We are a culture obsessed with rehabilitating the Civil War, trying to embody it and make it comprehensible. The piecework recovery of the Civil War is not left to only the professionals, but also a hobbyist industry.[27] This is a national community invested also in minutiae, helping to gauge the elephant through an infinite series of small observations. Unit files strive to account for every single individual who fought in the conflict. The descendants of Civil War veterans lovingly edit their family members' diaries. Civil War sabers, guns, paper ephemera, and so forth fetch top dollar on the collectibles market. Reenactors painstakingly reconstruct uniforms and weaponry, as well as mimic the actions of their national ancestors, in efforts to conjure the elusive bodies of the Civil War. There are Civil War magazines and e-mail groups, Civil War Round-tables and Lincoln Associations, and even children's toys such as Civil War Barbie. Hobbyists attempt to access the war's reality through a variety of means, but these means are most often geared toward capturing the war's materiality, whether through (re)collecting material traces of the era or tying one's own body to the event through genealogy or reenactment. Like trained scholars, Civil War hobbyists seek to fix the Civil War and the bodily states it still grounds. They want to know how those who lived through the Civil War really felt.

Yet a century and a half of hobbyist, scholarly, and artistic activity leaves us no closer to articulating the war, or to definitively answering impossible questions, than the writers who people my study, individuals who lived during the war and into the next generation. This book turns to the Civil War's diseased bodies to address the following questions: Why is the Civil War so important to us still? How does the depth of its grip on the national psyche reflect the larger, structural role it plays in postbellum society even today? Essentially, how did this nasty, bloody, four-year series of skirmishes and battles become "The Civil War," an event accorded almost religious reverence by subsequent generations? George M. Frederickson has recently suggested that the Civil War compels us because it "provides a persuasive argument for the uniqueness of American history" in the nineteenth century.[28] Although I find such national exceptionalism too sweeping, I do argue that in its incessant movement and in its reliance upon the power of bodily vagaries, the Civil War authorizes modern American history. Our consistent desire to claim the Civil War as historical truth, as national proving ground, is also our need to resist its shifting, representational nature and the profound consequences such instability has for national, disciplinary, and individual identities. The constant, intense attention given to the Civil War attests not only to its stability and coherence, but also to its essential slipperiness and, consequently, the instability of the identities founded upon its volcanic grounds.

Yet treatments of the Civil War do not founder on such uncertainties, but thrive despite—or rather, because of—them. I want to suggest briefly here that the incessant rewriting the Civil War elicits derives from its power as a historicizing trope. The deference we accord it, the concomitant breadth and detail we pursue in our study of it, and the comprehensiveness it seemingly requires of its devotees are what lends it its weight. Ironically, it is not only in the details that we ground the Civil War, but also in the volume of its effects. For example, in his introduction to James M. McPherson's best-selling, Pulitzer Prize-winning Civil War contribution to the "Oxford History of the United States," general editor C. Vann Woodward is compelled to address the 904-page length of *The Battle Cry of Freedom*: "That it should, despite its size, cover the shortest period assigned calls for some comment."[29] First, Woodward points us to McPherson's belief that "time and consciousness took on new dimensions" during the war years (xvii). Because time seemed to last longer during the Civil War, he reasons, there is more to be written. The Civil War is denser with history than any other American historical event. Indeed, Woodward, via McPherson, suggests that history *adheres* to the Civil War, that there is an undeniable magnetism between the two that effects a historical compression of sorts. Allusions to such Civil War congestion might seem at odds with an historical project that seeks to mete out the past so precisely. However, Woodward attributes this augmented sense of time to the notion that Civil War history is a scrupulous, self-perpetuating industry: "the more written, the more disclosed, and the more questions and controversies to be coped with" (xviii). By this logic, the war remains *only* rewritable, for any effort to address the event proliferates questions and the literature on the period rather than offering an endpoint to debate. Finally, none of these reasons seems to suffice, and Woodward concludes that the length of the volume is related to bodies: "one simple and eloquent measurement [of the magnitude of war] is the numbers of casualties sustained" (xviii). Written in 1987, Woodward's bodily reckoning of the length of McPherson's Civil War echoes Fox's 1889 efforts on similar fronts. Though neither of these historians deliberately ascribes the war's rewritability to bodily and psychic ills, focusing on numbers rather than natures, they represent the many nineteenth- and twentieth-century scholars who sense that the unwieldy shape and length of the Civil War project is tied to the problematics of corporeality. "This is hardly a normal period," Woodward notes.

Like General Fox, many literary historians and critics also continue to search for the "missing bodies," for the perfect and whole consolidation of texts that will complete the puzzle of the meaning of the Civil War. For example, though noting regional differences, early Civil War literary scholars tended to craft composite Civil War narratives, consolidating Northern and Southern accounts, war-era and historical fictions, in their ambitious reviews of the era's literature. Heroic efforts such as Robert Lively's *Fiction Fights the Civil War* (1957), Edmund Wilson's *Patriotic Gore* (1962), and Aaron's *The Unwritten War* (1973) treat the literature in toto. To a certain extent, the bulk of these studies derives from Americanists' anxiety about the lackluster quality of the literature inspired by our greatest historical event.[30] Their historicizing narratives fill up the space where emotional and historical truth are supposed to reside.

Recent literary critics have noticed the unstable bodies that undergird Civil War literature, and they focus on what I would call the rehabilitative strategies of many Civil War texts. Timothy Sweet, Kathleen Diffley, Elizabeth Young, and Gregory Eiselein, in particular, are attuned to wounded and improper bodies and the "disruptive Civil War moments" they engender. Read through the hermeneutic I lay out, they all engage in projects of rehabilitation, showing how the wounds of Civil War were purposefully exploited and/or recuperated through the rhetoric of the Civil War. These new critics fruitfully revise traditional literary genealogy; the addition of the narratives of women and African Americans, of commercial and magazine fiction, of photography and other media to the Civil War story has transformed the field.[31] Yet most Civil War scholars still subscribe to the gap theory that motivates the historical project at large. The urge toward material accountability permeates scholarly study of the period, as we concentrate on amassing Civil War writings themselves, expanding the body of the Civil War, but not essentially altering the parameters by which we define its potency. Neither does recent historical scholarship substantially challenge the basic premises of (ac)countability and (un)writability that both energize and vex Civil War studies.

I argue that such has been the case because the Civil War emerges as both a content and a mode of signification, an organizing topic that entails the theoretical underpinnings of postbellum American history. The content of the Civil War has produced its own narrative practice, a form premised on a preference for conveyances of the real founded on bodily experiences that resist such form. As I have begun to demonstrate, transcriptions of physical and psychological traumas are neither verifiable nor wholly imagined—to return to Scarry, they reside in the realm of the mutable body. Firmly grounded in this corporeal (il)logic, the Civil War narratives I examine overwhelm traditional generic distinctions, particularly between fiction and history. Any contact with the Civil War can conveniently collapse the already tenuous distinctions between the two; the war's sheer weight, the magnitude of its suffering, and the heft of its dead bodies press, condensing all representation into compact nuggets of history. Thus any text that treats the Civil War can become American history, even when it explicitly purports no such generic intention.[32] For example, Louisa May Alcott's *Hospital Sketches* has been praised by medical and Civil War historians as "perhaps the best account of what hospital life during at least one year of the war was really like," despite the fact that she clearly fictionalizes her experience.[33] In even more curious claims, many critics have dubbed Stephen Crane's *The Red Badge of Courage* as best able to represent Civil War combat experience, even as they acknowledge that Crane was not alive during the sectional conflict. This last example seems most significant, for I would argue that it is Crane's treatment of the Civil War—particularly, as I argue in Chapter 5, his delineation of war-era disease—that lends his fiction its semblance of truth. By the turn of the century, the war was firmly established as a grounding content, inviting considerations of textual facticity whether or not the text was determined to aspire to such standards.

Given this tendency, it is no surprise that Civil War writers themselves insist that their romanticized histories and autobiographical fictions deny quick categorization. Authors treated in this study, such as Alcott, De Forest, and Dr. S. Weir Mitchell, clearly fictionalize real-life experiences in their work; in her fictional *Hospital Sketches*, Alcott pleads that we believe "such a being as Nurse Periwinkle does exist . . . that these Sketches are not romance."[34] Yet the novella is derived from her avowedly nonfictional letters, and whole passages are transferred verbatim. Charlotte Forten, on the other hand, chose to publish her private writings—excerpts from her journals—in a public forum. Yet she too edited and shaped that version of real life when it appeared as "Life on the Sea Islands." The late-century historians and memoirists also treated in this study surely employed similar strategies in their efforts to fashion coherent narratives from their thirty-year-old memories. In addition, the serials in which many of these accounts first became available to nineteenth-century readers did not distinguish among the genres, publishing them side by side without generic labels. Such circumstances led Mitchell's anonymous short story "The Case of George Dedlow" to be read as fact by *Atlantic Monthly* subscribers. Sending money to the fictional "Stump Hospital" named in the story, Mitchell's readers insisted that the trauma of war was literally unimaginable, even as those who struggled to articulate the conflict suggested that it was *only* imaginable.

The historicizing force of the Civil War, finally, registers the assumed opposition between theoretical and materialist enterprises. As Scarry notes, "The turn to history and the body [is] the attempt to restore the material world to literature."[35] I add that it is not just literature to which this stabilizing weight must be returned; the obsessive reiteration of the Civil War suggests materiality is required on a much larger scale. Thus it is not surprising that George Frederickson notes quickly and intriguingly in a footnote to his historiographical review of the scholarship of nineteenth-century American history, "The explicit use of postmodernist theory is still rare in Civil War historiography."[36] His comment subtly implies that there is an opposition between the material realities of the war—the details that engross most Civil War scholars—and theoretical entanglements with the event and its representation, which many argue diminishes the horrifying and heroic. Wars are, indeed, sobering events, and civil wars particularly so, for they reveal the self-destructive, illogical impulses inherent in national and individual bodies.

The appalling circumstances of the Civil War inform American histories and identities, producing a national morality forbidding any cavalier treatment of "the glorious dead." Even before Abraham Lincoln consecrated the ground of warfare at Gettysburg Cemetery, the Civil War had become a sacred event. As Hayden White and other scholars have perceptively noted, there appears to be a "special class of events" that "must be viewed as manifesting only one story, as being emplottable in one way only, and as signifying one kind of meaning." [37] The practice of making unimaginable slaughters such as the Civil War solely historical—merely factual—forecloses the possibility that those deaths had no definitive meaning or that meaning more generally is relative. I do not find the American Civil War any less representable than any other event in human history. However, events whose apocalyptic natures are limned by the sheer magnitude of dead and brutalized bodies are nothing to be theorized for some. In the case of the Civil War, such seemingly frivolous and ancillary explorations entail a turning away from the monumental and meticulous accounting project that has preoccupied scholars for decades, and in the breach, those facts and figures—those bodies—may slip out of our grasp. And so too will go the carefully maintained sense of stability, coherence, and knowledge built upon the foundation of the Civil War. Again, heightened patriotism is not unique to the Civil War. However, the Civil War is unique in the way in which its representations embody the tensions between simple morality and endless inquiry, between fact and fiction, between the known and the speculative that inform subsequent study of American health and history.

The Civil War's Bodies

In embarking on this academic project, I find myself as subject to Civil War historicism as anyone else. However, my goal here is not necessarily to generate new knowledge about the Civil War, but rather to explore how the Civil War has become a lasting trope and to chart how that becoming is dictated by the vagaries of the human body. The three areas of interest I have delineated in this introduction do not lend themselves easily to linear arcs but are, rather, simultaneously at play in the texts I consider. Consequently, rather than mapping how one of the phenomena I have identified ended and the next began, I will explore how each of the following manifests itself in particular Civil War texts: the invisible ills that rock protagonists' and writers' worlds, the bodily rehabilitations that inform the production of disciplinary and cultural practices, and the incessant rewriting that seems to express the essential inexpressibility of those invisible ills.

Arguably, these complexities make the American Civil War our most cherished cultural palimpsest; each resuscitation adds to its signifying power. Although I eschew cause-and-effect logic, I do believe that the way in which the war has been claimed and represented at particular historical moments (even as the war was still being fought) has much to say about the culture that produced the representation and about the staying power of the sectional conflict. Recent historians such as Jim Cullen notice also that the Civil War has been "rewritten (or refilmed, rerecorded, etc.) to reflect the concerns of different constituencies in U.S. society."[38] Yet this process of historical revision has not been quite as arbitrary as such claims might suggest. The Civil War embodies a pliable, quintessentially American idiom of cultural disease; concurrently, it offers an imaginative space where Americans attempt to form rehabilitative strategies specific to contemporary needs.

That the writers whose texts I have chosen to focus on are more often than not Northern in their sympathies is not the result of geographic design. Rather, it follows from the bodily rehabilitations I seek to delineate. Within the corporeal rhetoric of the national body deployed before and during the war era, Southern aggression and the way of life that had prompted it was a diseased part that needed to be cured or excised. Thus the South was figured as an infected appendage, whereas the North maintained the original national identity. As Abraham Lincoln wrote of his approach to the war, "I have sometimes used the illustration . . . of a man with a diseased limb, and his surgeon. So long as there is a chance of the patient's restoration, the surgeon is solemnly bound to try to save both life and limb; but when the crisis comes, and the limb must be sacrificed as the only chance of saving the life, no honest man will hesitate."[39] Thus, texts produced by Northern writers are more likely to register their disease as loss, though many Southern writers depicted their own pain at the violent dissolution of the American body politic.

Ultimately, however, the South was restored to the North (a feat of reattachment unimaginable to doctors of the time) and by this logic the bodily integrity of the nation, though scarred, remained intact. In his renowned work on Northern intellectuals during the war, Frederickson reasons that because the North won the war, Northerners' cultural remembrances of it, and subsequent historical events, take national precedence.[40] Yet the notion of "America" as a unified identity is always fictional, a figment of our geographical imaginations; "North" and "South" are equally vexed designations. This is not to discount the reality that regional affiliations held for individuals; after all, Southerners were willing to die to establish the idea of an autonomous South. However, even though most of the authors who appear in this book identify themselves as Unionists, the people who populate this project—and the concerns that absorb them—traverse and transcend regional boundaries, just as their bodies did.

Similarly, the trope of the Civil War extends far beyond 1865. Though the war provides a convenient breaking point for literary and historical study of the nineteenth century, the bodily and textual diseases I identify should not be seen as transcending the times that preceded and followed them. Rather, the issues that crystallized most forcefully during the Civil War were undercurrents to nineteenth- and twentieth-century life that have come into focus at various historical moments. For example, Joan Burbick has argued cogently that as the American nation-state developed early in the nineteenth century, the "body of the individual citizen became the test case for the republic . . . the symbol of the very possibility of free human agency and human governance."[41] In the twentieth century, the 1929 stock market crash and subsequent deprivations of the Great Depression in the 1930s launched a renaissance of Civil War literature and scholarship, represented most notably by the craze for *Gone with the Wind* (1936) in both its novelistic and cinematic incarnations. This study is part of the most recent reclamation evidenced in the relatively recent popularity of texts such as Ken Burns's PBS series *The Civil War* (1990) and Charles Frazier's novel, *Cold Mountain* (1997). Though a comprehensive consideration of emergent postbellum representations of the war is far beyond the scope of one text, one need only recall the dead bodies strewn across the fields of Matthew Brady's groundbreaking photographs or the artificially blackened rapist who leers out at us from D. W. Griffith's *Birth of a Nation* to see how the Civil War immediately insinuated itself into the fiber of modern American modes of representation.

Although I remain grounded in war-era texts, I also aim more modestly to extend my explorations to the twentieth century. The bodily ills the Civil War expressed were most obviously troubling from 1861 to 1905, when the rehabilitative strategies that emerged were still unformed but also most vehement. Writers were especially prolific during two periods: the 1860s and a twenty-year period around the turn of the century (1885–1905). I have organized my chapters around these two periods—as distinct yet connected entities.[42] The turn of the century also marks the senescence and deaths of the Civil War survivors who were adults during the conflict, depleting the actual bodies that marked the disturbing reality of the war. It is during this time that remaining Civil War veterans and their children returned unerringly to the Civil War. In their medical texts, fictions, histories, and memoirs, writers again and again used the trope of the Civil War to articulate their sense of the modern world taking root—a world, I contend, marked by the bodily ills, psychological drama, and civil discontent that had alternately plagued and energized Civil War America.

Not surprisingly, the Civil War appealed to a wide variety of writers during this period. For example, the war continued to preoccupy wartime veterans such as S. Weir Mitchell and Susie King Taylor. Nonetheless, young, celebrated authors such as Stephen Crane and Paul Laurence Dunbar, who were born after the sectional conflict, also found in it a historical canvas conducive to the bodily dramas they wished to delineate. In some respects, the version of the Civil War that has occupied many twentieth-century writers and thinkers attributes the corporeal instabilities of the era to gender and racial confusion, consequently obfuscating the diversity of the Civil War of the previous century. In part, that is why students study *The Red Badge of Courage* in our literary classes instead of Dunbar's *The Fanatics*; why Taylor's memoir has disappeared in the shadow of U. S. Grant's; and why Mitchell is known only as the staid, sexist "rest cure doctor" and not as the experimental investigator of Civil War nerve injury. White, male authority—even that as ambiguous as Henry Fleming's knowledge of combat, as undistinguished as Grant's presidency, or as misguided as Mitchell's rest cures—offered the illusion of certainty premised on the universal health of white male bodies and minds.

Chapter 1 begins with one man's vexed efforts to establish authority through the Civil War. S. Weir Mitchell has become a pivotal figure in this study because his oeuvre so clearly illustrates the amorphous interstices that emerged as he attempted to firmly fix individual and professional meanings in rehabilitated bodies. A Civil War surgeon and later a famous neurologist, Mitchell was also a prolific novelist and poet consistently attentive to diseases that straddled physical and psychological realms—precisely the territory my project maps. Mitchell's medical texts theorize the concept of Civil War "nerve injury"—a diagnosis that linked a variety of physical and emotional ills that defied organic detection. Mitchell saw such ailments as indivisible from the Civil War; as he wrote in his 1885 novel about the national crisis, *In War Time*, "What is true of disease, is true of war."[43] The Civil War remained an abiding area of literary and medical interest for Mitchell, providing the historical foundation and psychological tension for his fiction during the 1860s and again in the 1880s and 1890s. Its nerve-injured victims launched his medical career as the "rest cure" doctor and remained the subject of follow-up studies decades after the war. Finally, it was the persistence of "malingering"—the notion that patients might feign their invisible ills and that doctors may not be able to tell the difference—that challenged

Mitchell's faith in the coherence and stability of the body and in the scientific basis of his professional identity. At heart, Mitchell's texts contend with his inability to know the ways of others' diseases, and serve as the lens through which later chapters should be read.

Caused by a gunshot wound or an emotional blow, nerve injury was a pathological condition with outward causes but primarily interior consequences. Elizabeth Stuart Phelps's best-seller, *The Gates Ajar* (1868), served a rehabilitative function for Americans dangerously debilitated by such war-time diseases. The alarming magnitude of illness, mutilation, and death sustained by the American citizenry during the war and the physical and psychological deprivations required even of those who did not serve on the front lines were partly responsible for the body consciousness ushered in during the war. Phelps's novel works in tandem with Mitchell's short story "The Case of George Dedlow," demonstrating how Civil War survivors made sense of living bodies literally and figuratively decimated by the war. Phelps's corporeal heaven promises the reconstitution of families and of selves dismembered by the carnage of war through the rehabilitation of mutilated, dead bodies. Such a solution acknowledges the surreality of earthly existence and the insufficiency of available rehabilitations by deferring stable embodiment to the afterlife.

Phelps's heaven not only repairs bodies but also restores the personal idiosyncrasies of the dead. Thus her work marks the coalescence of a corporate-historical culture that required the repression of individual biases, attachments, and passions—the topic of Chapter 3. The powerful United States Sanitary Commission (USSC) was a government-sanctioned, philanthropic organization dedicated to monitoring and improving the public health of the army. In practice it wielded sanitary science, which posited that self-discipline—enforced by military law—would ensure the continued production of sound "material," that is, soldiers for the army machine. Unsanitary disease was also described by the USSC as "soul-sickness," or an illicit, pathological display of self. As Joel Pfister claims in his work on anthropologists and psychologists of emotional life, "Social *regulations* of self (which promote the idea of self as naturally in need of regulation) are social *fabrications* of self."[44] The Civil War is a critical moment during which this inveterate notion of American selfhood emerged. De Forest's *Miss Ravenel's Conversion from Secession to Loyalty* (1867) dramatizes the costs of this brand of self-surveillance, along with the sanitized citizen soldiers—what one USSC operative labels "unconscious missionaries"—the war produced. Rebecca Harding Davis's novel of romance and war, *Waiting for Verdict* (1867), similarly charts the self-surveillance required of American citizens. Although many critics argue that romance plots such as those featured in De Forest's and

Davis's fiction are ancillary to matters of war, I contend that they firmly focus our attentions on individual desire, self-formation, and sacrifice, those issues central to the rhetoric of soldiering. Finally, Davis's extended treatment of African American characters—one, a nerve doctor practicing in Mitchell's native Philadelphia—converges with the USSC's postwar belief in the impossibility of ever curing the presumably unsanitary taint inherent in the bloodlines of the national family.

At the same time, ontological uncertainty and the perception of bodies in flux unmoored the physical bases of difference that were used to justify racism and sexism, or at least diverted national attention from them. Civil War texts portray not only the thousands of white soldiers who sustained life-altering injuries and the grief-stricken who survived them, but also African Americans who were property one day, citizens and soldiers the next, and single women whose severely circumscribed lives now extended to military hospitals and battlefields. These radical experiences convinced many of the possibility of future change. As social constructs that are always reliant upon embodied discourse— located, according to Robyn Wiegman, in a "pre-cultural realm where corporeal significations supposedly speak a truth which the body inherently means"—the strictures of gender and race were loosened by the prevalence of nerve injury, grief, and unsanitary disease, which compromised the stability of corporeal foundations.[45] The preoccupation with essential, psychological matters produced a leveling effect that not only forced Americans to examine how they felt but also allowed many to explore cultural roles from which they were prohibited during the antebellum era.

For example, Civil War service was perceived by many whites and African Americans as the antidote to African Americans' cultural disease— the presumed inferiority that marked and incapacitated the race. In Chapter 4 I turn to the diaries of Charlotte Forten and the newspaper correspondence of James Henry Gooding, two free African Americans who served the Union during the Civil War. Gooding embraced his service in the famous 54th Massachusetts Negro regiment, while Forten eagerly became a teacher in the South Carolina Sea Islands experiment. Both wrote at the pivotal moment of emancipation, when those who were considered constitutionally deficient legally became whole personages. As Americans adjusted to the transformation of African American bodies from capital to laborers in pursuit of capital, Forten and Gooding register their physical and mental well-being in economic terms. In both texts, racist commonplaces inform the meaning of Civil War rehabilitation. Gooding and Forten write that African Americans suffered the same injuries and losses as their white counterparts. However, they seldom dwell on the individual sufferings caused by the war, instead exploring the psychological wounds of racism as they were magnified by war service. White Civil War writers began with the premise of their racial integrity—a myth subsequently disproved by their experiences in the war. However, African American writers of the era related quite differently to dominant discourses of corporeality and disease. Civil War wounds could thus become the means of rehabilitation for Gooding's regiment; in agitating for the same clothing, weapons, pay, and battlefield experiences as white troops, African American soldiers worked for the habiliments and injuries that would signal their "manhood" to the nation. In Forten's case, her dangerous Civil War service initially ameliorates her persistent illnesses, which express her racial hurts and financial worries. Yet Gooding and Forten realized that the complicated web of biological and social sciences emerging at the moment of emancipation worked to reinscribe Civil War illnesses and deaths in familiar racist paradigms. African American Civil War service placed new emphasis on the meanings of African American corporeality, for Civil War-inflected wounds allowed for both discursive and political rehabilitation and for insistent belief in the disabilities of the race.

In particular, the reconciliationist literature of white historians across the nation that emerged during the Reconstruction era sought to rehabilitate postbellum bodies to seemingly inexorable antebellum racial and gender hierarchies. However, Chapter 5 reveals how a generation after hostilities had ceased, some writers returned to the Civil War for what it had revealed about the inherently unstable nature of white masculinity. During the Civil War, white men had unleashed their murderous passions upon each other, producing not only the national unity that consensual histories emphasized, but also the brutal deaths of hundreds of thousands of white Americans—a death toll that evoked the specter of race suicide. Crane and Dunbar recognized this fact and used battlefield experience to explore the "sickness of battle" which increasingly constituted white masculinity. *The Red Badge of Courage* (1895) and Dunbar's Civil War novel *The Fanatics* (1901) depict how the mindless, self-destructive violence that characterized the white men of their own generation—racial violence especially—emanated from their Civil War heritage. Many scholars, most notably T. J. Jackson Lears, have written about the resurgence of martial culture during the Progressive Era as a therapeutic prescription for enervated modern Americans.[46] I argue that the Civil War is reclaimed as the site of the modern senselessness that turn-of-the-century men were ostensibly trying to escape. Thus the "new" white masculinity of the Progressive period was not so very new; these works suggest that turn-of-the-century nervousness was only the most recent manifestation of a racial trait recovered through the Civil War.

Whereas Crane and Dunbar turned their attentions to the invisible ills that constituted postbellum white masculinity, many marginalized Americans reclaimed the rehabilitative power of the Civil War as their own. White women and African Americans were initially hopeful following the war's revolutionary political pronouncements. However, though the war remained an exciting, emancipatory moment for many Americans, its promise of equality and enlarged opportunity remained unfulfilled. Few achieved the full citizenship, financial viability, and physical autonomy that they hoped would follow close on the heels of this propitious national upheaval. As one postbellum Republican senator recognized, "There are many social disorders which it is very difficult to cure by laws."[47] The escalating racial violence and hardening of gender roles that occurred as the nineteenth century drew to a close were in some part a reaction against the Civil War and its unrehabilitated bodies. Yet many writers returned to the Civil War precisely because of the change those stubbornly unrehabilitated bodies promised.

I argue in Chapter 6 that Civil War nursing was remembered not only as a heroic way for women to participate in the war effort but also as a powerful cultural trope that both exploited and transformed the gender proscriptions inherent in the nursing role. The nursing bodies of these Civil War narratives evoke women's generative powers, rather than the weakness thought to emanate from their female reproductive organs. Although Alcott's initially empowered Tribulation Periwinkle succumbs to disease by the end of *Hospital Sketches* (1863), a generation later Mary Gardner Holland and Mary Livermore claimed that the Civil War did not reveal the disease of unfit mothers (the focus of contemporaneous eugenical theories) but that of impotent white men. Frances Ellen Watkins Harper's *Iola Leroy, or Shadows Uplifted* (1892) and Taylor's 1902 memoirs invoke female nursing as a legacy of the Civil War and of slavery which is useful to contemporaneous uplift movements focused on countering degenerate stereotypes of African Americans. Prohibited from the domestic realms of true womanhood, their nursing takes a more holistic and activist cast, for only by claiming the regenerative powers of their presumably unstable bodies could African American women assume their proper place in the national family.

In Chapter 7, Negro Civil War historians (as they were called at the time) George Washington Williams and Joseph Wilson use Civil War service to negotiate dangerous stereotypes about male, African American licentiousness in their respective texts, *The Negro Troops in the War of Rebellion, 1861–1865* (1888) and *The Black Phalanx* (1890). Historical method was increasingly ascribed permanence and stability by the emerging professional class of white historians, whereas the Civil War was reclaimed as the proving ground of individual fortitude and of a firm national identity. Thus, in writing themselves into Civil War history, African American writers were also able to delineate legitimate, rehabilitated selves. Historical visibility proved crucial in efforts to solidify the integrity of bodies that were perceived still as inherently diminished or underdeveloped. At the same time, the discipline of history-writing, embedded as it was in scientific notions of objectivity and verifiable human truths, placed impossible demands upon African American writers who wished to make scientific history serve their own ends. The racial identity of African American historians dictated the textual strategies they employed as they sought to write history and also highlighted the fact that all Civil War texts were founded on particularized bodily experiences and were impossible to verify.

The exciting and bewildering plurality of the war, as well as the instabilities such plurality evoked, have persisted into our own time. I end this project by briefly examining how the Civil War is still constituted through corporeal and historical discourse in late twentieth-century juvenile Civil War fictions and histories and in reenactments. The awkward, volatile, naïve protagonists of contemporary juvenile Civil War texts aptly dramatize Civil War rehabilitation: the movement from immaturity to full fitness, from plurality to consensus. For these white boy-soldiers the war becomes not only the seriously disturbing site of cultural and personal crisis but also an imaginative space where callow youths learn to become reliable men through the bloodless gauntlet of the Civil War. By the end of the twentieth century, a full-fledged reenacting culture had recast the Civil War as the mythic site of corporeal and social authenticity and of the racial integrity of white folks. "Living historians," the majority of whom are white, seek to claim the rehabilitative power of the Civil War by conjuring historical experience in their own bodies. Divested of its deadly consequences and the divisiveness that proved so disturbing to many Americans, the trope of the Civil War gained heroic proportions in twentieth-century national symbology. Yet the yearning for real suffering and for actual time travel to the Civil War that characterizes both fictional and reenacting odysseys points both to the reality of Civil War bodies in daily lives and to the unrecoverable nature of Civil War experience. The reliability of Civil War bodies and the authenticity of the stories that account for them can only remain a matter of faith.

We are still drawn to the Civil War for the cogency with which it encompasses issues demanding our current national attention: race relations, equal opportunity between the sexes, crises in masculinity, and general epistemological skepticism. Historically, the Civil War has provided images that are deeply wrought into the framework of our national identity. As the nineteenth century drew to a close, Northern veterans and their Southern brothers marched side by side in commemorative parades; African American veterans proudly recounted their exploits; former nurses congratulated themselves in print. In an age of economic turmoil, ethnic and racial divisiveness, and corrupt political leaders, the war became a cherished memory of self-sacrifice and cooperation, citizenship and patriotism, and meaningful political action. These are ideals to which the United States, as a culture, continues to aspire.

And so regional reconciliation, a solidified national identity, and notions of modern selfhood covered the very shaky ground on which they were founded. Like the hastily buried bodies left behind at the Battle of Gettysburg—decaying, half-buried bodies that made perceptible rises on the field of battle—the invisible ills of the Civil War, though renamed as they have been rewritten, continue to dot the American landscape. A reassessment of the modern basis of these diseases in the Civil War literature of the 1860s and the turn of the century is long overdue, for we are still engaged in the great project of bodily rehabilitation.

Chapter 1

Doctors' Bodies: Dr. S. Weir Mitchell and Patient Malingering

I like a look of Agony,
Because I know it's true—
Men do not sham Convulsion,
Nor simulate, a Throe—
—Emily Dickinson, #241

In 1863, Dr. Silas Weir Mitchell wrote to his sister of his increasing passion for the research he was pursuing in between his more mundane duties in a Civil War hospital. "I so much dread to find increasing practice or other cause removing from me," the young Philadelphian wrote, "the time or power to search for the new truths that lie about me so thick."[1] The "new truths" to which Mitchell alludes occupied his medical research and his fiction over the course of his long life. At Mitchell's death at age 84 his friend and fellow doctor, Owen Wister, summarized these interests: "Four years of mutilated soldiers and fifty of hysteria, neurosis, insanity and drug mania, unrolled for him a hideous panorama of the flesh, the mind and the soul."[2] It is precisely the interstices between flesh, mind, and that amorphous essence called soul that characterize Mitchell's imagination and distinguish his work. These issues coalesced early in Mitchell's career in his once celebrated but now forgotten war-era texts. During the Civil War Mitchell defined the new medical phenomenon that would shape the way he—and his whole generation—viewed the proper behavior of patients, the forms in which their stories could be told, and the role of the doctor: nerve injury.

Nerve injury during the Civil War was an all-encompassing rubric for a variety of ills and symptoms ranging from burning neuralgia to phantom limb pain to depressed or resistant behavior. Thus nerve injuries became the perfect vehicle for both literal and metaphoric discussions of the physical and psychological wounds of war. They were chronic and invisible. They flamed up and subsided at will. Most important, they foregrounded the tenuous distinction between "feeling" like oneself and enduring a growing sense of alienation from one's injured body and from one's self at war. The Civil War world Mitchell describes for his patients is a world viewed aslant, either numbly perceived through thick, insensitive skin or felt excessively and painfully through hyperaesthetic nerves. Thus Mitchell presents nerve injury both as an etiology and as a powerful cultural trope, one that would continue to accrue significance as the nineteenth century wore on.

Scholars have come to know Mitchell mainly through Charlotte Perkins Gilman's *The Yellow Wall-Paper* (1892) and Jane Addams's *Twenty Years at Hull-House* (1910), where he is revealed as the abusive inventor and implementor of the "rest cure," a therapy designed to relieve primarily upper-class female neurasthenics of a myriad of symptoms by enforcing stereotypically feminine behavior. Both contemporary praise and criticism of Mitchell focus on the mature, self-assured public figure he had carefully constructed by the 1880s when his expertise with nervous cases was highly sought. As his medical biographer, Richard Walter, writes, "Apocryphal stories continue to circulate, his name designates lectureships and prize papers, and his works are cited as references in the clinical game of roundmanship"—honors accumulated, however, relatively late in Mitchell's career. Recent articles in *The American Journal of Psychiatry* and *The New York State Journal of Medicine* celebrate the versatility of this poet-physician and invoke him as the beloved patriarch of modern neurology and even of American psychology. The preoccupation with Mitchell's late-century activities has commonly led most scholars to only two of his many medical texts: *Fat and Blood* (1877) and *Doctor and Patient* (1888). It is widely accepted that he formulated the rest cure in these two books.[3]

What is less well known about Mitchell's medical praxis but is equally significant is that the elements of the rest cure were developed for the treatment of Civil War soldiers suffering from nerve injuries. It was in *Gunshot Wounds and Other Injuries of Nerves* (1864) that he began to order "tonics, porter and liberal diet" for his patients, along with "shampooing [i.e., massage] and passive movement vigorously carried out" and electrical stimulus.[4] It is also here that we see the doctor's increasing resolve to carry out painful treatments despite the soldiers' "prayers and protestations" (*Gunshot* 25). Thus the foundations of Mitchell's later fame—the therapeutic aids of bed rest, forced feeding, massage, and electric therapy, as well as the vexed doctor-patient dynamic—were laid in the 1860s. Whereas women were to be returned to femininity through the therapy, these injured soldiers were to be rehabilitated into vigorous masculinity, ready to reenter their regiments and submit themselves to military rule. In both cases, patients suffering from symptoms that did not fit into existing categories or were unresponsive to known remedies were labeled "hysterical."

The distrust, even contempt, Mitchell felt toward his female patients was also apparent in his attitude towards Civil War soldiers; in all cases of hysteria Mitchell was hypervigilant, for he believed some patients feigned illness out of laziness or greed. Thus an important component of Mitchell's therapeutic protocol during both periods was distinguishing the real sufferers from the imaginary malingerers. In his own disease, Mitchell revealed the tenuous authority of the doctor and the medical knowledge at his disposal, admitting that doctors too are often malingerers feigning their roles. As a necessary correlative of the amorphous nerve injury, the concept of malingering became a trope in postbellum America for the ontological uncertainty of Americans who could no longer gauge how they felt. It also applied to those burgeoning professionals—such as Mitchell—who took upon themselves the task of deciding how Americans should feel.

Although designing a "system of therapeutics" was ostensibly his only goal in his medical texts, Mitchell was clearly embarking on an even more crucial project—one of hermeneutics (*Gunshot* 11). Civil War soldiers suffered from injuries that had never been recorded in medical history, presenting phenomena to Mitchell and his colleagues that were "naturally foreign to the observation even of those surgeons whose experience was the most extensive and complete" (*Gunshot* 10). In the introduction to *Gunshot Wounds* Mitchell explains that "never before in medical history has there been collected for study and treatment so remarkable a series of nerve injuries" (*Gunshot* 11). Again and again Mitchell expresses the difficulty of describing in "ordinary terms" bodies that are so extraordinarily diseased. Extant etiological vocabularies were simply unequal to the task of representing something that seemed to be inarticulable. He emphasized that this was not the "normal" pain found in civil practice, suggesting that what was suffered in the context of the Civil War was appreciably different—was felt differently, endured differently—from the pain of previous generations. Since feeling is subjective, we simply have no way of knowing if people had never felt in the ways they felt during the war, but because, as David Morris explains, "we experience our pain as it is interpreted, enfolded within formal or informal systems of thought that endow it with a time-bound meaning," we can assume Mitchell's patients endured, as he puts it, "a form of suffering as yet undescribed" (*Gunshot* 101).[5] Part of the Civil War doctor's task, then, was to create a system of meaning with which the doctors and patients could interpret their illnesses and their respective roles in the rehabilitative process.

Although Mitchell appointed himself the "historian" of the aftermath of modern warfare, his anxiety about the possibility of a valid history based on the narratives of diseased individuals and the observations of uncertain doctors is evident in both his medical and fictional work (*Gunshot* 69). The case history method evolving during this time explicitly linked medical and historical endeavors. Indeed, Mitchell makes history corporeal, siting specific psychic moments and historical events in bodily wounds—the scars of memory attested to the reality of corporeal experiences and of events long gone. Yet his efforts to substantiate truth-claims in the body proved untenable as his work on nerve injury proceeded. Viewed through the lens of nerve injury, the body itself became a mutable, even spiritual, medium. Even when an injury was visible, the true nature of another's feelings could only be a matter of faith. One's own body became uninterpretable when proximate to nerve injury as healer. In his late-century historical fiction especially, Mitchell continued to wrestle with the inadequacy of corporeal knowledge, an uncertainty he consistently expressed through the trope of the Civil War.

Finally, the malingering inherent in nerve injury signaled a change of consciousness Mitchell valiantly resisted. We can see him stretching to make the uncommon and incomprehensible—bizarre injuries; seemingly recalcitrant, even depressed, patients—fit into his medical prognoses, to make amorphous ills treatable. He reassures his reader, "Phenomena which one day seemed rare and curious, were seen anew in other cases the next day, and grew commonplace as our patients became numerous" (*Gunshot* 2). Mitchell crafts a bodily logic contingent on a vast quantity of diseased bodies. The considerable number of nerve injuries and the doctors' increasing familiarity with the "rare and curious" promised the possibility of knowledge and rehabilitation. It is through the meticulous layering of case history upon case history that individual bodies would become recognizable and, ultimately, treatable as they were amalgamated into a theoretical composite. Even if not properly cured, the idea that such diseases would become "commonplace" assured rehabilitation, for habituation to disease makes it normative. What remains unspoken is that insensibility could become the norm.

Most of Mitchell's significant medical work on nerve injury and malingering was written during his two-year stint as head army surgeon at Turner J. Lane Hospital, an institution created by his friend Surgeon General William A. Hammond to explore the increasing number of puzzling maladies produced by the war.[6] *Gunshot Wounds and Other Injuries of Nerves*, the first product of his war-era medical research, has been dubbed the major treatise of the nineteenth century on nerve damage. In the words of one recent critic, it was so "truly revolutionary" that it remained the definitive work on nerve damage for at least a generation, resurfacing in Paris hospitals during World War I.[7] Mitchell's pamphlet "On Malingering, Especially in Regard to Simulation of Diseases of the Nervous System," also published in 1864, was, like *Gunshot Wounds*, coauthored by Mitchell and his Turner J. Lane colleagues, Drs. Keen and Morehouse. This formidable trio confronts the difficulties of assessing personal character as a necessary aspect of medical practice, perhaps unwittingly presenting the doctor as an object of assessment as well.[8] Finally, in his anonymously published short story "The Case of George Dedlow" Mitchell's main character, who is both doctor and patient, confronts the psychic cost of wartime service.[9] Readers of the *Atlantic Monthly* were moved by the story of army surgeon George Dedlow, who after losing more than 80 percent of his body mass through the amputation of all of his arms and legs, experiences a short-lived spiritual reembodiment of his limbs at a seance. The imaginative resolution of Mitchell's story implies that rhetorical rehabilitations offered the only hope of recovery.

Two decades later, Mitchell's fictional imagination was still trained upon the Civil War. His first novel, *In War Time*, was serialized in the *Atlantic Monthly* in 1884 and subsequently appeared in book form. In it Mitchell returns to the Civil War hospitals and home fronts of his early career, places he revisited again and again in his fiction. It is in those historical and psychic spaces, as one of his characters proclaims, that men discovered "[what is true of] disease is true of war. It ruins some men morally, and some it makes nobler."[10] Perhaps not surprisingly, it is not the patients' demoralization or nobility that are the main focus of *In War Time* but, rather, the Civil War doctor's. Mitchell's Dr. Ezra Wendell clearly suffers from nerve disease, and the novel charts his incompetence and the mortal danger he poses to his patients. Mitchell's Civil War medical texts demonstrate that he was deeply invested in the emergence of a postbellum medical culture based on the practitioners' objectivity and the superiority of scientific methodology with its tenet of repeatable results. His fatally flawed fictional doctors often struggle with the disabling expectations this new medicine demanded. Wendell is rendered professionally and psychologically impotent by his inability to control his own senses and, then, consistently and fully rehabilitate his patients' bodies. Put another way, Mitchell's Civil War fiction demonstrates the futility of employing a method premised on producing objective results apart from the human beings who also embody those results. Doctors are always patients as well, subject to the science that they practice.

Thus Mitchell's Civil War texts provide a multifaceted picture of the convolutions of medicine, of narrative, of bodies, and of self that are completely integrated in the trope of the Civil War. This is not to say that his medical texts are primarily imaginative pieces or that they may be taken figuratively because the medical treatment and political views they espouse are largely outmoded. First and foremost, they must be read as serious efforts on the part of the medical community to cope with the very real injuries of Civil War soldiers and the doctors' abilities to serve their patients. Yet Mitchell himself seems aware that his texts not only attempt to heal patients but that they also construct crucial cultural narratives of body and selfhood. In particular, this chapter on Mitchell's war work reveals the psychological labor entailed in both the patient's recovery and the doctor's profession. The Civil War era, with its masses of diseased participants, established that all postbellum survivors would be long-suffering malingerers.

"When the Sensation Lenses . . . Become Destroyed"

In his war-era science and fiction Mitchell portrays patients at odds with their bodies, distanced, even alienated, from their unfamiliar, painful, and ultimately grotesque physical manifestations. In short, Mitchell explores how patients and doctors cope when "the sensation lenses" and the bodies that express them "become destroyed," as his George Dedlow puts it ("Dedlow" 8). Yet patients classified as nerve injured were impaired in an astounding variety of ways. In the most straightforward cases, the men described feeling detached, numb, and out of sync with normal body functions. The patients were fully conscious of what was happening to them, yet they did not feel at all, or felt partially or incorrectly. Mitchell focuses on men such as "Lieutenant G" who felt no pain when he was shot in his leg but eventually felt pain in the other leg (*Gunshot* 15). Another man could discriminate compass points equally well on injured and healthy tissue, "but when his eyes were covered, a large needle could be run nearly through the palm without pricking" (*Gunshot* 128). Their pains do not correspond to presumed physical sources and thus suggest that bodily damage does not hold as an originary source for nerve injury. There is not a necessary correspondence between the visible wound and the interior pain, as medical wisdom of the time would have it. What is clear is that these men do not feel the way they did before their war injuries.

Although some patients maintained a conflicted and alienating attachment to their pain and the corporeal or phantom body parts that expressed the pain, others were so overloaded with pain that they were overwhelmed by it. Mitchell describes patients to whom "touch is interpreted or felt as pain . . . the sense of tact not lost but practically defective, by the overwhelming influence of the pain" (*Gunshot* 95). These patients feel so much that it hurts; the faculty of touch is "constantly exercised" and obliterates all other types of sensation. The symptom of "too much sense" or hyperaesthesia may also be interpreted as an inability to feel. A patient's hypersensitivity to pain can cause one, in medical parlance of the time, to become "hysterical." As Morris phrases it, "Prolonged chronic pain threatens to unravel the self," ushering in not death, but insanity.[11] In *Gunshot Wounds* one patient is "nervous and hysterical to such a degree that his relatives suppose him to be partially insane" (89): "The temper changes and grows irritable, the face becomes anxious and has a look of weariness and suffering . . . at last the patient grows hysterical, if we may use the only term which covers the facts. He walks carefully, carries the limb tenderly with the sound hand, is tremulous, nervous, and has all kinds of expedients for lessening his pain" (*Gunshot* 103). Hysteria had not, of course, in 1864 attained the cultural significance that it would enjoy later in the century as a catchall for ills of the body and spirit plaguing modern Americans.[12] Yet this patient's hysterical body has come to be his entire sphere of existence, swallowing up all other concerns and perceptions. As Mitchell explains it, the diagnosis of hysteria is the only chance of "cover[ing] the facts" of this man's case, by organizing his disorder and offering the possibility of rehabilitation.

In describing such cases as hysterical, Mitchell contends that the body's uncontrollable susceptibility to sensation spills directly into social behavior. Mitchell wishes to rehabilitate the patient's body not only by measuring and standardizing how he feels but also by bringing him to his senses, restoring him to acceptable patterns of behavior. The seeds of a modern understanding of selfhood, in which the bodily economy is interpreted as out of control and in constant need of rehabilitation, were sown in Civil War hospitals. Not surprisingly, then, Mitchell concentrates on bringing the will to bear on the patient's body so that he will avoid becoming demoralized. Mitchell defers to martial law in his description of one patient, arguing, "Had he been abandoned to his own wishes, he certainly would have remained a helpless cripple; but it is quite sure that nowhere, except under military rule, could he have been relieved" (*Gunshot* 27). Self-discipline becomes a key component of the patient's physical rehabilitation. Because nerve injuries were so poorly understood, patients were often excoriated for lacking the will to overcome their physical maladies. Even today, when doctors do not have an organic understanding of a patient's disease, they may blame the patient for his or her inability to behave in expected ways. As Howard Brody persuasively argues, "There is a proper way to be sick . . . a proper way to carry out the role. . . ."[13] Since these injuries were being defined during a state of war, the military discourse helped to determine what was socially acceptable, even for the patient's muscles. Mitchell summons one patient's legs, insisting that an effort of will is "demanded to call them into action" (*Gunshot* 98). However, too many individuals failed in this effort during the Civil War for nerve injury to remain solely a matter of character. Mitchell and eminent colleagues, such as psychologist William James, spent the rest of the century grappling with the complicated relationship between the patient's bodily symptoms and his or her moral fiber.

As one might expect given this apparent crisis in character, patients who exhibited mental fortitude in disassociating themselves from their physical weaknesses were celebrated by physicians. Mitchell proudly recounts how "wounded men who are not weakened by loss of blood or excessive shock have a very natural curiosity as to the condition of the wounded part, and are apt almost immediately to handle it, and try to move it" (*Gunshot* 20). In this scenario, the injured body part—"it"—is rhetorically, and perhaps psychically separated from the individual. Early in *Gunshot Wounds*, the injuries are described rather mildly as "foreign" oddities; at a later point Mitchell comments upon the monkey-like appearance of a patient's atrophied hand, bestializing the injury; finally, the injuries are strongly described as "grotesque deformity" (10, 24, 70). The progression of Mitchell's imagery through the text signals his increasing frustration with the disease's resistance to treatment and the patient's inability to maintain corporeal integrity. As patients continue to suffer from their injuries, their humanity is systematically stripped away; likening their psychic realities to their atrophying limbs, Mitchell de-evolves the patients until they are no longer even animal-like, but monstrous. Although patients and doctors used this rhetoric for purposes of self-preservation, certainly one could not use such debasing language without imputing the individual.

Mitchell's stories of patients who do not feel pain and who exhibit courageous fortitude served an additional social function, that is, in Morris's words to persuade his audience "that they had nothing to fear from pain, at least when they suffered in a great cause."[14] This self-alienation was a necessary coping mechanism for a soldier who might be horrifyingly mutilated, let alone faced with the amputation of some body part. It gave the patient the illusion of an essential self that was protected from the ills that afflicted the self's shell. In its own way, this strategy combated midcentury physiological views of the reliable correspondence between the body and the mind. Certainly, their wounded bodies did not represent the physical self-portrait to which injured soldiers had been accustomed before the war. In many cases patients preferred amputation to deformity, perhaps believing that in excising the offensive, dehumanizing marks of war, they would be able to regain some semblance of their antebellum selves. Mitchell relates how he was "again and again urged by patients to amputate the suffering limb" as if it were apart from the patient's economy, a distantly suffering relation of whom the patient was fond but wished to put out of his or her misery (*Gunshot* 105). In addition, the amputated body, it was hoped, could provide a more accurate and healthy representation of the inner self than a whole but deformed body.

In "The Case of George Dedlow" Mitchell imaginatively explores the whole range of ontological states accompanying the physical undoing he encounters in *Gunshot Wounds*. Here Mitchell demonstrates the psychic and metaphoric death that can eventually accompany drastic changes in a person's physical experience of him- or herself or, as George phrases it, "how much a man might lose and yet live" ("Dedlow" 8). This is no conventional war story; we get only the sketchiest details of George's battlefield exploits. Rather, Mitchell concentrates on the "metaphysical discoveries" related to injury and loss of selfhood, presenting the gory details in order to "possess [the audience] with the facts in regard to the relation of the mind to the body" ("Dedlow" 1, 5). At the beginning of the story George describes his first injury in much the same terms Mitchell initially used in *Gunshot Wounds*. George is able to detach himself from his body, to look at his hand hanging loosely from his shattered arm and remark, "The hand might as well have been that of a dead man." He then proceeds to relate a thorough examination during which he determines the extent of the injury ("Dedlow" 2). However, sensation eventually does return, and the story illustrates that the feeling that persists after an injury is often reduced to pain when initiated through the gauntlet of the Civil War. The injured limb is "alive only to pain" and so is "dead" in every other sense ("Dedlow" 3). George begins to refer to his arm as if he were watching his own corpse, detaching from it and yet still feeling its miseries.

Initially Mitchell is eager to make George's pain meaningful. When George explains to a pastor that he feels fine "except this hand which is dead except to pain," Mitchell refers to nerve injury as a state not unlike purgatory or hell. The pastor makes that connection explicit when he warns, "Such you will be if you die in your sins; you will go where only pain can be felt. For all eternity, all of you will be as that hand,—knowing pain only" ("Dedlow" 3). Mitchell also suggests that George suffers for the sins of the Union; the doctor treating him in a prisoner-of-war camp is unable to relieve his pain with morphia because, he reminds George, "You don't allow it to pass through the lines" ("Dedlow" 3). Whether or not the pain is a divine or martial punishment, both the pastor's and the doctor's explanations make sense of George's pain, giving it a rationale and a predictable moral or spiritual meaning. The amputation of that arm functions not only as sanity-preserving detachment but also as expiation. Afterwards, George is calmly able to look at his amputated limb across the room and comment, "There is the pain, and here I am. How queer!" ("Dedlow" 3). The arm is no longer a body part; indeed, it is not even corporeal but instead signifies pure sensation for George. Who would not wish to rid one's body of pain? It is only through excision that his identity can be maintained.

Yet none of these solutions suffice, for George's body is endlessly vulnerable in the story. The continual pain does not transfigure Mitchell's patients or his fictional George or make their suffering meaningful; instead, it reinforces the fragile continuity between the previous and presumably coherent self and the new body consciousness.[15] Linking war, disease, and the (im)possibility of representation, George's eventual amputations and phantom pain suggest that re-membering war is either an absence of feeling—a death, a gap—or unremitting, excruciating pain. Once all of George's limbs are amputated, the pain does not end. In addition to throbbing or burning, George's phantom limbs now have the additional effect of keeping "the brain ever mindful of the missing part, and, imperfectly at least, preserv[ing] to the man a consciousness of possessing that which he has not" ("Dedlow" 6). Throughout his subsequent amputations, George's body-consciousness registers the dynamics of self and cultural history; he endures a pain that does not express the reality of his body or of the events he witnessed but only makes him aware of that which cannot be re-membered.

Consequently, when he awakes from the etherized sleep of the surgery during which his legs are amputated and "[gets] hold of [his] own identity," as he puts it, he claims he is "suddenly aware of a sharp-cramp in [his] left leg" ("Dedlow" 5). George is horrified to discover that his awareness is a false one as his amused neighbor informs him he "aint [sic] got nary leg." The longer he survives without his limbs, the more George feels his identity slipping away. "I found to my horror," he writes, "that at times I was less conscious of my own existence, than used to be the case. I felt like asking some one constantly if I were really George Dedlow or not" ("Dedlow" 8). Life is theorized as more than simply physical existence in Mitchell's writings; it is sentience, physical situatedness, a sense of individuality. Though George survives his injuries physically, psychologically he has been irreversibly lessened: "At the time the conviction of my want of being myself was overwhelming, and most painful. It was, as well as I can describe it, a deficiency in the egoistic sentiment of individuality. About one half of the sensitive surface of my skin was gone, and thus much of my relation to the world destroyed" ("Dedlow" 8).

He insists, as one medical ethicist has argued, "that life is not mere biological life . . . and human death is not, pure and simple, its biological termination."[16] Mitchell formulates a dynamic rather than static definition of the individual. As George explains, "A man is not his brain, or any one part of it, but all of his economy, and that to lose any part must lessen this sense of his own existence" ("Dedlow" 8). The body becomes the medium through which the world and the individual correspond along the course of "nerve threads"—as the body is diminished, communication lessens and so does one's sense of self ("Dedlow" 6). Without adequate materiality, this story theorizes, a human is no longer able to impress himself or herself upon the world or to be impressed by it. Indeed, George is unable to impress himself upon himself; he writes, "Often at night I would try with one lost hand to grope for the other" ("Dedlow" 7). In this story, Mitchell thus insists upon simultaneous correspondences and slippages between the body and the mind. George's corporeality must hold, no matter how imprecisely, the place for his identity, and, as the story's ending suggests, his ontological troubles can be healed by re-membering his body. But rehabilitation is achieved only in the realm of fiction. George's body is an incomplete signifier, and so George is a self unbounded—signification without substance or form.

As such, George's self seeps away, lacking the material sounding board, the friction through which he had been discernible. By the time he has lost all of his limbs, not only has George lost his identity, but he is also struggling to maintain his humanity. Rather than transcending his body, George becomes primarily identified through its absence. He is a "useless torso, more like some strange larval creature than anything of human shape. Of my anguish and horror of myself I dare not speak" ("Dedlow" 5).[17] He is unable to escape his decimated body—a body that makes visible the dehumanizing nature of war. His "useless" torso, shorn of its limbs by another human being, demands that we see the barbarity of war and the insensible self it ushered in.

Ultimately, Mitchell's medical rhetoric was unequal to the task of rehabilitating strange and debilitating nerve injuries like George's wrought by Civil War combat. His hermeneutical project was continually thwarted by his inability to read his patients and fit their symptoms into preexisting categories. The greatest test of the Civil War doctor's ability was the endless task of accurately and precisely taxonomizing nerve injury, because "it assumed all kinds of forms, from the burning, which we have yet fully to describe, through the whole catalogue of terms vainly used to convey some idea of variety in torture" (Gunshot 101). Further, the "causes are indeed so numerous and so perplexing related in individual cases that it is not always easy to assign to each its share in the production of defects of motility" (Gunshot 119). Mitchell sums up his frustration in despairing of describing seizures, for they have such a great variety of symptoms that they "know no law" ("Malingering" 384).

As George's dissolution demonstrates, these diseases unbound and unfixed the idea of a stable corporeality that was central to any notion of rehabilitation. Nerve diseases were particularly insidious; they could extend from the site of the injury to affect other parts of the body, to transfer "pathological changes from a wounded nerve to unwounded nerves." The very unpredictability of this malady, its ability to strike seemingly healthy and unaffected parts of the body, suggested not only the instability of life on the battlefield but also the war's ability to affect even those seemingly insulated from its brutality.

The vagaries of the nerves insinuated themselves into Mitchell's composing processes as well. Some of Mitchell's frustration stemmed from the phenomenal transformations taking place in medical practice at the time. It is important to keep in mind that medical writing of the 1860s was quite different from that of our own time. Yet Mitchell's Civil War work was part of a larger shift in medical praxis, as the "healing art" practiced by doctors such as Benjamin Rush was being transformed into a science. One medical historian explains that mid-nineteenth-century scientific writing was more leisurely, personal, and genteel than it was in subsequent decades: "With less editorial pressure, papers were frequently longer, more idiosyncratic and often autobiographical."[18] In a passage from his unpublished autobiography, Mitchell likens the writing of his medical articles to the mysterious process that overtakes him when writing fiction or poetry, where you "wait watching the succession of ideas that come when you keep an open mind":

I seem to be dealing with ideas which come from what I call my mind, but as to the mechanism of the process, beyond a certain point it is absolutely mystery. I say, "I will think this over. How does it look? To what does it lead?" Then comes to me from some inward somewhere criticisms, suggestions, in a word, ideas, about the ultimate origins of which I know nothing.[19]

Though I would not argue that Mitchell's scientific work is wholly fictional, the close connection in his mind between scientific and literary inspiration illustrates the transitional nature of his scientific work and the persistent difficulties of creating a precision between narrative and bodily experience. Debra Journet suggests that in "The Case of George Dedlow" "fictional techniques enable Mitchell to explore a phenomenon that he could not fully articulate within the scientific paradigms of his time."[20] Yet the etiology of nerve injury suggests that accounting for the idiosyncrasies of the human body is always a theoretical endeavor.

Most significant about Mitchell's self-reflexive passage on his medical composing process is that he cannot locate the "ultimate origins" of the theories he produces in his medical texts. Although one would guess, given the tenets of scientific praxis Mitchell advocated, that his patients' bodies would serve as the foundation and original material for Mitchell's texts, this candid passage suggests that the origins of his body theory emerged from the individual subconscious. Indeed, in "The Case of George Dedlow"—the work that most clearly muddies both the artistic and scientific intentions that animate Mitchell's writing—George metaphorically links bodily inscription and textual production. In recounting the story of his last injury in battle, George explains that the events of that day are "*burned* into my memory with every least detail" and reiterates "no other scene in my life is thus *scarred*, if I may say so, into my memory" ("Dedlow" 4, emphasis added). He uses the language of corporeal branding to express the permanent alteration his psyche sustained along with his body. Continuing his description, George also says that the moment of injury is "*printed* on my recollection" ("Dedlow" 4). Using the terms *burned, scarred* and *printed* interchangeably in this passage to express how injury impresses itself on bodies, psyches, *and* texts, Mitchell inextricably links the moment of bodily injury, the genesis of textual production, and the ability to access the past. The body literally is inscribed by historical events—each wound marks their reality. Yet the body's inability to remember—indeed, its volatility and substantial immateriality—indicates its lack of originative integrity for narratives of medicine and history.

The generic confusion "The Case of George Dedlow" provoked among its readers speaks not only to the amorphousness of medical authority at the time but also to the public's fears and desires about the authenticity of nerve injuries. In the opening paragraphs of the story, Mitchell purposefully exploits his readers, explaining that this story had "been declined on various pretexts by every medical journal to which I have offered" it ("Dedlow" 1). Thus he alerts readers immediately that the world of peer-reviewed scientific medicine denies the validity of the case history to come. However, he goes on to explain that although the story may not have any "scientific value," it has led him to new "metaphysical discoveries" that some readers have found valuable ("Dedlow" 1). Thus the text is supramedical; this introduction might have proven attractive to readers who found the medical community and their narratives of health inadequate and unable to account for the spiritual realms of experience so appealing to a country in mourning. The fact that Mitchell laces his story with accounts of actual battles and references to real regiments and hospitals also lends the story its veracity. Of equal importance, George Dedlow is a doctor, a professional identity that increasingly connoted authority.

Finally, though the narrator eschews the institutional world of medical science, he employs the scientific tropes of experimentation and repetition. George constantly situates his experiences in a larger context.

For example, after describing his thoughts and sensations during his first amputation, George writes, "At a subsequent period I saw a number of cases similar to mine in a hospital in Philadelphia" ("Dedlow" 4). And later, "There were collected in this place ["the Stump Hospital"] hundreds of these cases [nerve injuries]" ("Dedlow" 5). The instantaneous accretion of diseased Civil War bodies that Mitchell invokes validates the etiological explanations George subsequently proffers and ensures that the diseases he charts are genuine. Indeed, the most remarkable aspect of Mitchell's Civil War medical experience was that there were so many extraordinarily diseased people gathered together. In the hospitals surrounding Philadelphia alone there were 26,000 beds for the sick and wounded, and Turner J. Lane eventually housed 400 patients, all of whom suffered from some form of epilepsy, chorea, palsy, stump, or nerve disorder.[21] Medical historians are impressed by the meticulous case histories taken by Mitchell and his colleagues, thousands of pages detailing the stories of the men and their wounds.[22] The more material gathered, the more likely that one would be able to discern patterns. The apparently lawless diseases appear again and again, providing ample opportunity for experimentation, generalization, and finally rehabilitation.

Yet Mitchell later marveled that his readers had been so taken by his story. As he explained in his unpublished autobiography, "The unfortunate George Dedlow's sad accounting of himself proved so convincing that people raised money to help and visited the Stump Hospital to see him. If I may judge it by one of its effects, George Dedlow must have seemed very real."[23] By responding in such immediate and visceral ways, Mitchell's readers insisted that narrative treatments of bodily trauma were barred from the realms of fiction. Denied a generic classification or an author, readers assumed that the story conveyed new truths of the sort that Mitchell himself had wondered at day after day in the Civil War hospitals. In a way, the story became a phantom limb; Mitchell's subsequent statements would make it into a fraudulent version of reality, but his readers' responses suggested that it conveyed new and troubling information about postbellum bodies and identity. Indeed, the apparently seamless generic switch and bait suggests that all case histories are equally (un)able to communicate the reality of bodily experience.

The story Mitchell would later tell of how "The Case of George Dedlow" was produced and published echoes the mystical tone of his description of his medical composing process; it also smacks slightly of disingenuousness. He claims that he wrote the story on a dare: "A friend came in one evening and in our talk said, 'How much of a man would have to be lost in order that he would lose any portion of his sense of individuality?' This odd remark haunted me, and after he left I sat up most of the night manufacturing my first story, 'The Case of George Dedlow, related by himself.'"[24] For some unexplained reason, he then left the tale in the hands of a "delightful lady, Mrs. Caspar Wistar." When Mrs. Wistar's father, "Dr. Furness, a Unitarian minister," got his hands on the manuscript, he sent it to the editor of the *Atlantic Monthly* merely because he was "much amused." Mitchell then writes, "To my surprise, I received about three months afterwards a proof and a welcome cheque for Eighty-five Dollars." Thus the story's transference from nearly supernatural inception (the story "haunted" him) to anonymous publication to unforeseen compensation seems apocryphal itself. It is as if the story passed effortlessly—one might say divinely—from thought to print, unmediated by the mundane problems of composition, editing, and publication. Mitchell reveals that his medical and fictional narratives materialized from the "mystery" of "some inward somewhere," the "haunting" of bodily conundrums not far removed from those he saw in the Civil War hospital.

At the same time, Mitchell was keenly aware that empirical science was becoming the professional creed of American doctors.[25] Trained in this new milieu, Mitchell certainly felt pressure to present his new truths as persuasively as possible. Despite the amorphous nature of his composing process, the triumph of Mitchell's medical work lay in his ability to obtain objective detail by "ocular and microscopic examinations" and to posit a taxonomy of what paralysis "looks like, how it manifests itself in the skin" (*Gunshot* 36, 77). However, his patients' bodies and invisible symptoms continually subverted this scientific project. Mitchell had to vouch not only for the reliability of his observations but also for the authenticity of his patients' stories and the symptoms they presented. Again and again he attempts to convince his readers, and perhaps himself, of the veracity of the amazing bodily phenomena he witnesses. He argues passionately that one patient could not possibly be faking, for "he had never been in a hospital before" (*Gunshot* 104). The true difficulty of these types of injuries was that the body was an unreliable indicator of its own status—it gave even well-meaning patients false and unreadable symptoms, defied the known laws of physiology, healed itself seemingly without reason. A doctor could not establish nerve injury when patients knowingly or unwittingly presented falsified texts to the doctor. For both doctor and patient, then, these nervous maladies opened a fault or fissure in their worlds. Mitchell's desire to write a taxonomy of nerve injury contributed to the alienation of both physician and patient by providing physicians with new tools to systematize, objectify, and finally to appropriate not only the disease but also "the human experience and particular meaning the disease holds for the patient."[26] Doctors began to assume an adversarial relation to their patients, insisting that their diseases conform to the narratives of illness the medical establishment provided.

In *Gunshot Wounds* Mitchell briefly touches upon the issue of patient authenticity, an issue that grows to obsessive proportions in his pamphlet "On Malingering." In this correlative text, Mitchell and his colleagues put both doctor and patient on trial, outlining the various ways physicians can poke, prod, burn, faradize, cut, etherize and generally survey their patients in order to ferret out the dreaded malingerer.[27] What is most disturbing to the doctors is that malingerers purposely blurred the boundaries of illness, health, and self-representation that were already so fuzzy in medical discourse of the period. The notion of a "true self" at stake in this article becomes bound at points to contemporaneous anxiety about the disappearance of social distinction. For example, Mitchell writes that he is not alarmed that the otherwise "endur[ing] and tenac[ious]" malingerer would "pretend disease" but, rather, that he would carry on the double game of "an assumed character" ("Malingering" 371). Karen Halttunen has argued persuasively that the emergence of confidence men at midcentury resulted from an increasingly uncertain social system where, it was feared, men and women could pretend to a social status that they did not hold.[28] In pursuing malingerers, Mitchell believed that he would force patients to reveal an essential self that was, if not physically diseased, at least morally corrupted. For example, in etherizing a suspected malingerer in order to ascertain who is hidden beneath the hysterical exterior of one patient, "The tongue let out the thoughts, and the brain forgot to hold the eyes convergent, and then remembered it again with a sort of betrayed look most curious to see" ("Malingering" 391). Mitchell crows with success at his ability in this case to unveil the poser.[29] His rehabilitative work both returns health to the ill and stabilizes the identities of those who dare to feel something they should not given the way that social norms dictated bodily performances at the time. Mitchell's early experience with Civil War malingerers may have confirmed his suspicion of lazy inferiors, be they working-class men or upper-class women, which manifested itself most disturbingly in his domineering treatment of late nineteenth-century female neurasthenics.

On the whole, it was not malingerers themselves but the *possibility* of malingering that threatened the carefully constructed system of scientific diagnosis doctors were building at the time. Like the neurasthenia that would spread later in the century, the malingerer could infect others with his illness: "So long as one man succeeds . . . so long will ten others continue to imitate him" ("Malingering" 369). The doctors were loathe to admit that in cases of nerve injury only the patient possessed the "power of telling where exactly he has been touched" (*Gunshot*

115). In the face of such unflagging uncertainty and disempowerment, doctors desperately tried to regain control of the illness experience, initially devising a list of procedures and tests to be performed upon the patient to determine his health. When their tests revealed no organic condition, the doctors still cured the patients, though it was through the torture of "dry galvanism, actual cautery, setons and blisters" used normally to relieve neuralgic pain, as well as unnecessary anesthetics, that the malingerer was forced to reveal his true character ("Malingering" 371). Emily Dickinson's famous lines "I like a look of agony / Because I know it's true" cut only one way for these doctors. Whereas the pain their patients manifested as a result of their invisible wounds was always suspect, pain carefully administered by the physician and perceived "normally" by the patient could be an authentic indicator of their ability to feel. Mitchell advocates "faradizing" the skin with "a bundle of thin wires," for it is "the most intense and painful local excitant known to medicine, while yet it has not power to injure the part it thus violently irritates" (*Gunshot* 137, 141). Shocking his patients proved one of the Civil War doctor's most successful therapeutic strategies; malingerers treated in this way were immediately rehabilitated.

These tests were not foolproof, however; Mitchell and his colleagues desperately tried to create rhetorical control of the issue, removing nerve injury from the realm of medicine to that of law and morality by entering the "medical jury box," as they put it. The doctor was overtly transformed into a prosecutor armed not only with medical knowledge, but also with "ingenuity" ("Malingering" 371). Mitchell suggests that he should be aided by "detectives" who should "zealously follow [suspected malingerers] everywhere unseen . . . when they least suspect it . . . to see how they act when off their guard" (371). The doctors even recommend a "malingerer's brigade" as a punishment, made up of convicted malingerers marked visibly with a "peculiar dress" who are compelled to do the "hardest and filthiest duty" till they return to the battlefield as "honest men" ("Malingering" 369). Like Brody, who claims "a physician creates illness just as a lawmaker creates crime," Mitchell suggests that tracing the etiology of nerve disease relies as much upon the legal rhetoric that distinguishes criminals from innocents as it does upon physical exams and scientific observations.[30] Still the disease remained ambiguous. Malingerers managed to slip through the fingers of the law, unable to be court-martialed, for "it is yet impossible to swear to it, and even when it can be sworn to, it is often difficult to advance such evidence as will convince a court of non-professional men" of subterfuge ("Malingering" 369). Medical science ultimately failed the doctors in their case against malingering, for bodies did not provide adequate evidence for such purposes, and punishment and treatment remained elided.

Perhaps most surprising about the essay "On Malingering" is that doctors also became a subject of examination. They might also be malingerers, the authors suggest, employing desperate means to substantiate the diagnoses of these invisible nerve diseases and maintain control of the hospital. In trying to explain how doctors are qualified to make the important decisions between illness and criminality outlined in the work, Mitchell submits that he uses "his own sense, his habits of observation, and that peculiar tact in detecting imposters, which, whilst it seems an instinct with some, may be acquired" ("Malingering" 371). Ironically, the nerve doctor must rely upon his own senses, which—the doctors maintain throughout their medical literature—are always suspect during the Civil War era. In their effort to fix identity, the doctors became actors—or malingerers—playing their own parts in the elaborate game of one-upmanship. When approaching the potential cauterization of a suspected malingerer, the doctors "purposely, in his hearing, to the ward-master in the tone of a stage 'aside'" torture the patient with graphic descriptions of the "treatment" to come ("Malingering" 391). The authors themselves simulated various seizure types to see which signs could be mimicked and which were "involuntary." Finally, in some cases the doctors conspired to manufacture illness for the malingerer: "His body was perfectly free from disease, but we thought we would work a little on his imagination," Mitchell boasts as he begins to describe the painful examination to come.[31]

In "The Case of George Dedlow" Mitchell exploits the doctor's debility, for the patient is a doctor so spectacularly injured that he is unable to gauge the world around him, never mind assessing and treating patients. The doctor is the one who wastes away, who is incurable, and who eventually loses all sense of himself. George's case might be read as Mitchell's effort to tell the story of his own wartime illness.[32] Much had happened to Mitchell between the 1864 publication of his emphatic medical texts and the 1866 appearance of his anonymous foray into fiction. He had become a patient himself, forced by ill health to resign his nerve hospital, as he wrote to his colleague, William Keen. He would later explain curtly that he "broke down" in 1864. Mitchell complains to Keen that his winter of illness has been a "great hiatus full of aches and nausiaus [sic] doses—mustard plasters, slow, long, lazy days of convalescence and lots of not work done [sic]."[33] Most interesting is Mitchell's comment that after this long convalescence he was "just beginning to feel that [he] shall ever be [him]self again." Like George Dedlow, Mitchell lost something of himself in the war, but unlike his fictional character, Mitchell was confident that he could pull himself back

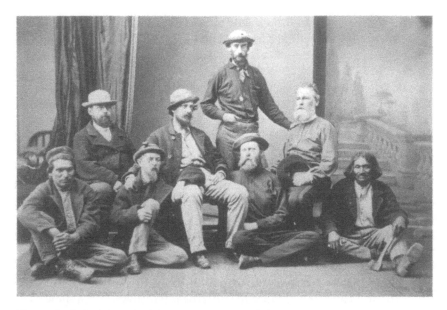

Figure 2. S. Weir Mitchell in Canada around 1870, possibly on a camp cure. Mitchell is sitting on a chair, fourth from the left. Courtesy of the College of Physicians of Philadelphia.

together again. Still, although Mitchell went on to be fabulously success-ful, it is clear that his own wartime disease continued to cause him pain (Fig. 2). He would abruptly abort his novel about how the news of Fort Sumter had been received in Philadelphia with the phrase "incom-plete—too painful for both sides." Even in 1905, commenting on the number and variety of injuries he saw during the war, Mitchell remarks tersely, "I sometimes wonder how we stood it."[34]

As we've seen, Mitchell's Civil War-era responses to the ambiguity of medical factuality and individual coherence varied widely, as widely as his ability to cure his suffering patients. Though Mitchell would later go as far as alienating the influential William James in proclaiming spiritu-alism bunk, the young, stunned George Dedlow finds it the only way to reconcile the scientific facts that rule his professional identity with the distinctly unscientific reality of his experience. Mitchell can only imag-ine full therapeutic relief from George's physical amputation and his psychic difficulty.[35] Even in his medical writings, Mitchell invokes the language of miracles and spiritualism in describing the recovery of his patients. For example, in some cases, Mitchell notes, nerve damage liter-ally causes a person's body to disappear: the "muscles waste," "tissue shrinks," and "vessels fade" until "nothing is left but bone and degenerated areolar structures, covered with skin" (*Gunshot* 70). The nerve damage eats away the individual's physical being. Mitchell's role, then, was to bring these "motionless, emaciated" sufferers back to life, so to speak, through his treatments (*Gunshot* 23). He wrote to his sister of the pleasure he felt conducting his "splendid Hospital work," for he was able to treat men who "have drifted hopeless and helpless from Hosp. to Hospital" by reenlisting their "dead limbs" and "moveless" lower torsos.[36] Mitchell then figures himself as a spiritual medium, bringing life back to the dead, manufacturing new, strong muscle and tissue out of thin air. He waxes poetic on the tearful thanks of men who identify him as their savior. Yet one senses that Mitchell feels little control over his healing abilities; the role the doctor plays in these miraculous rehabilitations is as suspect as that of a spiritualist.

Indeed, the sorts of bodies upon which Mitchell's medical knowledge is founded apparently reside in a spiritual plane. George Dedlow demonstrates that very little of the body is necessary to sustain sentience; he emphasizes that he has lost approximately four-fifths of his weight, that he sleeps and eats less, and that his heartbeat has slowed ("Dedlow" 7). His healthy limbs had connected George to the outer world in familiar ways and had provided the firm foundation of his individuality. But nerve injuries—and phantom limb pain in particular—proved the body's functionality beyond the grave; though impalpable, the body still registered feeling. Thus it is no surprise that George is compelled by the spiritualist follower who explains that nothing dies, that the soul "merely changes form" ("Dedlow" 9). Whether healthy and visible or amputated and invisible, George's body parts serve as mediums of communication, conveying feelings that were never completely translatable. Indeed, we might see phantom limb pain as another way of linking memory and corporeality, even when the latter has been compromised. "This pain keeps the brain ever mindful of the missing part," Mitchell writes, for it communicates the existence of that which one no longer sees but feels only in memory ("Dedlow" 6). The often observed "deformity" of the phantom limb indicates the imprecision of memory; the mutability of the phantom's presence represents history's evasiveness. George's reunion with his limbs at the end of the story imagines that corporeality can be communicated and that memory and the pursuit of history are consequently legitimate—that one can recapture and literally feel the existence of long-gone bodies and events. Thus the story grounds the possibility of personal memory and medical case history in the promise of corporeal rehabilitation.

Yet at war's end nerve injuries were still incurable, the soldiers unrehabilitated. Mitchell's final prognosis in the conclusion of *Gunshot Wounds* is that "the neural lesion may have been long well, and the ill it did live after it" (144). Mitchell's only real power lay in restoring some semblance of normality to the surface appearance of the body while coercing appropriate, obedient behavior. The disciplined, healed body seals the wound inside; the ghostly presence of long-gone limbs channels a corporeal reality that, Mitchell suspects, was never sure-footed. As he claims, "It would be in vain to amputate a member while the scar lies beyond it" (*Gunshot* 106). Though the injury had been metaphorically excised from the patient's body and mind through Mitchell's course of treatment, in reality the wounds of war remained in the patient in some unlocatable place.

"What Is True of Disease Is True of War"

After Mitchell's brief rest cure and the cessation of hostilities, he took up the compelling research he had begun in the nerve hospital; however, he found it impossible to make a living from this work. On July 11, 1868, Mitchell wrote to his sister Elizabeth that "the laboratory does not flourish," joking that his "cerebrum is softening." By July 1870 he admits defeatedly, "This year indeed every year now makes physiological research harder for those who cannot give their whole time to it."[37] At the same time, Mitchell discovered that he was consulted more and more about treating nervous maladies; *Gunshot Wounds* had gained prominence in its field and was expanded and re-issued in 1871 to wide acclaim. Capitalizing on the situation, Mitchell adapted his wartime therapies to treat upper-class female patients, consequently making a name for himself—and a lucrative living—as the world-renowned, charismatic "rest cure" doctor. Eventually, he gave up not only his research but also his general practice, focusing exclusively on cases of nervous disease. But despite his great success, he was still drawn inexorably to his war-era stints at Philadelphia's hospitals and to the professional and personal crises that first became evident during his tenures there.

Although Mitchell had published anonymous poems and short stories throughout the 1860s and 1870s, by the 1880s he was willing to claim his profession as part-time author, a self-described "literary physician who still remained loyal to medicine." *In War Time* was given a prominent position when it ran in the *Atlantic Monthly* during 1884; reviews and subsequent book sales were favorable according to Mitchell's biographer, Joseph Lovering. In this novel, Mitchell fully articulated the interconnections between medical narratives, fiction, and the Civil War that were evident in his earlier work. In particular, the affinity between his experimental medical texts and realistic fictions continued to animate his writing. Mitchell bragged that a therapeutic ethos pervaded his fiction; as he notably remarked, "There is a clinic" in every one of his books. He reveals to one correspondent that *In War Time* contains a "description of a case of locomotion ataxia," one that "conceal[s] the knowledge which a dr. has of these cases & . . . use[s] only enough to interest without disgusting."[38] He assures his intimate thus that his fictions are built upon the presumably firm foundation of medical science. Those "in the know" would surely recognize his characters' symptoms and be able to diagnose their diseases. Yet he confuses the work of the author, the doctor, and the medium or confidence man in this description as well, for he writes that he conceals the mechanisms by which he maintains the "interest" and credibility of his audience.

The congruence between his medical and fictional hermeneutics caused Mitchell a great deal of anxiety, which he expresses again and again in his private correspondence. In a letter to his great supporter, William Dean Howells, Mitchell explains, "I am twins and one is an amateur literateur in summer and goes to sleep in winter while the other attends to the literature of prescription."[39] Here Mitchell invents a professional schizophrenia to account for his dual interests and attempts to make them distinct from each other. Yet the fact that the "literateur" merely hibernates when the prescriptive writer takes over does not separate the two personae, for surely the dreams of the sleeper intrude upon the conscious self. Further, Mitchell twins his work, making the two "literature[s]" if not identical, at least fraternal. Mitchell's pride in his literary success clearly struggles with his need to downplay that success, for he senses that the plausibility of his fictional "clinics" might cast suspicion on the authority of his scientific work. In his autobiography, Mitchell writes that *In War Time* "had a large success, and trusting the good sense of the American people to know whether I was any the less a good doctor because I could write a novel, I continued to thus amuse myself."[40] Working in a still fledgling profession, Mitchell was keenly aware that he might be perceived as a dilettante for dabbling in the arts. He also implies that his facility with language and his ability to create credible characters and situations might undermine his medical authority. In transferring the language of medical narratives to literary ones and vise versa, the novels might confuse the distinctions between art and science, fact and fiction. As we have seen, lay readers perceived no difference between Mitchell's case histories and his stories. And because *In War Time* depicts in particular the duplicity and murderous mistakes of a very bad doctor, it seems logical that Mitchell might have worried that patients would turn from a practitioner who seemed to know the thoughts and motivations of a bad doctor so very intimately. Dr. Ezra Wendell might be read as the omnipresent nightmare of the waking doctor.

However, admirers chalked up Mitchell's detailed knowledge of the incompetent Dr. Wendell to his superior medical skills, his ability to discern the thoughts and motivations of his neurasthenic patients. Howells speaks for many when he claims, "There has seldom been a man in fiction so perfectly *divined* as Wendell," implying that Mitchell had merely fathomed the inferior Wendell's thoughts in godlike fashion.[41] According to Eugenia Kaledin, Mitchell delineated such diseased characters in order to "help his literary patients perceive the good life." In his journal Mitchell conflated disease and culture, writing that "good manners" could be "contagious."[42] Much in the same way that his war-era medical texts were meant to redress the demoralization of nerve patients, his novels of manners were prescribed as antidotes to what he perceived as an increasingly undisciplined citizenry. Dr. Wendell is a case in point. Though of supposedly good Anglo-Saxon stock, he is a weak, immoral spendthrift. His behavior is contrasted to that of the characters who make up his wartime community: his sister Ann, a Puritanical, unintellectual spinster; Alice Westerly, a strong, principled woman who is attracted by Wendell's dreaminess, but who is ultimately deceived by him; and Edward Morton, the man who suffers from the aforementioned "locomotion ataxia," but who bravely battles his illness and sacrifices his love in order to ensure his brother's happiness. These are just a few of the many characters who enact this very convoluted plot of love and betrayal, honor and disgrace, death and redemption. Yet Wendell unfailingly appears the weaker by comparison.

Perhaps what is most distinctive about Mitchell's diverse oeuvre, and what makes it a fit starting point for this project, is that his work imagines the Civil War as the primary site for explorations of the disruptions of the flesh and soul. Mitchell's son testified that in his deathbed delirium Mitchell ordered treatments for the suffering soldiers streaming in after the Battle of Gettysburg, and it is at this same martial crossroads that Mitchell began his first novel. As *In War Time*'s action begins, Dr. Wendell is attending to the wounded and dying in a long-gone Civil War hospital. Yet the narrative voice soothingly notes of those makeshift outfits: "The rest of the vast camps of the sick, which added in those days to the city population some twenty-five thousand of the maimed and ill . . . ha[ve] been lost, in the healing changes with which civilizing progress, no less quickly than forgiving nature, is apt to cover the traces of war" (*War Time* 1). One might argue that Mitchell implies Civil War rehabilitations are complete. At the very least, he rhetorically rehabilitates, stating that the "healing changes" of "progress" "cover the traces of war." To return to the etymology of *habile*, the wounds of war have been covered over, re-clothed. Yet significantly, Mitchell writes that the "maimed and ill" have been "lost," not erased or obliterated. The lost may linger; like neural lesions, they persist despite their inability to be located. Further, the "camps of the sick" may be gone, but their former citizens have not been exterminated, rather "heal[ed]" and redistributed during peacetime. Thus only the density of disease has been dispersed as that makeshift city's members were sent home. Indeed, Mitchell's story of war only briefly concerns itself with battles, soldiers, and hospitals; it moves immediately behind the lines, zooming past the hospital into the home of a Civil War doctor, and then into the homes of the doctor's civilian patients and acquaintances. Mitchell's novel flees farther and farther from the front lines, and yet disease, demoralization, and uncertainty pursue and infect all of the characters' doings.

In War Time was composed during the heyday of female hysteria and at the height of Mitchell's popularity; yet it is his fictional men who are permanently enervated, either by their wartime service or by their inability to serve in the war fully. Edward Morton, the invalid son of one of Wendell's hospital patients, claims, "All the man in me is going to shrivel up by degrees," for he has no opportunity to "die man-like in some wild rush of battle" (*War Time* 98). Conventionally, Mitchell initially posits that although both disease and battle diminish a man's body, disease emasculates that body, whereas battle lends potency to the body's impending dissolution. Prohibited from joining the army, Edward immerses himself in what Theodore Roosevelt termed the "strenuous life" to restore his manhood. In contrast to the "infantilazation and enforced debilitation" imposed upon female neurasthenics, men were sent to "hike in the Alps," engage in the sporting life at resort spas, or take "rough-riding camp cures," preferably "out West" somewhere.[43] Mitchell had prescribed such cures for neurasthenic friends and engaged in them himself. Yet Edward's exertions in Texas leave him permanently diminished, "unnaturally sensitive and nervous" (*War Time* 225). The masculine camaraderie and primitive conditions of such Western excursions were meant to replicate the invigorating deprivations of camp life at war. However, Mitchell reveals that the injuries that result from war are not ennobling or transforming either; rather they reduce men to hyperaesthesia. Edward's father, Major Morton, who has been manfully injured in battle, "can't think, for torment. [He] can only feel" (*War Time* 10). The long-term drain of his grave wound accentuates "all that was worst in Morton": he is increasingly "irritable and nervous" and ultimately undergoes the "moral degradation," as Mitchell calls it, that so often accompanies chronic illness (*War Time* 85).

Mitchell's most extended portrait of nervous disease is that of his main character, Dr. Wendell. Wendell is overemotional, one of the "unhappy people who are made sore for days by petty annoyances" (*War Time* 8). He is also hyperaesthetic, "exquisitely alive to the little annoyances of social life"; with eyes like "microscopes" and ears like "audiophones," his life is "one long misery" (*War Time* 89). And he is morbidly self-absorbed, using his "considerable intelligence" and imagination as funds for "self-torment" rather than as means of improving himself. Finally, he is violently moody. Mitchell claims that the shifting climate of Wendell's mind left him "without much steady capacity for resistance, and [he] yielded with a not incurious attention to his humors,—being either too weak or too indifferent to battle with their influence" (*War Time* 16). His "frequent changes of opinion" in diagnosis and treatment not only lose him clients, bur they also reveal Wendell's "mental unstableness" (*War Time* 235). Thus the doctor who suffers from the nerve injury he seeks to treat is bound to spread disease rather than cure it.

Most damning is Wendell's inconstancy, which costs his patients their lives. In the opening episode of the novel, one of Wendell's patients, a young officer, dies abruptly. Mitchell tells us that Wendell vaguely perceives that his moody impatience that day had prevented him from offering sufficient advice that might have made the young man more careful (*War Time* 17). Although he at first excoriates himself for his laziness, the realization that none of his colleagues notice his malpractice encourages Wendell to abandon his uncomfortable self scrutiny. Thus Wendell's neurasthenic self-indulgence goes unchecked, and his negligence continues to kill people. Near the end of the book Wendell's hysterical self-involvement leads him to hastily administer the wrong medication to Edward Morton, killing him instantly. Wendell is dimly aware of the way that his nervousness skews his world view, aware enough to notice with a dawning sense of "disturbing horror" that the "material importance of his favorite pipe," which he breaks, is "as important as the young officer's life" (*War Time* 18). The broken pipe also serves as a convenient and conventional metaphor for the compromised state of white masculinity.

Interestingly, given Mitchell's own vexed relationship to his literary work, he attributes Wendell's egomania to his aesthetic sensibilities: "The poets who live in a harem of sentiments are very apt to lose the wholesome sense of relation in life, so that in their egotism small things become large. . . . They call to their aid and comfort whatever power of casuistry they possess to support their feelings, and thus by degrees habitually weaken their sense of moral perspective" (*War Time* 18). In distinguishing poets who are seduced by the erotic and exotic headiness of a "harem of sentiments," Mitchell implies that there are literary types who are not weak and self-indulgent. Yet in making Wendell both a doctor and a poet, Mitchell explicitly links the literary and medical temperament. Mitchell's fascinating harem of sentiments even evokes the nature of his 1880s practice, when the famous rest cure doctor spent his time in the bedrooms of many women, attending to their overwrought sensi-

bilities and vulnerable bodies. Regardless of the character of that temptation, Mitchell posits that not only a nervous injury but also a literary
proclivity can reduce one's relation to the world and skew one's feelings.
The afflicted poet/doctor has no "wholesome" sense of the world, but
rather a partial or exaggerated relationship to it.

In describing the therapeutic protocol that Mitchell employed with
his nervous patients—and that we might use to discover the source of
Wendell's "moral measles"—David Rien suggests Mitchell's affinity for
Freud's notion of the subconscious (although Mitchell would later publicly denounce Freud's theories as immoral).[44] In Wendell's case, the
secret ailment that both typifies and triggers his nervousness is an early
show of battlefield cowardice. When serving on the front lines in West
Virginia, Wendell's regiment had come under heavy fire. "Dr. Wendell
very soon showed signs of uneasiness, and at last left his post," abandoning hundreds of injured men; Wendell is lucky that he is permitted to
leave the army quietly (*War Time* 303). This brief but key incident contrasts sharply with George Dedlow's thoughtless heroics, while illustrat-
ing that battlefield scenes provided concise, resonant shorthand for late-
century audiences. The legitimacy of self-concern is relative; what is an
instinct for self-preservation under normal circumstances is understood
as pathological in wartime. The Civil War becomes the source of subsequent diseases for Wendell. He frames his second immoral act—lying
about the cause of Edward's death—in terms of his previous "failure to
meet professional obligations" on the battlefield (*War Time* 393). The
discovery of his moral wounds, and the necessity of exposing them to
the view of those he loves, eventually destroys Wendell. We last see him
in an opium daze, shunned by his former society and proclaiming his
imminent death.

Yet *In War Time* does not allow itself to be resolved in a neat way. Critics who see Mitchell's fictions as prescriptions for a morally corrupted
culture contend that he "gave his stories happy endings because he saw
them as cases he refused to let suffer, situations he had rescued from
reality."[45] *In War Time* insists that Civil War disease resists both medical
and literary therapeutics. Indeed, the novel's most notable malingerer
is the Civil War doctor. It is perhaps understandable that the young,
unknown Mitchell who worked in Civil War hospitals would have
revealed Wendell's disease, just as he had exposed army surgeon George
Dedlow's foibles in 1866. One critic locates neurasthenia precisely "at
the intersection of personal insecurity about a career and the unsettled
and transitional status of the professions open" to young men of Mitchell's generation.[46] Mitchell's authorial aside on the great number of
"hapless persons" who were "more or less competent" and glad enough
to extend their "feeble tentacula" to grasp the eighty dollars a month

offered them as contract surgeons indicates that the tremendous number of casualties sustained during medical treatment may have been due to a compromised medical corps (*War Time* 3). And according to Mitchell, the exigencies of wartime medicine only encouraged laxity. "It is difficult not to become despotic," Wendell reflects, for when "no keen critic followed him, or could follow him, through the little errors of unthoughtful work" he is happily free to continue his "slipshod" technique (*War Time* 363, 45). Recall that Mitchell had called for detectives to help him discover the dreaded malingerers in his hospitals. His description of Wendell's inability to police himself suggests that perhaps doctors were the ones in need of constant surveillance.

But by the 1880s, Mitchell was an internationally renowned neurologist, seemingly secure in his rest cure and his profession. Presumably he had conquered his war-era ghosts. And yet they intrude upon his psyche, invading his fictional worlds. Perhaps Mitchell suspected what an 1892 survey of wounded veterans would confirm: an army of neurasthenic, insomniac victims denied his curative powers. The erratic success rate of nineteenth-century doctors, their susceptibility to mood swings that might affect their work—in short, their humanity is interpreted by Mitchell as the disease still plaguing modern Americans. Mitchell's professional reputation rested upon the forcefulness of his character, the certainty of his diagnosis, and the rigidity of his cures. However, in 1884 as he composed *In War Time*, he had been treating neurasthenia for two decades with, at best, mixed and, at worst, disastrous results.[47] Scholars of neurasthenia note that doctors themselves were frequent sufferers of the disease. Mitchell wrote often of his own erratic nature to intimate correspondents. In one letter he confesses to his young son John: "I have on me my Sunday mood which is grim enough & has been so for years—Yet why I can hardly tell—since on the whole life ought to satisfy me—but does not—Indeed I have had great luck to have had to work always for otherwise the sensitive side of me would have so grown that I might have come to be a morbid sort of man."[48] Though neurasthenia would remain a viable diagnosis well into the 1920s, in the 1880s scientists searched in vain for the organic source of neurasthenic symptoms and behaviors.

Certainly, Mitchell's fictional alter-ego, Wendell, engages Mitchell's personal demons and professional ambivalence. Yet Wendell's incompetence, his halfhearted efforts at doctoring, relieves him of the responsibility of curing his patients and ultimately explains his failures. Ironically, although the doctors' disease makes rehabilitation impossible, it also makes rehabilitation possible. To clarify, in this circle of logic, rehabilitated Civil War doctors could act with an objective, robotic precision and potentially effect their patients' rehabilitations—which would then ensure the patient/doctors' cure, and so on. Thus the Civil War can represent both the potential for sure corporeal knowledge and the tragedy of lost chances. Mitchell's fictional doctors admit that watching the sick leaves "vague but lasting mental impressions which may wear out with time, or be deepened by future circumstance and which are, as it were, memorial ghosts that trouble us despite our unbeliefs in their reality" (*War Time* 53). The bodies of their unrehabilitated patients— the reflections of their own inherently diseased subjectivities—linger around the doctors like amputated appendages. The experience of the Civil War hospital becomes representative of the persistence and inadequacies of medicine and of memory itself. Though time may rub away the sharp edges of trauma, they continue to "trouble," generating a surreal, interior world of half-truths and self-doubts. Even scientific pursuits reiterate this new lawlessness. When Wendell looks in his microscope searching for cures and answers, he sees

a wild world of strange creatures; possibly, as to numbers, a goodly town full of marvelous beasts, attacking, defending, eating, or being eaten: some, merely tiny dots, oscillating to and fro; some, vibratile rods; and among them, an amazing menagerie of larger creatures, whirled hither and thither by active cilia too swift in their motions to be seen. (*War Time* 165)

Mitchell suggests that medical research only confirms that the "invisible" worlds that he knew defined Civil War disease reflected, and more important, naturalized, the frenetic, combative nature of wartime and postbellum worlds. Like ghosts, these microscopic beings are alien, "strange" and "beast[ly]" "creatures" that come and go at will. Their constant, chaotic motion reinforces the idea of a reality too impalpable and elusive, always slipping away before one can get a fix on it.

The brief episode concerning Wendell's hysterical confederate patient, Captain Gray, dramatizes the war's incessant, ghostly return. Gray is brought to the Union hospital as a prisoner-of-war. As an officer, he is treated with respect and housed with a Union officer, Major Morton. Although Gray's prognosis is initially bright, he soon becomes convinced that he will not pull through. He explains to Wendell that he has a "queer sensation of confusion in my head, and—then I can't change my ideas at will. They stick like burrs, and—I can't get rid of them" (*War Time* 31). Frances Gosling notes that men's hysteria was most often characterized by such "obsessions or 'fixed ideas.'"[49] Those relentless thoughts eventually begin to eat away at Gray. After a conversation between the rebel and his Northern roommate about the battle at which they were both injured, Gray becomes convinced that Morton is the very man who shot him. At first, Gray claims that he is comforted by the fact that it is a "gentleman" who has been the cause of his misfortune. However, a new disturbing idea takes hold of him, a "brain echo" that, like a "silent song[,] comes and goes a thousand times" (*War Time* 41). The inarticulable pain of Civil War injury became an endless repetition—not the repetition of scientific cure, but the recurrence of Civil War trauma. Mitchell's Civil War texts return to the site of failure, where the only thing consistently produced is disease. The doctors insist that only Gray's silence will cure him; but Gray continues charging, "He shot me!, he shot me!" Unable to quiet the voices, dispel the ghosts, or stop the continuous loop of his moment of injury, Gray develops a fever that ultimately kills him. Like Shakespeare's Macbeth, who utters the phrase Gray repeats in his final delirium—"To-morrow, and to-morrow, and to-morrow"—Gray has "supped full of horrors," too glutted to move on to the future.[50]

The Civil War was a lifelong obsession for Mitchell, a gnawing wound, a persistent ghost, an incurable disease. In January 1914, the year Mitchell died, a colleague wrote of his life's work after the war, "Whatever his thoughts henceforth deep down was that memory perpetual. His tales and poems, no matter what be their subjects, all come from a spirit over which has passed the great vision; every drop of ink is tinctured with the blood of the Civil War."[51] Mitchell's work illustrates what becomes apparent in the work of others—that the Civil War is itself "memory perpetual": it is not necessarily a one-time, fixed event, but rather a trope that embodies the notion of memory as a constantly reoccurring but unpredictable presence. Writing itself for Mitchell and his contemporaries becomes Civil War writing—a rewriting, a constant return, an obsession with the corporeal. The bodies of war and text mingle here in the bloody ink that inscribes Mitchell's texts. That those bodies proved as tenacious and ephemeral as the memories they summoned and the texts meant to account for them is the legacy of the trope of the Civil War.

Chapter 2
Dead Bodies: Mourning Fictions and the Corporeity of Heaven

'Tis not that Dying hurts us so—
'Til Living—hurts us more—
But Dying—is a different way—
A Kind behind the Door—

The Southern Custom—of the Bird—
That ere the Frosts are due—
Accepts a better Latitude—
We—are the Birds—that stay.

The Shiverers round Farmers' doors—
For whose reluctant Crumb—
We stipulate—till pitying Snows
Persuade our Feathers Home.

—Emily Dickinson, #335

"A man would seem to be out of his senses deliberately to doubt what the world thinks to be simple truths," wrote C. F. Sprague in an 1867 *Atlantic Monthly* article entitled "What We Feel."[1] Yet as the Civil War drew to a close, more and more Americans not only began to question "simple truths," but they also discovered that they were, indeed, "out of [their] senses." Sprague reveals to his audience that even "greenness, the sweetness, the fragrance, the music, are not inherent qualities of the objects themselves, but are cerebral sensations, whose existence is limited to the senses" ("We Feel" 740). In doing so, he charts an alarming crisis of self-consciousness that had emerged during the previous half-decade of fighting. During the Civil War a fissure became perceptible between "what we feel"—what average Americans had taken to be the commonly experienced physical realities of their daily lives—and "cerebral sensations"—the way individuals experienced and intellectualized increasingly unfamiliar realities. Sprague writes that postbellum Americans are "deceived" by the limitations of their perceptions and the duplicity of even the most pleasant sensations for, he claims, "many appearances in nature are only simulations which we have no means of detecting" ("We Feel" 741). Sprague follows Mitchell's lead, outlining a world without locatable physical boundaries, one in which treacherous bodies have lost the ability to indicate reliably the nature of an equally deceptive universe.

Most disturbing is that Sprague's observations indicate that sensory stability had never existed in the first place, only that people had been unaware of the multiple realities that existed beyond the grasp of human sense. As this chapter demonstrates, mourning fiction novelist Elizabeth Stuart Phelps was just one of many writers who similarly imagined a world beyond sense, a reality outside the reach of human perception that would hold the promise of individual coherence and of stable knowledge broadly conceived. Sprague's scientific text serves as an apt introduction to Phelps's *The Gates Ajar* (1868), which, because it treats Civil War mourners rather than soldiers, traditionally has not been read as a Civil War novel. Though Sprague does not write about the Civil War at all, his essay illustrates a ubiquitous postbellum concern with the nature of reality and the body's ability to discern it, a concern that war writing such as Phelps's epitomized. According to Sprague, the physical sciences are based on the belief in a realm that dispels any apprehensions, a stable "Nature" of certainty and truth. In pursuing knowledge about the nature of the world around them, Sprague and other scientists merely seek to recover accurate feeling. It is fallible bodies that limit one's ability to discern the fullness of the world. For example, Sprague contends that a rose "exists in nature as a physical structure, and its existence is evident to us through the various sensations it creates in different nerves of our bodies, and through them alone" ("We Feel" 744). He reveals thus the unnerving interstices between the outer world and inner perception, the insubstantial meeting of the "ethereal wavelets" emanating from the natural object and the "nervous sensation" of bodies through which solid Nature is mediated and (mis)translated.

Of course, such debates about the nature of reality and perception are not unique to the Civil War. Indeed, Sprague himself writes that he is intrigued by "one of the ancient philosophies [that] maintained that all Nature is but the phantasm of our senses" ("We Feel" 744). However, although he finds the spirit of this old dictum compelling, he does not find the specifics suited to his postwar world. Nature is not the "phantasm" for him; on the contrary, Sprague has faith that Nature is the reality. Rather, it is phantasmic bodies that make inaccurate seemingly stable perceptions of the world. Sprague translates the words of the old philosophy into the new science, maintaining, "We frequently make the mistake of endowing matter with attributes which it does not possess, and which are resident only in the impression communicated to us by forces emanating from it. And we can understand that there may be forces in nature as powerful as those which we perceive by our senses, but which are utterly unrecognized by them" ("We Feel" 744). Sprague explains that human bodies and minds conspire to create comforting corporeal fictions to account for a physical world that must always remain just out of reach. At best, we perceive the world as an "impression" on our bodies. In using this term, Sprague seems to invoke a sort of accuracy, for an impression can be a copy of the original. At the same time, he could be seen as auguring impressionism, which values the associative and evocative over the presumably realistic. Regardless of how (in)accurately the perceptible world is felt, Sprague maintains that there is a world of sensation that might be all around but which limited and mortal bodies are unable to discern.

Though published more than two years after the Southern surrender at Appomattox—and apparently situated many worlds away from war—Sprague's article contends with the epistemological erosion ushered in by the long, demoralizing Civil War. Both soldiers and civilians had been asked to subsume individual, material, and bodily needs in the service of victory. And yet they were constantly faced with the grisly realities of dead, wounded, and suffering bodies; those who survived the war seem besieged by vulnerable, disruptive flesh (whether their own or loved ones') and unnerving psychological deprivations. The insensibility that Sprague reports was associated as much with emotional traumas suffered far from the frontlines as it was with sensory impairment, pathological or not. Clearly the material realities of daily life had changed during the war, but so apparently had bodies themselves. Rather than fault the world around them for its inadequacies, writers and thinkers of the era sited disillusionment and sorrow in the already illusory human body. As we have seen, amputations and other serious injuries complicated the sufferers' abilities to ground themselves in physical reality. This chapter explores how the emotional scars born by veterans and mourners alike similarly blunted their faculties. Unable to "feel" themselves, Civil War–era Americans lost the experiential boundaries of their individual identities. The end result was a country full of diseased individuals who were uneasy in their own skins.

Enter popular author and sometime correspondent of Dr. S. Weir Mitchell, Elizabeth Stuart Phelps, whose corporeal heaven was devised to rehabilitate disabled earthly bodies. Phelps, like Mitchell, has not been fully embraced by the American canon—indeed, each has been dismissed at one time or another as prosaic or conservative. Still, I believe that Phelps produced one of the most comprehensive and germane texts of the Civil War era in her attention to the profound and manifold sense of loss that the war evoked in those who survived. As I will explain, Phelps, like Mitchell, addresses the dissolution of human bodies, but she also focuses attention on those who were prostrated by the destruction of loved ones in the war. *The Gates Ajar* was phenomenally popular during the nineteenth century, remaining a best-seller for decades. In it Phelps traces the emotional sufferings of a woman who experiences the loss of her beloved brother as both corporeal and psychological disease. Phelps's protagonist, Mary Cabot, feels as if the physical loss she has sustained during the war has caused her to lose her sense of individuality and selfhood; her psychological wounds are expressed through the deterioration and distortion of her own physical senses.

Indeed, Phelps's imagery evokes nerve disease, extending the ailment's reach beyond the confines of the Civil War hospital. Civil War survivors, both veterans and noncombatants, could thus be likened to Mitchell's wartime patients, one of whom "walked sideways; there was one who could not smell; another was dumb from an explosion. In fact, every one had his own grotesquely painful peculiarity" ("Dedlow" 7). Mitchell describes patients who apparently suffer from neurological disorders, but their illnesses are also metaphoric for the distorted ways in which many postbellum Americans perceived their worlds. As Mitchell's work demonstrated, the source of such pain was unlocatable, but Phelps's novel insists that the disease's origin is irrelevant. Whether one was disabled by shells or shock the symptoms of insensibility persisted and required ministration. Such sentiments clearly struck a chord with Phelps's readers: *The Gates Ajar* garnered Phelps record sales and hundreds of grateful letters. Ultimately, Phelps's work suggests that the staggering death toll and the number of critically injured prompted a reappraisal of the meaning of embodied existence for both the dead and the wounded survivors of the Civil War. Personal loss, religious disillusionment, and a growing skepticism about the national mission are experienced as and expressed not only through the amputated bodies of soldiers such as George Dedlow but also through the jangled nerves of Phelps's grieving protagonist. Mary's physical afflictions resist national efforts to heal the bodies that bear the psychosocial wounds of war.

Yet even as she reclaims Mary's pain, Phelps demonstrates that the repression of individual desire and the self-sacrifice required by soldiers and civilians during the war produced a "vacant place" that could be recuperated only through the spiritual rehabilitation of distinctive bodies. Like Mitchell, Phelps recognizes that psychic healing is contingent upon physical integrity—though Phelps suggests that the rehabilitation of a dead loved one's body may effect the living's cure. Whereas Mitchell designs scientific remedies for his patients, Phelps offers a spiritual solution: the promise of a corporeal heaven. Thus Phelps discloses a new world to her readers, one where the ontological instability of her protagonist is defunct. Heavenly bodies are perfect versions of earthly forms, completely under the control of the individuals who inhabit them; in keeping with the logic of nerve injury, they also symbolize emotional well-being.

Although Phelps's corporeal heaven provides some comfort for those left behind, it does not completely ease Civil War survivors' distress—after all, those who had not died during the war needed to continue on earth. Comparatively, Mitchell's treatments did not offer a definitive cure for the crippling ailments that plagued his patients. Even Sprague, a scientist, acknowledges that the newfound inadequacies of the human senses signaled pessimism about the possibility of knowing ourselves on earth. Though not properly a mourning fiction, Sprague's text is elegiac as he realizes the loss of sensual security. He staunchly maintains the sufficiency of the natural world, but he does not offer any solutions for the deficiency of the human form. Indeed, individual perceptions of one's own seemingly solid body are as specious as one's understanding of the world outside the self: "A looking-glass does not possess, as a constituent part, the image of a human face; but that face, when put before it, appears to be a part of the glass; and if no looking-glass had ever existed except with a certain face before it, that face would be just as much a part of the glass as the color green is of grass. They both reflect" ("We Feel" 741). Like the color green, one's sense of self is a mirage, a simulation of the "real" and original face that exists outside the reflection of the glass. However, limited faculties do not allow one to perceive one's self originally, but *only* a reflection. Efforts to know selves fully and authentically are thus doomed to failure. Though Civil War survivors are not dead, Sprague's theory of a wholly reflective Nature does suggest that postwar Americans are unconscious of the marvelous world outside of reflection.

Science and spirituality are oddly linked in the immediate postbellum period, for Phelps's corporeal heaven fleshes out Sprague's theories. Her text grapples not only with the self in the glass but also with those who are no longer sensible to postbellum survivors—the many dead of the Civil War. Like Sprague, Phelps imagines a parallel, contemporaneously existing world where full sensation and, consequently, full knowledge reside. Whereas Sprague argues for a plane of invisible but omnipresent sensations to which humans must remain insensible, Phelps imagines a postwar world populated by the ghostly presence of the dead who speak to her living characters who cannot hear. Her life on earth is reflected by a perfected, earthly heaven where loved ones await the living. Jean Baudrillard's recent work on simulation and reality echoes the earlier thinking of Civil War-era writers such as Sprague and Phelps, for the correspondence the latter two imagine between life on earth and its uncanny perfection initially seems, as Baudrillard puts it, "Natural, naturalist, founded on the image, on imitation and counterfeit, that are harmonious, optimist, and that aim for the restitution or the ideal institution of nature made in God's image."[2] Sprague's Nature and Phelps's heaven are figured as utopic realities; presumably, bodily and spiritual imperfections make life on earth only a simulation of the mourned-for perfection of God's heavenly realm. However, the power of such utopias are maintained only when the "dissociation from the real world is maximized." The difference between the limitations of cerebral sensations and the full range of sensations is nearly inarticulable for Sprague. On the contrary, Phelps makes life on earth and life in heaven commensurate, the latter being merely an unbounded projection of the possibilities of the former. Though life on earth presumably is the reality, Phelps suggests that heaven is the idealized model for earthly existence. One might argue that heaven imagines earth into existence, and so mortal life becomes a reflection of the "real" afterlife. Yet the existence of heaven, corporeal or not, is unproven. In confusing the real and the simulation, and in turning the presumed real—life on earth—into an imperfect version of the unattainable original—heavenly afterlife— Phelps has made the real into a "utopia that is no longer in the realm of the possible . . . that can only be dreamt of as one would dream of a lost object."[3] Earthly rehabilitation is unrealizable and heavenly perfection, perhaps, an impossible dream. The suffering of the Civil War is attached to the deficiencies of corporeality, and through those deficiencies, to an epistemological uncertainty that persists beyond the war and beyond the grave.

The Corporeity of Heaven

Mitchell's last, ambiguous image of George Dedlow deserves one more look, given the way that he too relies on the imagined corporeity of the afterlife to heal afflicted bodies and minds. After sustaining treatment at the Stump Hospital for a year, the still despondent George is brought to a spiritual medium by a man who belongs to the "New Church." George's companion assures him that nothing ever dies, that "in space, no doubt, exist all forms of matter, merely in finer, more ethereal being." "You can't suppose a naked soul moving about without bodily garment," George responds, "The thing should be susceptible of some form of proof to our present senses" ("Dedlow" 9). Suffering from a waning sense of selfhood, George experiences the return of his legs at a seance, achieving a spiritual embodiment that allows him to feel like himself again. "Suddenly I felt a strange return of my self-consciousness. I was re-individuated, so to speak" ("Dedlow" 11). Though the moment of rehabilitation is short-lived, the story ends with George feeling hopeful that he will be rejoined with his "corporeal family" in "another and a happier world" ("Dedlow" 11).

Phelps produced a seemingly disparate, but surprisingly resonant response to the unprecedented carnage of the Civil War in *The Gates Ajar.* Phelps's and Mitchell's thematic convergence is providential. Though unacquainted in the 1860s, twenty years later the two struck up a lively, albeit short-lived, correspondence revolving around their common efforts to write the "Great Medical Novel" (Mitchell's *In War Time* [1884] and Phelps's *Doctor Zay* [1882]), the intricacies of treating "the human body and soul," and nerve disease—in Phelps's case, chronic illness.[4] These common interests had already appeared in *The Gates Ajar.* Searching for comfort at a sermon on the nature of heaven, the protagonist of *The Gates Ajar,* Mary Cabot, who has lost her beloved brother only days before his release from four years in the Union army, finds only "glittering generalities, cold commonplaces, vagueness, unreality, a God and a future at which [she] sat and shivered."[5] She longs for the tangible and specific, for a heavenly future that reflects and validates earthly lives rather than repudiates them.[6] The specter of a bodiless existence is horrifying to Mary, just as it is to George Dedlow and the patients on whom Mitchell patterned him. Luckily, Mary's Aunt Winifred Forceythe arrives to draw vivid and comforting pictures of Mary's brother Royal going about his business in heaven in an earthly, physical manner. Winifred audaciously suggests that the material wishes and the idiosyncratic potential of each individual are fully realized in what has traditionally been taken to be the most spiritual of places. Although Winifred acknowledges that Roy will be an angel, she adds, "He is not any less Roy for that,—not any less your own real Roy, who will love you and wait for you and be very glad to see you, as he used to love and wait and be glad when you came home from a journey on a cold winter's night" (*Gates* 53).

The Civil War's significance to Mitchell is unmistakable: he is heralded as the preeminent Civil War doctor, and his war fiction deals unambiguously with military men. The war that raged as she composed *The Gates Ajar* also had a lasting impact on Phelps; her final short story, "Comrades" (1911), dramatizes the Memorial Day observances of an aged Civil War veteran and his truest and strongest "comrade," his wife, "Peter."[7] And yet *The Gates Ajar* has not been read as a novel of and about the Civil War. Traditionally, Civil War scholarship has been concerned largely with the physical actions of male combatants, the material minutae of warfare. Virtually all *Gates* scholarship reinforces this view of the Civil War. Many critics find that instead of dealing explicitly with war, Phelps deflects "military into social history." Ann Douglas contends that Mary is able to accept the consequences of war only by denying its reality. Phelps's own admission that she wrote the novel to comfort "the bereaved wife, mother, sister, and widowed girl . . . whom the war trampled down" apparently substantiates such claims.[8] Phelps's critical disassociation from the Civil War signals a more general, ahistorical response to the work of nineteenth-century American women writers, a problem of which writing during the war era is a particular example. As Jane E. Schultz suggests, the perception that "only men make, fight, and matter in wars" has resulted in the invisibility of those women who did participate in the war. I would add that it has also masked women writers' dialogue in Civil War-era debates, leaving those aspects of their texts invisible to subsequent critics. Until recently, those who had recognized or anthologized Civil War-era literature by women had clustered women's works together, limiting them to home-front concerns and labeling their diverse responses as the "women's view" of the war. Elizabeth Young's recent work begins to rectify matters, relocating an impressive variety of women's writing in their Civil War context.[9] Yet the essential difficulty of examining "women's" Civil War writing is that the gendered qualifier brackets women's writing from the mainstream of the Civil War.

Both the interest in Phelps as a prototypical feminist and the damaging consensus that *The Gates Ajar* is largely a religious tract have also stripped the novel of its historical context. The relatively few extended treatments of *Gates* situate it within the dominant religious trends of her time or within female-dominated consolation literature, largely circumventing the historical context in which she wrote. As Lori Duin Kelly reminds us, "It was as a religious writer that Phelps was best known to her contemporaries, and it is largely for her religious writing that Phelps is remembered at all today."[10] Some critics, perhaps viewing Phelps's attention to religious orthodoxy as conservative and hoping to give her image a critical makeover, have steered clear of her theological entanglements or given only cursory treatment to *The Gates Ajar*, opting instead to study (and reprint) books in which she reveals herself as a "writer of books for women."[11] Phelps would consider such pronouncements surprising; in an often-quoted section of *Chapters from a Life*, an autobiography written in old age, she recalls how "religious papers waged war across that girl's notions of the life to come, as if she had been an evil spirit let loose upon accepted theology for the destruction of the world" (118). Certainly the novel's clear debt to the Spiritualist practices and beliefs sweeping midcentury middle-class homes did not set well with sanctioned theologians. I argue that Phelps's novel shows that the "destruction of the world" was fait accompli; it was her creation of a rehabilitated heaven that was her most radical act.

To this end, *The Gates Ajar* offers not only sentimental consolation but also a rigorous exploration of the ontological systems stirred by the Civil War and its aftermath. Steeped in, as Barton Levy St. Armand phrases it, an "American Protestant ethic at its most neurasthenic," Phelps responds to a lifeless, enervated faith with a visceral, re-embodied alternative.[12] St. Armand's reference to contemporary theology as neurasthenic is apt, for it allies Phelps's grieving protagonist with Mitchell's nerve-injured soldiers. It is not surprising that the symptoms of Mary's grief mirror those of nerve-injured patients: Phelps's mother and father apparently suffered from nervous conditions, and she describes herself to Mitchell on January 25, 1887, as "a 'professional invalid' in 'good and regular standing for about half [of her] life.'" Read alongside Mitchell's ground-breaking medical texts and fiction, Phelps's work takes on new significance as part of a philosophical debate on the relation between the body and the individual at war. In her depiction of grief Phelps speaks to the difficult issues confronting Civil War doctors and their patients: locating the source of amorphous pain, assigning truth value to the invisible suffering, generating the authority to articulate one's experience of these invisible phenomena, and devising effective treatments for the crippling ailments.

In her concentration on suffering, mourning, and the afterlife, Phelps is not, as one critic has suggested, conducting "exercises in necrophilia," nor is she morbidly fixated upon the deaths of her relatives, as many of her biographers insist.[13] *The Gates Ajar* is no more and no less macabre than Mitchell's story, with its grisly amputations and tortured protagonist. Phelps uses the afterlife as a transitional state suited to her explorations of a culture in perpetual flux. The gates to heaven are not wide open but "ajar," suggesting the unsettled situation of the period. Contemporary clergy too recognized the unrest, accusing Phelps of instigating the "overthrow" of "church and state and family" (*Chapters* 118). This charge notwithstanding, I contend that she is both responding to the cultural crisis precipitated by the war and creating one with her novel. Although *The Gates Ajar* may indeed have consoled a generation of believers who were devastated by the effects of the Civil War and unable to find comfort in traditional religion, its phenomenal popularity, not only in the United States, but also worldwide, attests to its larger therapeutic value. Some critics—most notably Nancy Schnog—have already assigned therapeutic significance to Phelps's fictional ethos. Others have read its curative potential in narrowly personal terms—as "therapeutic self-indulgence" for Phelps as she struggled to come to grips with her mother's death.[14] Phelps and Mitchell are the first in a long line of American writers and thinkers who found that rehabilitating Civil War bodies was a means of expressing both the personal transformations and social revolutions of their changing culture.

The nature of wartime death is central to the Civil War's signifying power. The massive casualty rates, previously unimaginable injury and dismemberment, and, ultimately, the lack of corpses to bury and mourn disrupted mourning rituals and prompted a reappraisal of the afterlife. *The Gates Ajar* clearly attends to a society in mourning. A staggering 623,000 Americans died in the Civil War (slightly fewer deaths than in all subsequent American wars combined). A half-million soldiers returned home physically wounded. At least 30,000 amputations were performed, generating grisly tales of the piles of arms and legs left outside hospitals and making amputees who remained dramatic reminders of the war's physical carnage. Many of the corpses never made it home. Thousands of unknown soldiers were buried in the South, and the War Department estimated that at least 25,000 were never buried at all.[15] All of these conditions disrupted a culture of death that emphasized the importance of tending the dying body, witnessing the moment of death, gathering keepsakes, and finally envisioning loved ones in heaven as they had appeared in life.

In many antebellum novels such as that other midcentury best-seller, *Uncle Tom's Cabin* (1852), the expiring body is celebrated and beautified by its death; family members gather around the angelic child, Little Eva, in order to glimpse the glories of heaven through her dying body. Material keepsakes gathered from the body were often an important part of mourning rituals; for example, hair that might be woven into watch-fobs, flower arrangements, and jewelry. There was also a midcentury vogue for memorializing the dead in photographs and paintings, as well as for displaying the dead body in glass-topped caskets. The embalming techniques perfected during the Civil War and the increasing skill of the newly appointed funeral directors, who would attend to the corpse cosmetically and compose its limbs in the most lifelike poses, allowed the corpse to "enact its own final genteel performance with bourgeois propriety," as Karen Halttunen has observed. Finally, as Martha Pike points out, the hexagonal wooden coffins of antebellum America became ornately decorated rectangular caskets, lined with silk and customized with brass nameplates; such vessels were in keeping with the original meaning of *casket* as a repository of jewels and other valuables to be preserved.[16] Thus, by midcentury Americans apparently found the dead body valuable in and of itself. What had once been an integral part of the individual—the mortal coil—came to represent the whole individual economy it had once housed. The dead body and/or its constituent parts became a synecdoche for the person in his/her former totality.

Yet Phelps's novel studiously avoids the corpse, which is the silent, motivating center of the novel. Instead, her heroine Mary focuses on the sights and sounds that surround her only contact with Roy's body: "He came back, and they brought him up the steps, and I listened to their feet,—so many feet; he used to come bounding in. They let me see him for a minute, and there was a funeral. . . . I did not notice nor think till we had left him out there in the cold and had come back" (*Gates* 4). Neither Roy's death nor the status of his corpse is described. Roy's body is perceived by Mary as a physical sensation in her own—the sound of feet on her stairwell. It is striking that the most popular consolation fiction of the nineteenth century displays none of the usual accoutrements of the contemporaneous death culture. For obvious reasons, postmortem images of soldiers would not have been comforting or, in many cases, even possible. The belief that death was "a sweet deliverance from life" served well the bereavement typology of suffering, angelic children gently fading away in illness. There was little sweetness or comfort to be found in the startlingly quick, violent deaths of grown men at war. Gary Wills's brief but explicitly grotesque description of the "thousands of fermenting bodies, with gas-distended bellies, deliquescing in the July heat" or poking out from shallow graves after the Battle of Gettysburg dispels the carefully maintained mourning fictions of middle-class culture.[17]

Yet Phelps does not simply deny the physical difficulties of wartime death. She writes circumspectly of the dead, attempting to assuage the anguish of readers who might be doubly afflicted with a dead body that is mangled, diseased, or simply missing. Consolation rhetoric suggested that dying loved ones—though thin or pale—remained essentially the same as when they were healthy. There was comfort in the thought that God had taken them and that they would enter whole into heaven. But in a time when tens of thousands of family members, friends, and lovers had disappeared—had been absent for months and even years before their deaths—many mourners found no comfort in the thought of a disembodied soul floating about in heaven. In memorializing Roy's physical being, Phelps attempts to achieve what Daniel Aaron has called "fictive solidity."[18] Mary remembers "the flash in his eyes," his "pretty soft hair that [she] used to curl and kiss about [her] finger, his bounding step, his strong arms that folded [her] in and cared for [her]" (*Gates* 9). Phelps builds an "altar of the dead," a rhetorical monument to Royal as she felt him in life. Yet she must still contend with the actual disintegration of dead soldiers' bodies. Consequently, Aunt Winifred insists that "*something* of this body is preserved for the completion of another," enough at least "to preserve identity as strictly as body can ever be said to preserve it" (*Gates* 116).

Many of Phelps's contemporaries were very literal-minded about the necessity of the body for the afterlife. In Louisa May Alcott's 1863 *Hospital Sketches,* a young amputee humorously muses upon the "scramble for . . . arms and legs" on Judgment Day; he supposes, "my leg will have to tramp from Fredericksburg, my arm from here, and meet my body, wherever it may be."[19] Phelps, too, resorts to humor in her oblique acknowledgment of the difficulties of dismemberment. However, she displaces anxieties about the possibility of a Christian afterlife onto what was certainly considered in her time a foreign, barbaric Other. In admitting the difficulty of transferring one's body to heaven after it has been mutilated, Phelps writes, "imagine for instance, the resurrection of two Hottentots, one of whom has happened to make a dinner of the other some fine day. A little complication there! Or picture the touching scene, when the devoted husband, King Mausolas, whose widow had him burned and ate the ashes, should feel moved to institute a search for his body!" (*Gates* 115). It is perhaps not too great a leap to read Phelps's Hottentots as warring countrymen. Significantly, in the second scenario King Mausolas's dead body has been consumed as part of his culture's mourning rituals. It is his grieving widow who is compelled both to ingest his physical remains and then to relocate them. Such "barbaric" practices are not so different, Phelps subtly suggests, from those of her own culture, which required women to sacrifice their loved ones to a national cause; like Mausolas's widow, Mary "feels moved" to search for her brother's body.[20]

It is thus extremely important for Mary to be able to imagine her brother as embodied in heaven; otherwise he would become savage, unrecognizable, and unlocatable. Dead bodies are rehabilitated in *The Gates Ajar* in the sense that they are reclothed in heaven with ideal earthly forms. Winifred assures Mary and Phelps's army of readers, "For ought we know, some invisible compound of an annihilated body may hover, by a divine decree, around the site of death till it is wanted," thus ensuring the heavenly reconstitution of the earthly self (*Gates* 115). Bodily rehabilitation is even more necessary during times of war when precious human bodies are so vulnerable, so cheap. Yet Mary must not only imaginatively reconstitute Roy's body, but she must also situate it in her geographic imagination. She supposes all of the people wandering around heaven must have "local habitations" and live "under the conditions of an organized society" (*Gates* 140).[21] It is impossible, Phelps insists, to transcend the limits of the human imagination; even existence as a soul—the faith in some essential self that survives life on earth—needs the physical boundaries of the body in order for it to be articulated and have resonance in human minds.

Phelps's preoccupation with heavenly embodiment inevitably leads

her to confront contemporaneous theological debates on heavenly existence. The Christian concept of the afterlife endlessly complicates the
relationship between physical and spiritual existence.[22] The idea of resurrection—the soul that does not die, the body that must—especially
confounds many Christians, even the clergy, Phelps argues. Mary is devastated by her local minister's account of heaven in an eagerly awaited
sermon on the topic. According to Mr. Bland, "Heaven is an eternal
state. Heaven is a state of holiness. Heaven is a state of happiness." Bland
goes on to list the "employments" of heaven, among them glorifying
God and studying God's infinite mind. Finally, he concludes, "I expect
to be so overwhelmed by the glory of the presence of God, that I may be
thousands of years before I shall think of my wife" (*Gates* 69–70).
Although this is meant to be a comic moment, it also shows that the
minister's notions of heaven are just as constrained by the limits of
human knowledge as the middle-class, embodied heaven Phelps eventually posits. Phelps helps her readers to see traditional notions of heaven
anew: "Vague visions of floating about in the clouds, of balancing—with
a white robe on, perhaps—in stiff rows about a throne, like the angels
in the old pictures" are no more ridiculous than Winifred's tidy cottages
(*Gates* 117).

Winifred argues that we will not live a "vague, lazy, half-alive disembodied existence," as Mary had supposed (*Gates* 113). She uses the Resurrection as proof that the tendency of Revelation is to show that an
embodied state is superior to a disembodied one. At one point she tallies
the number of times the word "body" appears in descriptions of our
heavenly state: " 'There are celestial *bodies*.' 'It is raised a spiritual *body*.'
'There is a spiritual *body*.' 'It *is* raised in incorruption.' 'It *is* raised in
glory.' 'It *is* raised in power.' Moses, too, when he came to the transfig-
ured mount in glory, had as real a *body* as when he went into the lonely
mount to die" (*Gates* 119). More than anything else, Christ's ascension
whole into heaven convinces Winifred of an embodied afterlife: "His
death and resurrection stand forever the great prototype of ours," she
insists (*Gates* 121). Her references to Christ carry added weight in a culture that consistently figured fallen war heroes as Christ-figures sacrificing their lives in a holy cause. In an 1862 sermon, for example, Octavius
Frothingham, a Boston minister, likened dying soldiers to Christ
because their deaths, too, would regenerate society. In one of Walt Whitman's best-known war poems, the speaker uncovers the face of a dead
soldier, proclaiming, "Young man I think I know you—I think this face
is the face of the Christ himself, / Dead and divine and brother of all,
and here again he lies."[23] It is no coincidence that the dead brother is
"Royal," and the grieving woman is named Mary—at once the mother
and lover of Christ and the archetypal figure of female mourning. Yet it

is not Christ as God that Winifred invokes, but Christ as man. In response to the concern that we shall "lose our personality in a vague ocean of ether" after death, Winifred explains: "He with his own wounded body, rose and ate and walked and talked. Is all memory of this life to be swept away?—He, arisen, has forgotten nothing. He waits to meet his disciples at the old, familiar places; as naturally as if he had never parted from them" (*Gates* 203). Winifred privileges Christ's humanity and his earthly connections over his divinity. Thus Phelps challenges those patriotic Transcendentalists who, George Frederickson has shown, eagerly adapted their contemplative theories to the war effort. Whereas influential thinkers such as Ralph Waldo Emerson were heralding the divinity within all people, Phelps concentrates on the humanity that had been sorely tested during the war.[24]

Phelps goes still further in her indictment of these powerful cultural convictions. *The Gates Ajar* demonstrates that received socioreligious doctrine provided an utterly inadequate worldview in this time of war. Ultimately Phelps's novel evolves into a carefully crafted theological argument for an interpretive strategy of the Bible that makes the afterlife material and, consequently, knowable. There is a pointed acknowledgment of the subjectivity of language and, more specifically, of biblical exegesis. Winifred complains, "No sooner do I find a pretty verse that is exactly what I want, than up hops a commentator, and says, this is n't according to text, and means something entirely different" (*Gates* 90). Phelps strives to prevent such dialogue from degenerating into spiritual meaninglessness and to find something comforting and tangible in Christianity.[25] Aunt Winifred becomes the novel's theological mouthpiece: her marriage to a minister and her own role as a missionary in Kansas give her theological authority, whereas her first-hand experience of the death of her husband makes her a credible representative of mourning. And her own battle with physical frailty—the breast cancer that takes her life—gives her the conventional apprehension of heaven that was so often bestowed upon the ill and dying. Winifred's vision of the afterlife is infinitely more comforting to all of the characters in the book. When his wife is fatally burned, even the misguided Mr. Bland is faced with the inadequacies of his faith and turns to Winifred for guidance.

Winifred locates "the mystery of the Bible . . . not so much in what it says, as in what it does not say" (*Gates* 93). In the gaps and silences, in the "dark corners" of theological sophistry lies the hope for reintegration and rehabilitation. Heaven is initially represented as the supreme abstraction; it is a blankness or silence to Mary. She lies in bed at night longing "for a touch, a sign, only something to break the silence into which he [Royal] has gone." "Has everything stopped just here?" she wonders (*Gates* 21). Mary relies on corporeal sensation as proof of Roy's existence beyond the gates; in a twist on traditional empiricism, accurate sensation becomes the means of assuring knowledge of invisible truths. Winifred is able not only to identify ideological and emotional vacuums but also to embody them, articulate them and fill them with the sensation for which Mary yearns. She creates what she calls "synonomes," that is to say, heavenly experiences and items that are similar or equivalent to earthly pleasures. Though earthly and heavenly existences are not the same, the former signifies the latter, making it comprehensible. Winifred explains that she treats her young child Faith just as "the Bible treats us, by dealing in *pictures* of truth that she can understand." She makes Mary's neighbors "comprehend that [in heaven] their pianos and machinery may not be made of literal rosewood and steel . . . [but] whatever enjoyment any or all of them represent now, something will represent them" (*Gates* 186). Aunt Winifred thus boldly builds a material argument with no empirical evidence, insisting that in the Bible God has not given us "empty symbols," but instead "a little fact" (*Gates* 78). Phelps's corporeal heaven is not an empty promise, as the Civil War had proved to be for many grieving Americans, but a factual reality, a material reward befitting the material sacrifices required by those remaining on earth. Her heavenly "pictures" combat the photographs of Matthew Brady and Alexander Gardner, which were simultaneously circulating images of blasted landscapes and decomposing bodies throughout the country. As Alan Trachtenberg explains, photography allowed the culture to create "a collective image of the war as a sensible event," "felt" even by those who remained far from the battlefield.[26] The Civil War was the first modern occasion for such imagery. Phelps merely responds in kind with her palpable heaven.

Literal, tangible interpretation of abstract concepts is the hermeneutic program forwarded by Aunt Winifred throughout the book. Even the act of naming her child Faith, which Mary claims is an inappropriate moniker for such a "solid-bodied, twinkling little bairn . . with her pretty red cheeks, and such an appetite for supper," heroically assigns physical being to an abstraction. In Winifred's corporeal theology, conversion is achieved through physical contact. Her "little soft touch"—not her words—preaches most convincingly against Reverend Bland's inchoate sermon and converts Mary to her way of thinking (*Gates* 71). When Winifred chides the local clergy for their inability to "tell picture from substance, a metaphor from its meaning," she insists upon the material and historical base of knowledge, resisting the psychological and experiential restraints of religious orthodoxy (*Gates* 77). Winifred's theology fosters individual authority, empowering the uneducated and disenfranchised to find spiritual answers in their lived experiences, rather than

demanding their submission to incomprehensible, abstract explanations. Anne C. Rose argues that midcentury Victorian Americans still
identified the Bible as an "essential point of reference," finding not
firm meaning there but "consoling allusions and personal uplift."
Phelps's novel supports Rose's contention, suggesting that postbellum
Americans had necessarily become skilled readers not only of the Bible
but of the texts of their own lives. The war seemingly enabled Phelps—
and her whole generation—to make such claims to authority, to
approach "reading" as a "strenuous, self-productive experience."[27] It
was their proving ground.

Phelps's insistence on Winifred as an "interpreter" of the afterlife,
Winifred's insistence that "the absent dead are very present with us,"
and her usurpation of masculine authority, ally Phelps with the Spiritualist movement, which Anne Braude argues was ubiquitous during the
middle of the nineteenth century. Not surprisingly, Spiritualism flour-
ished during the Civil War period: planchettes (the triangular pieces
that moved over Ouija boards) began to be mass-produced in the
United States during the war, the first national convention of this eminently antiauthoritarian movement finally occurred in 1864, and women
Spiritualists began to speak more frequently in public forums in the
early 1860s. Mary's spiritual crisis mirrors exactly those that Braude contends often provoked an interest in Spiritualism: "the desire for empirical evidence of the immortality of the soul; the rejection of Calvinism
or evangelicalism in favor of a more liberal theology; and the desire to
overcome bereavement through communication with departed loved
ones."[28] Braude explains that, before the Civil War, few found science
and religion incompatible. After all, the invisible mechanisms of elec-
tricity were as unbelievable to many as the invisible spirits that supposedly communicated to Spiritualist mediums. It is thus perfectly plausible
that Mitchell, a trained scientist and man of medicine, can only imagine
full therapeutic relief for his suffering protagonist in "The Case of
George Dedlow."

Most important, Spiritualist beliefs literalize the implicit foundation
of both midcentury spiritual and medical therapeutics: healed bodies
represent healed souls. As Braude writes, "While orthodox clergy portrayed the human soul as inevitably prone to sin, orthodox physicians
portrayed the human body . . . as inherently prone to disease."[29] Leading Spiritualist Andrew Jackson Davis believed that bodily affliction
reflected spiritual discord; healing bodies would restore spiritual health.
Both Phelps and Mitchell speculate on this Spiritualist truism. George's
belief in his self-healing power and Winifred's faith in a reconstituted
heaven put bodies back together again, undiseased, unbroken; in doing
so they ease distressed minds. Winifred's spiritual and psychological

ministrations "heal" Mary, Dr. Bland, and other sufferers in the novel, whereas George's Spiritualist encounter enables him to continue living in his ravaged body. All find "comfort" in their "fancying," as Schnog has shown; yet spiritual healing is located very particularly in bodily rehabilitation. In *The Gates Ajar*, Winifred's Spiritualist-inflected rehabilitation "cures the rift between the living and the dead" felt both in Mary's psyche and in her body.[30]

In part, such spiritual solutions combated the rhetoric used to marshal Northern enthusiasm for the war effort, a rhetoric that buried individual grief and denied the particularity of the slain soldiers. As many Civil War scholars have argued, religious and political leaders used "jingoistic Christianity" to drum up support for the Holy National Cause: "The onset of battle was God's judgment on men who abandoned the Christian Sparta to feast on the fatted calf."[31] Leaders reverted to the rhetoric of the Puritan enterprise, in which New England was the "City on the Hill." To endanger the nation that God had ordained with a special mission was to obstruct God's purpose. Julia Ward Howe's "The Battle Hymn of the Republic" is the most famous example of this rhetorical conjunction. Such sentiments were disseminated by everyone from local ministers to journalists to justify the soldiers' self-sacrifice to the national project. One minister, presiding over a regimental farewell ceremony, assured listeners that "your country has called for your service and you are ready. . . . It is a holy and righteous cause in which you enlist. . . . God is with us."[32] Gail Hamilton's 1863 essay "A Call to My Country-Women" clearly focuses such claims toward women. She exhorts her readers to "consecrate to a holy cause not only the incidentals of life, but life itself. Father, husband, child,—I do not say, Give them up to toil exposure, suffering, death, without a murmur;—that implies reluctance. I rather say, Urge them to the offering; fill them with sacred fury; fire them with irresistible desire; strengthen them to heroic will."[33]

Certainly Mary could find no comfort in a sermon such as eminent theologian Horace Bushnell's "Obligations to the Dead," which absorbed the individual suffering of soldiers into a great "hecatomb offered for their and our great nation's life." The soldiers' dead bodies strewn across the fields of battle are metaphorized by Bushnell as the "spent ammunition of war," "the price and purchase-money of our triumph."[34] Lincoln's widely publicized Gettysburg Address is perhaps the most egregious example of the obfuscation of Civil War bodies. Gary Wills argues that in this speech, trumpeted by most scholars as the pinnacle of rhetorical delicacy, Lincoln transfigures the "tragedy of macerated bodies" into the "product" of the democratic experiment. Gary Laderman adds that Lincoln "succeeded in incorporating the Union dead in the shared history, destiny, and physical landscape of the nation" by making them into a "monolithic totality." Whether individual bodies were incorporated into economic profit, the national soil, or the foundation of history, as Timothy Sweet has pointed out, "the system of the body politic recuperates wounding and death in war by omitting any description of [the individual body] and focusing on ideology."[35] The impersonal and disembodied national narrative of wartime death provided no consolation.

And, Phelps insists, the well-meaning condolences of personal acquaintances were equally injurious. In *Chapters from a Life,* she writes of spending between two and three years preparing for the novel by reading everything that had been written on mourning.[36] Denying traditional rituals, she uses her knowledge to mount an explicit assault against them. In refusing to accept callers or to attend church, Mary shreds the delicate social scripts of consolation and bereavement to which antebellum culture subscribed. What is more, she aggressively denies the religio-national truths that existed to help the bereaved make sense of death. Immediately after Roy's death, she is a self-described "Pagan" telling the church deacon who offers her the usual comfort, "God does not seem to me just now what he used to be." Deacon Quirk replies that he is sorry to see her in such a "rebellious state of mind" (*Gates* 14–15). Yet Phelps's imagery suggests that Mary's resistance to contemporary consolation is much deeper than the passing rebellion of grief. Mary describes how Deacon Quirk looks at her "very much [as he would] a Mormon or a Hottentot, and I wondered whether he were going to excommunicate me on the spot" (*Gates* 16). The racial and cultural privilege assumed by "civilized," white Christians such as Quirk, who condemn so-called Hottentots is clearly endangered by the barbaric war and by responses such as Mary's. Mary is therefore figured as exotic and debased, separated from her community by her insolence and the public nature of her spiritual battles. Phelps's only other reference to Hottentots occurs when Mary comments upon the difficulty of resurrection for people who make dinners of each other. The novel thus implies that the mourning rituals and religious orthodoxy forced upon Mary by her community threaten to devour her.

Mary's allusion to herself as a Hottentot also allies her with disorderly bodies. Her illicit grief resurrects the dead soldiers, incorporating their silent pain and suffering. Her emotional anguish is spatialized and felt in the body: the telegram announcing Roy's death "shut me up and walled me in," Mary claims (*Gates* 4). The consolation system is then figured as a physical assault upon Mary's person; it is not experienced as similar to the attacks Roy sustained in battle, where a solid blow provides the "relief of combat," but as feminine, as "a hundred little needles piercing at us" (*Gates* 6). Ironically, this is exactly the sensation described by Mitchell's neurasthenic soldiers, who complain of "prickling pain" along with "jagging, shooting, and darting pain." Taken together, Phelps's and Mitchell's texts suggest that all who suffered doing the war were similarly afflicted. Just as Mitchell's soldiers and Mitchell himself feel the world differently during and after the war, Mary's visceral understanding of the familiar is altered. Like Mitchell's hyperaesthetic patients, for whom touch is felt or interpreted as pain, Mary experiences the world as too much, as sensory overload.[37] As she describes it, "The lazy winds are choking me. Their faint sweetness makes me sick. . . . I wish that little cricket, just waked from his winter's nap, would not sit there on the sill and chirp at me" (*Gates* 30). The children's voices outside "hurt [her] like knives," conjuring up the instruments of amputation (*Gates* 2). Condolences are figured as probing and invasive, as surgery; Mary's callers violently penetrate her being, reaching in to "turn her heart around and cut into it at pleasure" (*Gates* 7). Her inconsolable grief is not expressed appropriately through gentle weeping and lamentation; it threatens to obliterate and destroy her.

All that is left, Mary says, is the "vacant place" in her home—and in her psyche—where Roy used to be. As we saw, George Dedlow's amputations symbolized this loss of individuality and integrity. Royal's death prompts a similar crisis for Mary and results in a psychic amputation: a part of her has been metaphorically cut off and must be reconstituted in order for her to rediscover herself. In framing their losses as the decimation of their "corporeal families" (as George calls his limbs), both Mary and George indicate that their connection to community and self is disrupted by the war. Mary's tenuous position as a self-described "old maid" makes her reliance upon Roy for identity even more acute. In a culture that valued women mainly as caregivers, Mary has lost one aspect of her existence in losing her brother. As Schnog observes, she is now "the sole inhabitant of a depopulated domestic realm."[38] Yet Mary's connection to Roy is much deeper than is usual between siblings—so intense that she describes him as a double, as part of herself: "Why Roy was so much more to me than many brothers are to many sisters. . . . We have lived together so long, we two alone, since father died, that he had grown to me, heart of my heart, life of my life. It did not seem as if he *could* be taken, and I be left" (*Gates* 8). Thus Mary mourns not only Royal's loss but also the loss of her self.

Essentially, Civil War-era protagonists yearn for a sense of authentic selfhood that would combat their mounting anxiety over their inability to feel and thereby define themselves. Three years after the publication of *The Gates Ajar*, Phelps wrote that religion consistently required of women a sacrifice that paralleled that required of soldiers: "to live for others; to make complete abnegation of themselves and to have no life but in their affect." Such a notion of Christian duty, Phelps insists, is "the most insidious and most hopeless injury which society worked upon women . . . [a] perversion of the great Christian theory of self-sacrifice."[39] St. Armand, among others, argues that Roy's death precipitates the loss of Mary's religious faith and perhaps signals Phelps's own doubts.[40] I would counter, however, that Christianity is recuperated by the end of the novel. *The Gates Ajar* dramatizes not precisely a religious crisis but an ontological one; Americans understood themselves and their places in the world differently after the Civil War. Roy's death removes all claims upon Mary's continued self-abnegation and conveniently serves as a metaphor for the material and psychological changes of the war. Like George, Mary initially has very little self-consciousness, for she is flattered that Aunt Winifred "seems to love me, not in a proper kind of way because I happen to be her niece, but for my own sake. It surprises me to find how pleased I am that she should" (*Gates* 58). During the course of the novel Mary must discover her own self-worth; it is her own individual idiosyncrasies, and not just her capacity to fulfill feminine stereotypes, that confer value.

Aunt Winifred's heaven is crucial in this effort. To Mary, its most appealing feature is that there will be no "fearful looking-for of separation" (*Gates* 81). Mary's concern with separation signifies not only physical separation from her brother but a sort of self-alienation precipitated by the all-out ontological assault of the war. Mary Louise Kete's notion of "sentimental collaboration" nuances Mary's dissolution. Kete argues that the sentimental mode of midcentury mourning literature is "not interested in autonomy or liberation but in the restoration of constitutive bonds, which make subjectivity possible."[41] Thus Winifred's heaven returns Mary to herself, so to speak, by returning Roy. What is most comforting is that Roy will be Mary's "own again,—not only to look at standing up among the singers,—but close to me; somehow or other to be as near as—to be nearer than—he was here, *really* mine again!" (*Gates* 54). Mary's intimacy with the heavenly Roy, her ownership of him, will enable her to become completely self-possessed. I don't think that, in emphasizing Mary's desire for possession, Phelps meant to invoke an exaggerated capitalism of the sort so caustically attacked by Mark Twain in his *Extract from Captain Stormfield's Visit to Heaven*.[42] Yet there is a sense that all of the things that people used to define themselves—possessions, relationships, desires, even fears—had been sacrificed or repressed in furtherance of the war effort.

Most alarming, Phelps argues, was the loss of privacy. Deacon Quirk preaches that in heaven "disguise and even concealment, will be unknown. The soul will have no interest to conceal, *no thoughts to disguise.* A window will be opened in every breast, and show to every eye the rich and beautiful furniture within!" (*Gates* 71). The most frightening part of traditional heaven is its nakedness, or as Mary phrases it, its "blankness" and formlessness. The exposure of an ethereal heaven is equated in Phelps's ethos with raw nerves exposed to harsh winds. Again, her psychic pain is figured in the language of nerve damage. Thus the embodiment of heaven also expresses a desire for enclosure, which can be read as privacy. Yet it is not the enclosure of mourning rituals and consolation visits for which Mary longs; recall that she feels the house transformed into a prison after she receives the news of Roy's death (*Gates* 2). Mary longs for spiritual habiliment (as Winifred phrases it, the "'garment by the soul laid by'") for its ability to shelter her and define her (*Gates* 114). Aunt Winifred is quite adamant on this point, providing the imaginative protection Mary seeks: "I would rather be annihilated than to spend eternity with heart laid bare,—the inner temple thrown open to be trampled on by every passing stranger" (*Gates* 79). Heaven will shelter the interior spaces of the soul; more important, it will maintain the illusion of individuality and coherence that both Mary and George so desperately crave.

Mary is not completely passive in her journey toward self-discovery; it is not enough for her to merely await her passage to heaven. *The Gates Ajar* plumbs the "psychology" Phelps found so fascinating in her schoolgirl studies of theology (*Chapters* 69). Not only do readers learn to interpret the text of the Bible, but Phelps argues they must be able to interpret themselves within the psychosocial paradigms that emerged after the war. She insists on the need for self-analysis—a rigorous interrogation of authority and dissection of the religious and philosophical givens upon which midcentury Americans built their identities. Mary admires Winifred because she "has done what it takes a lifetime for some of us to do; what some of us go into eternity, leaving undone; what I am afraid I shall never do,—sounded her own nature. She knows the worst of herself, and faces it fairly" (*Gates* 95). Though this Calvinist-inflected self-examination is decidedly Puritanical, the alienation and self-denial practiced during the war create protomodern detachment from its spiritual implications. Phelps's clinical protocol in examining the injured psyche is similar to that followed by Mitchell's nerve-damaged patients. Like George, Mary too manufactures distance between herself and an alternate self, the youthful "Mamie." "This poor, wicked little Mamie, why, I fall to pitying her as if she were some one else, and wish that some one would cry over her a little. I can't cry" (*Gates* 20). Certainly Mary and George's psychic fragmentation is a survival mechanism designed to excise unbearable pain. But Phelps also implies that the "sounding" of the dark depths of the soul that war and death forced will lead to self-knowledge.[43]

And yet, both authors suggest that earthly bodies continually subvert such efforts. Mary's desire for corporeal enclosure and integration directly combats the psychological fragmentation Phelps and Mitchell ultimately treat. As we saw in Chapter 1, Mitchell's real and fictional hospitals were populated by such broken individuals; even Mitchell himself inhabits the wounded bodies he ordinarily treats. Phelps outlines the end result of this incoherence in her "promiscuous theory of refraction":

We should be like a man walking down a room lined with mirrors, who sees himself reflected in all sizes, colors, shades, at all angles and in all proportions, according to the capacity of the mirror, till he seems no longer to belong to himself, but to be cut up into ellipses and octagons and prisms. How soon would he grow frantic in such companionship, and beg for a corner where he might hide and hush himself in the dark? (Gates 80)

Sprague's mirror had reflected back a facsimile image of the individual self. Like Alcott's joking amputee and Mitchell's harried protagonist, Mary insists that postbellum bodies are felt so incompletely that they are unrecognizable. Bodies are refracted by the movement from original to reflection and become fragmented and unreliable. Both Mitchell and Phelps suggest that Civil War survivors suffered from some sort of postbellum psychological trauma akin to shell shock and post-traumatic stress disorder. Civil War nerve injury, I contend, defined a generation just as powerfully as its twentieth-century counterparts, characterizing postbellum Americans' ways of knowing. According to Eric T. Dean Jr., though post-traumatic stress disorder was not a recognized disease after the Civil War, many disturbed veterans were diagnosed as suffering from "War Excitement" or "Exposure in the Army"—terms that formed part of the lexicon of nerve injury. Others suffered from "Nostalgia," a "stark terror" of combat so strong it induced the sufferer to demand immediate evacuation from the battlefield.[44] Like the characters in Phelps's novel, Nostalgics suffered from a sickness for home—the illusion of an antebellum home that can only be recuperated in heaven.

In a culture that would soon find itself masterfully expanding through industrialization and imperialism, nerve injury represented the contemporaneous inward-turning of its citizens. Both Phelps and Mitchell dramatize how neurasthenic pain creates a narrow, self-involved world for its sufferers. As postwar America feverishly worked to temper the brutal reality of war, traumatized survivors turned inward, where the reality of war had been forced to reside. Phelps's heaven publicly erases the traces of war from the soldiers' reconstituted bodies; their wounds are borne instead by the bodies of survivors such as Mary and George. Thus Phelps insists that modern bodies express the displacement, alienation, and insensibility—the unstable subjectivities—of postbellum society.[45] Phelps and Mitchell do not seek to mend, obfuscate, or transform but rather to expose the "crisis of representation" Sweet feels characterizes postbellum depictions of war. War is not "unwritten" in these texts, as Daniel Aaron has notably argued; it is, rather, ubiquitous, inscribed on the nerve-injured bodies of the living waiting to be deciphered.

Phelps's corporeal heaven will finally acknowledge and heal Mary's suffering. There the dead will be not only embodied but also clothed in a superior version of themselves. "There is to come a mysterious change, equivalent, perhaps, to a re-embodiment," one character insists, "when our capacities for action will be greatly improved" (Gates 114). The new bodies shall be "vastly convenient, undoubtedly, with powers of which there is no dreaming. Perhaps they will be so one with the soul that to will will be to do,—hindrance out of the question" (Gates 124). Bodies will become mere manifestations of individual will, neither diseased nor constrained by social mores. In Phelps's heaven, individuals regain control of themselves through imaginatively regaining control of their bodies.

Given the way that the Civil War and heaven are intertwined in her fictional imagination, it is no surprise that Phelps, like so many of her war-era contemporaries, returned to the metaphoric site of the Civil War. She wrote three "Gates" novels during her career. Though the subsequent novels are not true sequels to the first in that they do not continue to develop the characters or plot of The Gates Ajar, they do take up the philosophical and corporeal theories the first novel introduced. In 1883, for example, Phelps moved eponymously Beyond the Gates, from shadowy glimpses of heaven through gates ajar, to detailed description of a palpable location—from conjecture to knowledge. Indeed, she explicitly links scientific, spiritual, and emotional desires in this second novel, imagining they are commonly met in heaven. Whereas in The Gates Ajar heaven is only a potentiality, in Beyond the Gates Phelps fulfills Sprague's wildest dreams, for she creates a heaven where unfettered scientific discovery and complete knowledge are possible. Phelps's new protagonist is a forty-year-old spinster named Mary; though not the "Mary" of The Gates Ajar, she is perhaps an extrapolation of the first Mary, fifteen years older and gifted with the family the war had taken from Mary Cabot. In this disjointed character development Phelps continues the refractive effect she first explored in The Gates Ajar.

When this new Mary dies from an extended illness, she finds that those who inhabit the afterlife describe themselves as "neither unscientific nor unphilosophical."[46] And though heaven is thought to be the most ethereal of places, Mary finds that the reverse is true: the "secret of all abstract glory" becomes "attainable facts" (Beyond 45). Indeed, Mary employs the language of science and physics to convey the *reality* of heaven, its knowability: it is not spirits or angels but, rather, "a force like the cohesion of atoms that helps [her] to eternal hope" (*Beyond* 108). Heaven makes scientists of us all, kindling the "fire of discovery" in Mary and offering "endless variety and experimentation" (*Beyond* 53, 186).[47] In order to discern this place, Mary discovers that she has a body that is not "greatly changed," for she has "form and dress" just as she had on earth. Yet she also discovers that she "move[s] at will and experience[s] sensations of pleasure and, above all, of magnificent health" (*Beyond* 44). Heaven effects the full rehabilitation that Mary Cabot had craved. This second Mary writes further that even though she feels the "nervous and arterial and other systems . . . to which [she] had been accustomed" in her earthly body, she senses the heavenly forms' unspecified difference from "their representatives down below" (*Beyond* 54–55). Thus Phelps makes explicit what had remained implicit in *The Gates Ajar*: heaven holds the promise of solid and original corporeality, whereas earthly bodies merely suggest what only exists on high. At the end of the novel Mary comes back to life, secure of the empyrean knowledge waiting just beyond the gates.

And yet Civil War survivors continued on earth. Phelps insists in *The Gates Ajar* that heaven has become the "reality," the "substance," whereas life on earth is the "shadow," "the dream" (*Gates* 194). Ultimately life will be the most life-like in heaven; postbellum America is, then, a surreal shadow of its lofty ideal. As her novel suggests—and Mitchell's work concurs—life on earth is insubstantial, felt incompletely and thus only partially embodied. If heaven is reality, Mary Cabot's life, like those of Mitchell's nerve-injured patients, is characterized by the surreal, self-haunted "weightlessness" that T. J. Jackson Lears recognized in urban life several decades later.[48] Even before the onset of full-blown industrialism, Phelps demonstrates that the Civil War showed Americans the fragility of human life, exposing faith in individual significance as a sham. Belief in purposeful, individual agency withers during the Civil War; confidence in the recuperative ability of national rhetoric and the verity of religious truths also wanes. As Phelps would write to Mitchell on November 18, 1887, regarding her unstable health, "I suffer more from the future even than from the present." The postbellum future of a similarly diseased, prostrated culture seemed to promise little in the way of individual recompense.

As Mitchell settled into his postbellum practice in the summer of 1871, he related a seemingly innocuous but pertinent professional anecdote to his sister, Elizabeth. Mitchell had "flirted with popular literature" that year in his little book, *Wear and Tear*; like George Beard's more famous *American Nervousness* (1881), Mitchell's book denounces the disturbing enervation of postbellum Americans. Americans clearly craved such work for, Mitchell writes Elizabeth, he had received letters and visits from folks "from Maine to Georgia" upon the publication of *Wear and Tear*.[49] Mitchell proceeds to relate one particularly "droll scene" from his practice when a Pennsylvania lawyer who admired his work made an office visit. Mitchell notes that the lawyer's correspondence to him had been addressed to "Wear Mitchell," ironically conflating Mitchell with the diseases he treats. "Was it a joke?" Mitchell wonders. Yet he had written *Wear and Tear* to work out his own professional and mental exhaustion.

The lawyer complains that he is "awfully deaf & his head out of kilter." Thus he presents the ailments of any number of postbellum Americans: he suffers from sensory impairment, hearing the world through muffled ears that presumably cushion his perception of external hurts. The lawyer has adjusted to the quiet rhythms of his own insulated environment. The cure is a simple one here: Mitchell syringes the lawyer's wax-filled ears. Yet the treatment proves more painful than the disease, for the lawyer "suddenly heard—not as you or I do, but a whisper across the room—his own voice was terrible and the street noises thunder." Everything is too loud; even his own articulated thoughts hurt him. "Normal" unimpaired hearing has become unbearably frightening. He runs back to Mitchell's office "faint and begg[ing] to rest awhile before returning into the tremendous row of the street." With all of his faculties restored, the lawyer finds that the world has become too much for him. The country—and people like this lawyer—had survived the cataclysm of the war and its tragic aftermath, inured to feelings that were likely to cause trauma. Subsequent experiences were recast through the all-encompassing world of war and the sensory impairments it engendered. Ironically, Mitchell has effected a full cure for this patient; yet he feels the worse for it. As Emily Dickinson notes, "Tis Living—hurts us more—" than dying. Normal feeling—the promise of accurate perception—had been lost.

The carnage of the Civil War and its effect on all Americans became a trope expressing the numbness and detachment associated with modern sensibility. Thus mourning fictions such as *The Gates Ajar* should not only be read in conjunction with *Uncle Tom's Cabin* and *Agnes and the Key to Her Little Coffin* but also with Stephen Crane's *The Red Badge of Courage* (1895) and Ambrose Bierce's *Tales of Soldiers and Civilians* (1892). Comparing Mary Cabot's rebellion with Henry Fleming's psychological permutations, her heaven with Bierce's spectral landscapes, reveals *The Gates Ajar*'s shadows and depths and its resonance with the fiction of the modern period. The war lent itself particularly well to representations of dramatic cultural upheavals and to more probing explorations of embodiment and self-consciousness—those hallmarks of modern society and identity. In her 1887 correspondence with Mitchell, Phelps writes that it is high time "we reminded each other of what all but soldiers and mourners forget," for the experiences of George Dedlow and Mary Cabot were entirely pertinent to the daily experiences of turn-of-the-century Americans.[50] In 1868 Phelps deftly foregrounded the gap between abstract social systems and beliefs and the physical and emotional realities of life in America, which crystallized during the Civil War.

Chapter 3
Sanitized Bodies: The United States Sanitary Commission and Soul Sickness

The Battle fought between the Soul
And No Man—is the One
Of all the Battles prevalent—
By far the Greater One—

No News of it is had abroad—
Its Bodiless Campaign
Establishes, and terminates—
Invisible—Unknown

—*Emily Dickinson, #594*

I begin this chapter by returning briefly to the initial route of Northern forces at Bull Run. Strolling around Washington after the debacle, future secretary general of the United States Sanitary Commission (USSC), Frederick Law Olmsted, focused on the soldiers returning from the field and described them as clustered together, "pale, grimy, with bloodshot eyes, unshaven, unkempt, sullen, fierce, feverish, weak and ravenous."[1] Their officers, he noted, were detached from the corps under their command—mean and brutish men who had gathered at the local Willard's Hotel to drink and carouse. Olmsted used the aftermath of Bull Run to comprise his *Report on the Demoralization of the Volunteers* (1861), a document that criticizes the government's grasp of sanitary science. Consequently, Olmsted argued for the establishment of the USSC, a philanthropic organization meant to serve as a liaison between the United States government (namely, the incompetent Army Medical Bureau) and bewildered and underserved civilians and soldiers. Olmsted treats the dreaded "demoralization" as a diagnosis, explaining that when soldiers are mistreated by callous superiors, denied proper food, shelter, or clothing, and given only repetitive and menial tasks to perform while awaiting battle, they will become "soul sick."[2] The cure? Sanitary science, the goal of which was to nurture "the greatest military vigor and good discipline, to render the national forces in the highest degree effective, reliable, and physically and morally strong."[3] In this seminal document, discipline is thus allied with military success, and both are contingent upon a mutually constitutive complex of physical health and self-control. Reliability, that hallmark of solidifying scientific method, grounded the USSC's approach. Proper management of wartime "material"—described interchangeably as men or supplies in the USSC's subsequent documents—would produce repeatable results and, ultimately, Union victory.

Like S. Weir Mitchell (himself a USSC inspector), the USSC directors were anxious to identify and combat the invisible ills that stole into army encampments and decimated the soldiers' ranks. "The perils of the actual battlefield are nothing," Commission President Reverend Dr. Henry Bellows wrote, compared to the "irrational and viewless enemies" that threaten the army's health. Ailments such as malaria, fever, and pestilence are the "inglorious but deadly foes" before which our "brave boys will flinch; before their unseen weapons that they will fall!" Bellows insists (*Succinct* 11). Although the USSC's efforts to identify and prevent such physical diseases are laudable, the invisibility and great variety of ills that beset their subjects pressed the limits of the commissioners' knowledge and tolerance. In their many assessments of camp and hospital sanitation, they began to link the "special wants and perils" regarding diseases such as malaria to the "special causes of home-sickness and of insubordination, [and] camp vices" (*Succinct* 16). Physical diseases that subsequent generations would know were caused by germs were perceived as being of the same etiological order as the distress and misbehavior caused by loneliness, dissatisfaction, or so-called immorality. All manifested themselves in polluted bodies and unmanageable behaviors. Bellows further claims not only that soldiers may be weakened by inadequate living conditions and exhaustion, but that they may also be "prostrated with relaxing disorders" caused by underexertion while awaiting battle (*Succinct* 10). Thus under the auspices of the USSC's beneficence, physical needs became indistinguishable from moral failings, the strain of overwork the same as the stress of underemployment. According to this science, virtually all soldiers were in need of sanitation. USSC rehabilitations were geared literally and almost exclusively toward reclothing the body—covering it, nourishing its flesh, and attending to its fevered brow and broken limbs. By this logic, a sanitary body and vocabulary reflected a healthy soul.

And yet, as Mitchell's work showed, a healthy body could harbor a dissolute nature. In response, the USSC developed a rhetoric of actuarial science able in theory to make visible moral and spiritual well-being.

In 1864, even before the war had ended, USSC operatives asserted that the achievements of the USSC would "best be told by the Actuary of its Statistical Bureau, and by the journals and balance sheets of its Relief Department, or by the hundreds of hospital and regimental surgeons, with whose daily service and wants the Sanitary Inspectors had made themselves familiar" (*Succinct* 14). Thus the numbers of dead and wounded counted by the statistical bureau, the amount of money expended by the Relief Department, and the professional assessments of those treating the soldiers—statistics in general—would stand in for the physical and psychological well-being the soldiers were unable to convey. Anomalous dissolutes could be statistically insignificant in such vast company. Sanitary science translated into the military effectiveness of the Northern forces, and vice versa.

As the tide of the war turned toward Union victory, the USSC was eager to proclaim the perfection of their sanitary practices. The commissioners argued that their organization's history should be documented using the same sanitary science methods they applied to the cure of soul sickness. Such "systematic business" worked equally well, they implied, for the curing of diseased souls and bodies as it did for the subsequent telling of those cures; indeed, those narratives were necessary preludes to the cure itself. In professing a new precision between bodies and texts, the USSC created the illusion that they could turn the tides of war through their textual activities. This theory explains the immediate and extensive documentary project undertaken by the USSC. At points, USSC operatives admit that the "woes that were suffered by the wounded . . . can never be adequately described" (*Succinct* 80). Still, the USSC audaciously claims that it is able to indicate "with comparative certainty the Sanitary perils, weaknesses, or wants of the National forces" through such bodily accountings; in other words, it can enumerate intangibles—desires and drives—through the tallying of numerable bodies (*Succinct* 48).

Although physical descriptions and economic reckonings of the soldiers' bodies are scrupulously detailed in the extensive documents of the USSC, invocations of individual, emotional lives are rare. This is no coincidence. "Perils, weaknesses, or wants" were not only the symptoms of an unsanitary condition; they were also the cause of impurity and disease, the very vulnerabilities that needed to be eradicated. Disease was not merely the product of camp life, but of a much more insidious, preexisting condition. Western philosophical traditions have long considered bodies as things apart, as entities in need of control and discipline. These Civil War texts inaugurate ways of understanding the idiosyncratic psyche of each individual as diseased by definition. As members of a military body, soldiers are always asked to sacrifice individual care and concern in the name of corporeal and national unity. This was a commonplace practice long before the Civil War. However, in the texts I treat in this chapter, the incorporation of the wartime North not only secured Union victory but also exacerbated the disabling war-era diseases it was meant to relieve. Sanitary science revealed both the possibilities of martial rehabilitation and the notion that soldiers who insist on maintaining their individuality are distinctly unrehabilitatible.

In suggesting that the Northern military forces functioned by an ethos of incorporation—that is, reducing individuals to the states of their corps—I also acknowledge the economic and managerial values that were employed on a large scale during the war. Alan Trachtenberg has detailed how the rise of the corporation in the Gilded Age spawned "subtle shifts in the meaning of prevalent ideas, ideas regarding the identity of the individual, the relation between public and private realms, and the character of the nation."[4] Wartime culture already required that each individual's distinct emotional life be sacrificed to the cause; the USSC emerged as an institutional mechanism for codifying and enforcing such dictums. The documents of the USSC in particular insist that bodily desires, familial attachments, and individual emotions were enervating to the men and their war work, and military disobedience was more than a sign of insubordination—it was pathological. In this way, of course, the myth of a locatable and stable individualism was maintained—soldiers needed to know what constituted the self in order to eliminate it. USSC rehabilitations were not geared toward personal well-being but were pursued solely to repair bodies and cleanse minds so that they could be returned to their deadly work.

The USSC was as concerned with disciplining civilians as soldiers; indeed, most scholars agree that the USSC was formed initially to monitor the flow of charity from the home front to the frontlines and to coordinate the works and travels of overzealous mothers, sisters, and wives. Consequently, the ethos of sanitized bodies and de-individuated minds saturates war-era fiction. Both Rebecca Harding Davis's Civil War novel *Waiting for the Verdict* (1867) and John William De Forest's well-known war opus *Miss Ravenel's Conversion from Secession to Loyalty* (1867) establish bodily diseases—not frontline exploits—as the foundational narratives of Civil War fiction. Properly sanitized bodies become the sites of victory and national union. Critics have often puzzled over the prominence of the romance plot in many Civil War novels, complaining that such insignificant, home-front (read feminine) concerns do not express the grandeur and heroism of camp life and battlefield. Kathleen Diffley has attempted to understand the political significance of Romance, arguing that such plots "helped transfer Reconstructive allegiance at the altar of civil responsibility."[5] I argue that the lovesickness that dominates each novel is commensurate with the soul sickness the USSC diagnoses. De Forest's and Davis's protagonists' efforts to eradicate individual attachments and their struggles with debilitating personal histories speak to the goals set by the USSC. Although soldiers in USSC history or fiction are rarely allowed to express human emotions within the context of their war work, thwarted lovers are allowed to run the gamut of emotion. Each novel exploits the romance plot to this end. Yet in the final analysis, love is by no means idealized: some love remains unrequited, and the concluding marriages are largely unsentimental. Thus, to use one USSC benefactor's terms, the texts produce "unconscious missionaries," citizen-partners whose unions ensure stolid prosperity, not ardor or the threat of lusty dissension. Whether or not matters of the heart are dictated by the body (e.g., through primitive sexual drives) or merely expressed there is unclear in these novels. But what is clear is that love and intimacy reveal bodies as permanently disruptive forces.

The rhetoric of sanitation is particularly fraught when one examines the racial and regional bloodlines of the national family current at the war's outbreak. Because the Civil War was an internecine conflict, ostensibly geared toward reuniting the estranged regions (at least on the North's part), the racial slurs, ethnic stereotypes, and general hate-mongering typical during foreign wars was not as attractive or effective as it might have been. And when one applied social Darwinist theories of "survival of the fittest" or eugenic theories of degeneracy to the family war, the outcome did not bode well for the racial fate of white America. Within this logic, which I take up at length in Chapter 5, white men would be proven unfit and/or degenerate, regardless of which region won. The notion of unsanitary diseases caused by the extraordinary circumstances of war and army service allowed white Americans to maintain the racial integrity of the national family, while validating the "surgical" maneuvers necessary to heal the nation. Davis re-invests racial rhetoric, making her battle of brother against brother that of mulatto versus white versus black man. The language of sanitation reanimated the rhetoric of race—already so contingent on notions of purity and cleanliness—in this crucial era of emancipation. The individual concerns, family attachments, and bodily desires of African Americans, particularly of the enslaved historically denied such individuality, are found to be in need of cleansing just as there is the chance that they could be indulged. Indeed, excessive emotion was ultimately naturalized through the familiar imagery of "dirty," inherently diseased African American bodies.

Unconscious Missionaries

As I discussed in Chapters 1 and 2, Mitchell and Phelps were both committed to the notion of a singular selfhood, which was achieved through re-membering bodies. Their corporeal rehabilitations respond directly to the corporate enterprises detailed in the official documents of the USSC, which also diagnosed diseases and proffered treatments specific to a martial citizenry. However, the self-fashioning offered up by the USSC is the fashioning of no self at all, but rather the continual labor of unfashioning. Soldiers were asked by the USSC to wage a "bodiless campaign," to borrow Emily Dickinson's language, ordered not to feel in order to carry out the disaffecting and barbarous work of war. Sympathy, fear, humor, homesickness—all were figured as self-generated disease that must be wiped out by the new mechanisms of Sanitary Science. Soldiers were reduced to insensate material, their sole function being to serve the corporate mission of army, nation, and God. The multitude of USSC documents insist that sanitary science as perfected during the war would be eminently useful to Civil War and postbellum society. As one USSC operative asserts, "If five hundred thousand of our young men could be made to acquire something of the characteristic habits of soldiers . . . the good which they would afterwards do as *unconscious missionaries* of a healthful reform throughout the country, would be by no means valueless to the nation" (emphasis added).[6] Civil War missionaries, by their unthinking, unfeeling, insensible example, would induce others to devote themselves to the national mission.

As a national endeavor, the Civil War was always a corporate undertaking. The USSC assured its audience that "the management of all details in the current expenditures of the Commission, is conducted with the same rigid exactness and rules of accountability that prevail in commercial life" (*Succinct* 245). Cultural scripts of capitalism overlay the descriptions of war work in comforting and profitable ways. They helped to ease anxieties when the army became the only feasible career option for some men, for economic depression and unemployment during the war's first years made even a private's meager pay attractive.[7] Financial need lent additional ardor to the patriotism that fired recruiters as well. As the war wore on, the army became so desperate for soldierly material that it embraced adolescent boys and others who were not physically fit for camp life. The USSC estimated that fully twenty percent of the volunteer force was composed of such "weak material" that was hustled through physical examinations in the fervor of recruitment. In one case, a Chicago regiment was paraded past the doctor and passed en masse.[8] The USSC protested the "great number of under-aged and unsuitable persons mustered," for they were "a mere source of weakness, demoralization, and wasteful expense" (No. 1; No. 43). Subsequent sanitary policies suggested, however, that nearly the whole military populace suffered some form of debilitation, whether or not it had escaped the attentions of the initial examiners.

Meanwhile, the wealthy and influential could pay a fee to avoid service. The ethos of substitution has a long military history and fairly clear class implications. Only the relatively wealthy could afford to rent a body to stand in for their own. Both bounty prices and substitution fees reinforced a unique system of fungibility: one man was surely as good as another. Like many of the aspiring professional class, Mitchell evaded war service, capitalizing on the absence of other doctors to expand his private practice. In August 1864 Mitchell complains, "Folks have paid up well but bless me how it goes, $375 for a carriage & $400 for a substitute."[9] De Forest did serve the Union but had the means to raise his own regiment, thereby securing himself a captain's rank.[10] Although war successes were measured by the accounting of interchangeable bodies, the nation's and individual states' magnanimity was repeatedly expressed through monetary amounts. In 1864's propagandistic *The Philanthropic Results of the War in America*, the anonymous author offers the $37,701,991 advanced by the states to the national government during the first year of the war as palpable proof of the loyal sentiment of their citizens.[11] Substitution and bounty practices, as well as self-sacrificing benevolence, implied that human and monetary capital were, if not coequal, at least commensurate.

Those wishing to garner support for the USSC in particular and for the war effort more generally needed to negotiate the dehumanizing rhetoric of sanitary science without alienating those who clung to the belief in their individual worth. As scholars have documented, Civil War authors turned simultaneously to the tropes of sentimentalism and realism in their efforts to narrate the war credibly and camouflage the nature of warwork.[12] Sentimentalism allowed writers to suggest the emotional lives of the soldiers in coded tropes their readers presumably would understand, while the "realism" of sanitary science let them fulfill their audience's appetite for sensational detail. All USSC operatives walked this narrow line, one, for example, insisting that "succor" should be given to the wounded: "Not as if a hard master were driving a bargain with them . . . but as if the love and pity of mothers, wives, sweethearts, and sisters, were exercised" (*Succinct* 24). This writer is acutely aware of the exploitive nature of the labor soldiers performed, and invokes the language of domestic sympathy to mask the former's potency.

Although both sentiment and reality apparently appealed to readers, as evidenced by the skyrocketing sales of papers and magazines that utilized the two genres successfully, both, ironically, were predicated upon the erasure of individual soldiers' psyches and experiences, and their reduction to voiceless, compliant bodies. As Mark Seltzer writes of the fate of bodies in turn-of-the-century machine culture, "What from one point of view appears as the reduction of persons and actions to sheer physicality or materiality, appears, from another, as the abstraction of bodies, individuals, and 'the natural' itself."[13] In the USSC's accounting of soldiers' bodies, they are made into "statistical persons," both materially fixed and translated into the abstract realm of the type. In this way, unwieldy bodies were made to seem static. On this front, realistic and sentimental rhetorics are strangely allied. In so-called sentimental renderings of the soldiers' bodies, they are spiritualized, initially lured by and eventually subsumed in these seemingly gentle fictions. De Forest is one of the many writers who fabricates euphemistic death scenes where "none of the wounded men writhed or groaned, or pleaded for succor . . . all sooner or later had settled into the calm, sublime patience of the wounded of the battlefield."[14] His description is no different than that of the sanitary scientist, who describes the "patient and even cheerful endurance" of dying wounded who use their failing powers of speech, not to "groan, or even [to] sigh," but to "give final expression to the sentiments of the loftiest patriotism" (No. 42). In these scenes the suffering individual is distinct and severed from the national body he inhabits. Or rather, his mangled, wounded, or diseased body is the only iteration of suffering allowed. An impassable boundary is erected between visible bodily disease and mental distress. The soldier's quiet acquiescence validates the sacrifice he and his loved ones have made in the name of the Union; his death does not interfere with the constant movement of the war machine.

And yet those back home were fully aware of the physical hardships endured by soldiers as part of their military service. The USSC was created in 1861 precisely to rectify the physical abuses that Northern soldiers bore: tainted water supplies, rotting and/or nutritionally deficient food, unsanitary hospitals, filthy campsites, lack of clothing, and so on. As many documents emphasize, one of four soldiers died of disease during the war—disease caused by "unsanitary" conditions; this was a statistic that clearly could be lowered if troops and officers followed the teachings of the USSC. The USSC concluded that these problems were often self-generated. Reports from the field complain that the men do no use their "sinks," urinating and defecating all over the camp; that they eat food in their tents and attract vermin; that they tie their horses near their quarters and neglect to remove the dung; that they refuse to wash themselves or their clothing (Nos. 17, 26, 36). Such unhygienic conditions obviously led to contamination and expedited the spread of disease. Thus USSC documents, which appeared in many popular venues in efforts to raise funds for the largely charitable organization, waffled between tender sympathy for the troops' hardships and a taskmaster's scorn for the troops' misbehavior.

The initial document of the USSC's official papers succinctly expresses the way that sentimentality and dispassionate science worked together to mollify home-front discontents and standardize the flow and form of home-front relief. USSC Document No. 1 describes the organization as "the great artery which bears the people's love to the people's army." In using the "heart" as a metaphor for the USSC, the writer points to both the organization's ideological function of bringing home-front love to the battlefield and the structural function of the USSC as a channel for supplying lifeblood, that is, functioning soldiers, to the warfront. Yet the mawkish tone of this and similar imagery is deceiving. By the end of the war, the USSC admits that it does not strive for the "ultimate end [of] humanity or charity"; rather "it is to economize for the national service the life and strength of the National soldiers" that USSC officers persevere (No. 69). "Disabled soldiers" are rehabilitated so that they are "surely and quickly restore[d] to the ranks" for future use (No. 46). The USSC dehumanizes soldiers, circulating and legitimating a cultural discourse of mechanization and economy, one that Trachtenberg has already charted, noting that "the diminishment of warfare to industrial work results in the conversion of workers into mechanical parts, into mirror images of their machines."[15]

Sanitary science was ultimately cost-efficient. The loss of a soldier became a calculable sum commensurate with his military experience: he was worth "the cost of his enlistment, his pay and his rations, while he was an inefficient recruit, the bounties that must be paid to replace him, and the pension which his death or disability charges on the public; and to these must be added his worth to the nation as a producer, had he survived the war, and returned to the industrial pursuits of civil life" (Nos. 69, 56). Like modern actuaries, the USSC officials figure human life in terms of corporate investment and potential labor. Death is a "pecuniary loss to each of the citizens" rather than an emotional loss to his family. In their ongoing efforts to solicit funds for their reforms, the USSC appealed primarily and explicitly to "Various Life Insurance Companies." Indeed, the Life Insurance Companies of Massachusetts, New York, and New Jersey were early and generous contributors to the commission's cause, offering cash and counsel (*Succinct* 22, 242). Their pleas to the insurance companies are couched in sentimental language—for example, they insist that generous donations will offer "the best proof of the solid claim we have on the liberality of the rich, the patriotic, and humane"; however, the main subtext of this document is that contributing money now will preclude large policy payouts in the future (No. 5).

The USSC crafts a complex but subtle chain of logic whereby military discipline is equated with good health, good health is transformed into individual productivity, and coordinated productivity yields general efficiency and economy. The first link in the chain, however, is an insidious one to the mental health of the soldiers. As the USSC phrases it, military discipline requires the relinquishment of local affiliations, home ties, and individual desire. Military discipline was the crucial element of the USSC's philosophy of improvement; indeed, it was a matter of life and death, though not for the reasons one might suppose. Document after document insists that the "first sanitary law in camp and among soldiers is *military* discipline," adding that "laxity of discipline" is the most destructive "disease" in the army (No. 2). The USSC attests that "sanitary" regiments from New England and New York were

inured to toil, obedient to discipline, observant of sanitary laws, in person and quarters, and were an efficient contented body of men. By the side of these were regiments from the—army corps, who were discontented, and occasionally accused of a tendency to insubordination, neglectful of conditions essential to health. Among these there was a much greater percentage of sickness than in other portions of the army similarly situated. (*Succinct* 217)

When sanitary laws were followed, the inspector claims, the troops benefited with not only better health but also a "marked improvement in efficiency and discipline" (*Succinct* 217). When the regulations pertaining to cleanliness were not enforced, the USSC insists, the whole nation's health was in peril. Such seemingly transparent and exact equations gave the illusion that individual health and, subsequently, the fate of the union were simple matters of self-discipline.

According to the USSC, the lack of leadership among the officers crippled efforts to teach the soldiers to discipline themselves. One USSC inspector caustically remarks that the army "rashly assumes that intelligent men know how to take care of themselves" (*Succinct* 11). If the soldiers cannot watch themselves, then they need to be watched; thus the "health and comfort and efficiency of the men is mainly dependent on the uninterrupted presence, the personal watchfulness, and rigid authority of the regimental and company officers" (No. 20). De Forest's cowardly Colonel Gazaway is an example of a commanding officer unable to control his urges and, by extension, the men under his command. "Every feeble source of manliness in him had dried up by his terrors," De Forest sneers. "He gave no orders, exacted no obedience, and would have received none. . . . [It] bordered upon mania or physical disease" (*Ravenel* 306). Gazaway gazes away rather than within; his inability to control himself is predictably feminized, externalized, and even pathologized. His personal paralysis clearly hinders the orderly chain-of-command of the war machine; as the USSC cautions, when an officer neglects duties, "the body to which he is attached becomes simply in a certain degree less effective" (No. 51). Gazaway's fear infects his corps. In the absence of a forceful commander, USSC operatives took it upon themselves to externalize this model of surveillance, giving the "constant attention and care of intelligent and educated inspectors charged with the sole duty of watching over the sanitary condition of camps" (No. 22).[16]

Thus the true diseases of war, embodied by Colonel Gazaway, are the fears and desires that constitute one's individuality and that obstruct martial discipline. They can lie dormant in anyone. The USSC attempted to expedite psychic repression, claiming that soldiers would be harmed by material reminders of home and their individually referential power. Indeed, it was the necessity of stemming and systemizing such unwanted affections that initially provoked the formation of the USSC (*Succinct* v). In justifying why they will not distribute goods sent from home to the individuals to whom they are sent, the USSC proclaims, "Let the homes of the land abandon the preparation of comforts and packages for *individual* soldiers. They only load down and embarrass him. If they contain eatables they commonly spoil; if they do not spoil, they enervate the soldier; if made up of extra clothing they crush him on the march. All this kindness kills" (No. 48). The belief is that soldiers literally will be encumbered and harmed by cherished personal possessions. The soldier will be both "weightier," that is, more fully in his body, and more "weightless", that is, more mobile and disconnected, when thinking and moving en masse.[17] The symbolic result of such policies is that one USSC inspector finds a discharged soldier wandering around the city who claims he has "lost" himself. "He had apparently had a fever, which had affected his brain and he had strayed off, and was unable to recollect where he belonged or what his regiment was." The man pleads with the inspector to "take [him] home to [his] mother," for he has forgotten where to go (No. 39). Still, the USSC maintains that their unwillingness to "receive contributions with any restriction on their destination" is done in the name of "national unity" and in order to flush out the "State or local pride" that is antagonistic to the war effort. Such selfish passions were, of course, the disease that had infected the national body in the first place. Southerners' insistence on state's rights and the maintenance of their peculiar political, economic, and familial institutions had caused the internal disease enfeebling the national body politic.[18]

Such evidence, not surprisingly, corresponds with the conclusions the USSC wishes to draw even before the war is over. Indeed, just such evidence was crucial to the stabilization of the scientific narratives they constantly refine, for the USSC's capacity to spread the new gospel of sanitary science at this time was contingent upon their ability to craft Civil War history. The USSC argues not exactly from cause and effect, but from reciprocity, suggesting that the commission's work has "imperishably associated the history of that work, and the people's sympathy and aid, with the history, valor, and prowess of those armies" (*Succinct* 142). It is unclear in the documents whether the USSC caused Union victory, or if Union armies caused USSC ascendancy. Regardless, it is clear that the USSC believes its scientific mission "inscribed" itself, to use their term, on all it touched. The USSC writes history on and with sanitized bodies. USSC tactics can stabilize current events, producing a series of snapshot-like images of what is going on; it can rehabilitate seemingly useless material, helping readers to see it anew; and it can shape the future, determining the outcome of wars. One sanitary commissioner proclaims that with their "hygienic agencies" the USSC "'modified history'" (*Succinct* 129). Sanitary science's presumed triumph over the human body is the foundational myth upon which victory, defeat, and subsequent reunification are founded.

Dispassionate in tone, often anonymously authored, and thick with charts, statistics, reports, and other authenticating materials, USSC documents adhere to scientific method, influencing the form of subsequent medical, military, and economic histories. In the *Succinct History* of the USSC—published while the war and the USSC's work was still in progress—the introduction acknowledges that they have cobbled together various documents in efforts to convey "a truthful and connected view of the whole scheme" (*Succinct* iii). Implicit, then, is the fragmentary nature of their narrative, their work, and the reality they seek to validate. Relying on rehabilitated bodies as foundational material is a perilous proposition. I believe that the sheer bulk of their statistical and reportorial work is meant to quell any doubt of their effectiveness and control. The vastness of the human material used during the war; the tremendous task of keeping the men fed, clothed, and in fighting condition; and the silent but ever-present dead seem to have produced a similarly vast, tremendous, and ever-present attention to detail. In keeping track of the number of stockings and pickles they have on hand, the USSC imagined it could keep the war manageable. The seemingly infinite inventory is a project, I suggest in my introduction, in which we are still engaged.

Bodiless Campaigns

De Forest's novel of the Civil War covers the same terrain as the documents of the USSC, but from the soldier's point of view. His narrative conforms to the conventional and seemingly sentimental Civil War romance, where fiery Southern belle Lillie Ravenel enacts national reconciliation through her marriage to disciplined and level-headed Northerner Edward Colburne. De Forest's dramatic tension derives from

Lillie's imprudent first marriage to the dashing but intemperate career soldier, John Carter. Lillie's father—a doctor, a mineralogist, and a Northerner by temperament and sympathy—sides with Colburne throughout. De Forest concentrates on how the good martial worker, Colburne, cultivates mental domination over body, emotion, and even cognition. However, Colburne battles not only to overcome martial soul sickness in the novel but also to defeat his lovesickness. De Forest illustrates how the two etiologies are intricately bound, both requiring complete self-abnegation, a cooling of hot blood, and the sublimation of feeling into the war.

We learn early on that being a stoic and obedient soldier involves much more than simply conforming one's body and outward behavior to the mandates of the army. Ironically, De Forest's volatile John Carter is a model soldier and leader measured by the USSC's standards. The narrator tells us that "Carter disciplined his green regiment into a state of cleanliness, order and subserviency, which made it a wonder to itself. He had two daily inspections with regard to personal cleanliness, going through the companies himself, praising the neat and remorselessly punishing the dirty" (*Ravenel* 102). Carter rules his regiment like a sanitary despot, even executing without compunction those who do not bend to his and the army's will. For example, Carter lightheartedly promotes a sentinel who has shot and killed a fellow soldier returning drunk from a weekend pass. " 'Bully for him—he died happy,' laughed the Colonel" (*Ravenel* 221).[19] However, Carter is "at bottom and by the decree of the imperious nature, very volcanic. As we say of some fiery wines, there was a great deal of body to him" (*Ravenel* 165). De Forest consistently connects Carter's nature and the cataclysm of the war to volcanoes, echoing the sense of cultural and personal unease that shook many to their very cores. As such, Carter's body is not disciplinable; it is a force with which to be reckoned, for there is a "great deal of it"— indeed, his body is dangerously excessive. Warren Hedges argues that Carter is a "white dissolute"—a white man of unimpeachable racial and class standing who, nevertheless, acts like a stereotypical black man in succumbing to his fleshly appetites.[20] His drinking, inability to manage money, and infidelity to Miss Ravenel spell his doom.

De Forest's titularly conspicuous Miss Ravenel becomes the projection of this inner battle. As her name suggests ("rave," "ravenous"), she possesses an unrestrained and promiscuous personal economy. Though Miss Ravenel has no philanthropic tendencies, USSC minions often wrote that the formation of this commission was necessary to rectify the "want of system and organization" in the charitable activities of just such women. Indeed, their frenzied patriotism, it was argued, could lead to "waste[d] zeal" that would "produce as much harm as good," whereas others claimed that it caused a "danger, after all, that some would suffer" (*Philanthropic* 27). It seems clear, as Judith Ann Giesberg points out, that commission men made themselves into heroes by demonstrating how they had mastered the presumably uncontrollable tide of women's energies.[21] De Forest's text is of its time, for as a woman, Lillie is the site of desire, emotion, and physicality, "more completely, and more evidently under the power of influences which she can neither direct nor resist, and which made use of her without consulting her inclination" (*Ravenel* 372). She is individuality embodied, an unstable, nonconforming nature buffeted about by the shifting winds of her environment. Northern ideologues co-opted the rhetoric of femininity, investing the foolhardy South with those same undesirable traits.[22] Miss Ravenel's "conversion" signifies victory not only over the uncontrollable, feminized South but also over the "feminine" desires with which each soldier grappled.

In reading the novel as depicting a war on individuality, one is able to make sense of the romantic plot that virtually all De Forest scholars deride as detracting from the valuable war story. Early in the novel Colburne's beloved mother dies, and in his grief he turns to a passage from Edgar Allen Poe:

Thank Heaven! The crisis,
   The danger is past,
And the lingering illness
   Is over at last,
And the fever called Living
   Is conquered at last.

His grief incapacitates him, and for a time "it seemed to him as if life were but a wearisome illness for which the grave was but a cure" (*Ravenel* 72–73). Although the poem suggests that Colburne's mother has been released from her earthly suffering, it also sets the stage for his subsequent lovesickness for Lillie Ravenel. The passage allies sentience with disease, love with inevitable illness and demoralization. The USSC required that "the fever called Living" be conquered, not at the last, but much earlier. And Colburne is stricken again when Dr. Ravenel writes to inform him that Lillie is engaged to Colonel Carter. Colburne metaphorizes his pain in the image of a dying person:

No matter, for instance, how long we have watched the sure invasion of disease upon the life of a dear friend or relative, we are always astonished with a mighty shock when the last feeble breath leaves the wasted body. Colburne had long sat gloomily by the bedside of his dying hope, but when it expired outright he was seemingly none the less full of anguished amazement. (*Ravenel* 212)

This deathbed scene echoes not only his mother's death but also the deaths of his fellow soldiers. De Forest thus links the conquest of the soldier's body to the death of affection. Love is an invaded body that will weaken the individual and national corps. This scene is a turning point, for Colburne is subsequently able to detach himself from his emotional life, priding himself in his "soldier's indifference" (*Ravenel* 257). Indeed, it is the folly of personal passion and vice, and the triumph of obedience and impassiveness, that emerge as the lesson of the war in De Forest's novel.

Within this context, De Forest's plodding Colburne is the true military hero, for he internalizes control to the extent that even thought is exterminated.[23] As Colburne watches one of his men blown apart by a shell, the only thing that goes through his mind is the army regulation outlining how to dispose of the body (*Ravenel* 263). Dogma replaces analysis. The formerly intellectual Colburne "lost [his] taste for reading even for all kinds of thinking except on military matters" (*Ravenel* 341). The battle with the desiring self was not, however, the only contest waged in the mind of the soldier. Army rhetoric further persuaded him that warfare itself was primarily psychological. Carter proclaims that "all victories are won . . . by the terror of death rather than by death itself" (*Ravenel* 29). In effect, he argues that it is self-generated fear, not the guns of the enemy, that kill soldiers. Veterans warn, "Don't let your men get to blazing away at nothing and scaring themselves with their own noise" (*Ravenel* 179). As the USSC had initially observed, the "invisible ills" that stole into army encampments were the most "deadly foes" at war. According to veteran and historian, William Swinton, hand-to-hand combat was rare during the Civil War, for the enemy was often a butternut uniform seen from afar through a cloud of smoke, the sudden "boom of hostile guns and the clatter of the hoofs of the ubiquitous cavalry."[24] Even before the war has begun, De Forest's potential soldiers agree: "But do you suppose that we in these times ever fight hand in hand? No sir. Gunpowder has killed all that" (*Ravenel* 29). Denied the body of the enemy, the army and the USSC targeted the enemy within (a logical strategy, given that this was a civil war). Like the body of the unregulated regiment, the psyche of a self-conscious, terrified soldier would suffer from a diseased internal economy that would put not only his body but also the whole national project in peril.

De Forest suggests that internalizing the battlefield helps to obscure the contradiction inherent in being asked to defeat the barbarous South through barbarous acts of warfare. The scientific ethos advocated on this front by the USSC is represented in De Forest's novel by the actions of the eminently logical man of science, Dr. Ravenel. His first kill is symbolic of the mental distance the Civil War soldier must supply. Ravenel sticks his gun through a tiny hole in a fort wall to shoot at the enemy. The explosion of his gun is "followed by howls of anguish from the exterior, which gave him a mighty throb, partly of horror, partly of loyal satisfaction. . . . After all, it is only a species of surgical operation," he tells himself (*Ravenel* 312). The thick wall of the fortress that hides the humanity of the faceless "enemy" must be imagined by the soldier on the battlefield. Such imagery bolsters the notion that soldiers waged "bodiless campaigns." Wartime murder is elided with surgical operations, conventionally linking the sterile, productive procedures of the operating room with the battlefield curatives necessary to heal the ailing body of the nation.

Still, the heinous work of soldiers and doctors needed the sanitizing gloss, the incorporate tactics of the USSC. It is significant in this regard that Dr. Ravenel is not a soldier, but a man of science, schooled not only in medicine but also in mineralogy.[25] His science offers the illusion of emotional distance; Ravenel travels the country eagerly seeking "new species" for study and analysis. In focusing on types, not particulars, such scientists are able to maintain a clinical stance. Thus when Ravenel is given control of a Southern plantation, he "proposed to produce, not only a crop of corn and potatoes, but a race of intelligent, industrious, and virtuous laborers" by "analytically acquainting himself not only with the elements and possibilities of the soil, but with those of the negro soul" (*Ravenel* 235–36). The scientific method employed upon humans and soil is much the same here—in each case, Ravenel will plumb the depths of his specimens, ferreting out contagion and instability in the name of knowledge and ultimate productivity.

Most important, De Forest links human nature and firmament, suggesting that only a medical doctor who is literally grounded can get to the core of disease. Late in the book, after the war, De Forest steps outside the narrative and offers a metacritical commentary on the composition of his war story:

Not long ago, not more than two hours before this ink dried upon the paper, the author of the present history was sitting on the edge of a basaltic cliff which overlooked a wide expanse of fertile earth, flourishing villages, the spires of a city, and, beyond, a shining sea flecked with the full-blown sails of peace and prosperity. From the face of another basaltic cliff two miles distant, he saw a white globule of smoke dart a little way upward, and a minute afterwards heard a dull, deep *pum!* of exploding gunpowder. Quarrymen there were blasting out rocks from which to build hives of industry and happy family homes. But the sound reminded him of the roar of artillery; of the thunder of those signal guns which used to presage battle; of the alarums which only a few months previous were a command to him to mount and ride into the combat. (*Ravenel* 319)

Significant here is the way history writing is linked to blasted foundations and then irrevocably to the Civil War. The transcription of the Civil

War is given immediacy and fluidity, as the narrator tells us the drying of the ink is coincident with eruptions of the earth. History is inscribed but not yet fixed, implying that it is still subject to smudging. Although these are not natural volcanoes but rather manmade quakes, they immediately evoke the cataclysm of the war. The twinning of the basaltic cliffs further invokes the foundational demolitions of ground and war on which "hives of industry and happy family homes" are subsequently based.

That Civil War history becomes the lens through which De Forest's narrator views postbellum society suggests that the discipline of disease was not only a short-term, military concern. Rather it was an issue of national import, for the USSC insists that "the mere presence in any country of an army extensively infected, is a center of poison to its whole people" (No. 2). And if discipline is not instilled in the vast army populace, the USSC calculates, those who have been "demoralized for civil life by military habits," will be a "trial to the order, industry, and security of society" (No. 49). Early on in the war they estimated that one hundred thousand men would be "demoralized for civil life by military habits" whereas another one hundred thousand would suffer from "impaired vigor," acknowledging the insufficiency of their scientific curatives (*Succinct* 233). USSC principles were not abandoned, however, for much work remained in reconditioning discharged soldiers as postbellum missionaries to the general public—as the USSC put it, they wished to "economize our battered heroes." Writers were then faced with the challenge of imagining the callous, mechanized workers in postwar society. Many projected a peaceful, romanticized transfer of material from one sector to another. Conventional historians such as Swinton claimed, "When the pageant was ended the troops were mustered out of service, and the men, doffing the Union blue, were quietly reabsorbed into the body of society." In "A Great Public Character," published in the *Atlantic Monthly* the same year that *Miss Ravenel's Conversion* appeared, James Russell Lowell takes another tact, recasting the martial worker as a "soldier-citizen" and reassuring his readers of the value of inner surveillance beyond the battlefield. Lowell argues that "fit honour should be paid to him . . . who comes off conquerer on those inward fields where something more than mere talent is demanded for victory."[26] De Forest's Colburne conforms to these images, for he has grown so ambivalent that "he troubled himself very little about the world" (*Ravenel* 45). Our final image of Colburne celebrates the fact that he has not been singled out for military honor, for it will "give strength to his character and secure to him perfect manliness and success. . . . The chivalrous sentiment which would not let him beg for promotion will show forth in a resolute self-reliance and an incorruptible honor. . . . His responsibilities will take all dreaminess out of him, and make him practical, industrious, able to arrive at results" (*Ravenel* 484). Colburne fulfills the USSC's promise that an investment in continued sanitary training would eventually prove beneficial to postwar society, for the soldier could immediately assume his role as "producer" when he "returned to the industrial pursuits of civil life" (No. 69).

Ultimately, the system of discipline and efficiency that the USSC devised would be brought to bear on the national citizenry at large. In an impassioned letter to President Lincoln arguing for their reforms, the USSC maintains, "In the theory of our Government, every citizen is a soldier at the command of the President, and it is the duty of the President in time of war to command the soldier-citizen" (No. 47). They continue in an epistle directed at those "who stay at home," to put forward the "conviction of the grand economy of the Union and of the necessity of sacrificing local, personal, and transitory interests to the policy of the Union" (No. 5). Sectional affiliations and passionate prejudices led to disunion, warfare, and death; De Forest's subdued, converted heroine, Lillie Ravenel, and her benumbed, ambivalent new husband, Colburne, serve as models for the next generation. Divested of their personal passions and interests, the pair would pose no threat to the national corporation. Commissioner Bellows presciently notes, "What chloroform is to surgery, humanity is to war. It does not stop bloodshed, but it spares needless suffering."[27] USSC humanitarianism served as a powerful cultural anaesthetic, inducing unconsciousness in its army of participant-observers who, ideally, were insensible to the lifeblood seeping from their bodies.

Sanitizing the Lifeblood

The language of blood that Bellows invokes was central to the USSC's ideology. Again and again, USSC agents speak of the commission as a great artery—a structure for carrying fortified blood supplies from the heart to the outlying organs in need of replenishment. That the "blood" was often impure or "impoverished" made the USSC's sanitation work even more complicated (*Succinct* 199). Rebecca Harding Davis takes up the circulation of blood as it dictates the dual and interconnected plots of romance and of racial passing in her 1867 novel of the Civil War *Waiting for the Verdict.*[28] Here Davis brings the rhetoric of purity and sanitation to the fore; blood links bodies irrevocably to personal history, sanitary illogic to ontological uncertainty. It is on all levels a novel of the heart, spending very little time on the frontlines, preferring to focus its energies on the romantic and psychic battles fought on the homefront. In her historical fiction, lovesickness is decidedly meta-phoric for the invisible ills plaguing Civil War-era Americans.[29]

Two of the novel's three romance pairings use matters of blood to block the path to love. The novel begins with a chance meeting between two children: illegitimate, poverty-stricken Rosslyn Burley and the mulatto enslaved, Sap, who reappears later in the novel as the white doc-tor, John Broderip. The novel focuses primarily on the difficulties bad blood poses when Ross and Broderip fall for their respective love inter-ests. Ross's plebian roots and illegitimate status may taint the supposed purity of aristocratic Southerner Garrick Randolph's bloodlines. And John Broderip's hidden black blood would prove insuperable to stolid, New Englander Margaret Conrad's preference for racial purity. Thus this novel becomes less a story of army battles and more an emotional drama charting battles with the self and one's idiosyncratic desires and needs. Later in life Davis pronounced the "histories we have of the great tragedy" grossly inadequate, for they "give no idea of the general wretchedness, the squalid misery that entered into every individual life in the region given up to the war" (*Bits* 116). Ironically, she turns her attention to what she calls the more unsavory "facts," the "unpleasant details of our great struggle" in her fiction, offering a sort of psychologi-cal portraiture that she implies is more accurate in conveying this check-ered past than the most carefully contrived scientific history.

Waiting for the Verdict asks: Can or should one's socially unacceptable love for the individual overcome matters of type and race—of blood? "It is the man that a woman accepts in a true marriage, I think, and not the faults or—or diseases of his ancestors," one character tentatively offers (*Waiting* 151). The novel investigates the notion of individuality the USSC seemingly accepts and rejects—is one determined by the purity of his or her blood? Or is he or she a unique and particular individual apart from the dictates of heredity? How does succumbing to one's desires—to one's fantasies of singularity—affect the social order? Illegiti-macy becomes a matter of great import, for it is the primary source of ontological knowledge in the novel. The ability to authenticate one's ori-gins and learn personal history is a powerful self-stabilizer. Blood is the source of this knowledge. And that is why the enslaved, such as Broderip's brother, Nathan, and his wife, Anny, the third romantic pair in the novel, are always denied the particularity of blood bonds and familial love. Ultimately, the slipperiness of this primary blood knowledge—the impossibility of certifying the source and effects of so-called sanitation—suggests that all knowledge of self is unstable. Unconscious missionaries are not just repressed soldier-citizens; they are not seduced just by their lovers but also by the presumed certainty of the racist and classist logic of blood, willing to repudiate their emotional lives in the name of sanitation.

Like the USSC's rhetoric of sanitation, Davis's language of blood is meant to convey a stable set of meanings. Blood is seemingly undeniable, irrevocable, a "stain" that is permanent. In the opening confrontation between the misfit children, Ross and Sap, blood is immediately established as a primary signifier of value, temperament, and health. The aristocratic Mr. Strebling, who we later discover is Ross's biological father, claims that "half-breeds are terribly diseased in body and mind!" (*Waiting* 11). Thus Sap/Broderip's race is not only morally offensive but also pathologically dangerous. Moreover, the disease encoded in mixed blood bodies is contagious. The "dirty yellow skin" of Sap produces a natural antipathy in Ross, Davis observes; indeed, it "made her sick" (*Waiting* 7). Sap's unsanitary bloodline is unambiguous and easily identifiable—here it is visible on his body. Even poverty-stricken white girls are made sick by their proximity to such uncleanness. Like the USSC, Davis conflates Sap's moral heritage, his bodily integrity, and the state of the community that harbors him. Ross is equally fixed by her bloodlines, as Strebling claims that her supposedly instinctive hatred of Sap is a "sign of good blood" (*Waiting* 10). One might argue that Davis uses children in this early scene to establish the "natural" and foundational logic of blood and sanitation, a logic that is confused as the children become adults.

Given contemporaneous notions of evolution, particularly recapitulation theory, which posited that African Americans and other "inferior" races suffered from arrested development, one might also argue that Davis allies the certainty of blood with the children's immaturity. As the novel progresses, Davis employs blood in multiple and various ways to highlight its illegitimacy as a stable marker. Blood is cultural capital ("blood like his to pay their ransom," 52), the characters' inborn racism and racial difference ("physical disgust in her blood to the black skin," 51), a precious life-fluid ("thirst for their blood," 57), age ("the blood of his youth," 82), immorality ("miserable, bloody work," 93), ethnicity ("Bourbon blood," 121), desire and restlessness ("an unknown heat in his blood," 94), violence ("the war, terrible and bloody," 124), class ("on'y de meanest sort ob white blood dat comes into our veins," 180), labor ("made out of our sweat an' blood," 350), and means of legitimacy and commitment ("write your freedom and mine with his blood," 359). Like the flow of supplies channeled through the USSC, blood circulates continuously through Davis's fictional communities. Davis, like the USSC operatives, strives to make the rhetoric of blood, if not blood itself, organized and sanitized, good for healthful public consumption.

In this regard, Davis, too, grapples with the challenges of unsavory personal histories and passions, "diseases" from which even the most seemingly privileged suffer. Ross claims that when men and women come face to face they always see "stains, which no water will wash away" (*Waiting* 116). Thus personal intimacy always leaves a dirty residue and endangers the purity of those who engage in loving relationships. For example, the subplot regarding Garrick and Ross's courtship and marriage ostensibly tackles the (im)possibility of cleaning away the grime of an "unclean childhood" (*Waiting* 183). Garrick firmly believes that "coarse sights and sounds, such as [the lower classes] know, leave marks which never wash away. . . . Vulgar training is the damned spot that will not out" (*Waiting* 103). Presumably, then, Ross's childhood contact with commerce and poverty would show on her body or reveal itself in her behavior. However, this theory does not hold; Garrick proves a poor reader of Ross's body, which gives false testimony to her history and inheritance. Garrick finds Ross "easily read," thinking her a "princess of the blood," only to discover later that she is the product of an enervated aristocrat—a "flaccid, feeble fellow"—and an ill-fated, easily seduced plebian (*Waiting* 95, 96). Yet Garrick finds that "her singular purity and fairness shone among the coatings of soot, and foulness of the room about her," making her "pearl-like" (*Waiting* 102).

In order to maintain provisionally the logic of blood, Davis makes Ross's simple, good-hearted grandfather, Joe Burley, the "smut and stain" Ross must renounce in order to obtain Garrick's love. Joe exhorts Ross to "forsak[e] father an' mother an' house" in order to fit herself for union with the presumably purebred Garrick (*Waiting* 115). Her relations—both to family and world—are filthy, but somehow Ross is not. The logic of blood falters here, for Ross becomes a sort of genetic anomaly, transcending the blood relations that seem to fix everyone else. As Don Dingeldine notes, animal husbandry laces the novel, bringing theories of scientific breeding to bear on discussions of human origins.[30] The bloodlines of horses and dogs are no different than those of people, the novel suggests at times. But there is nothing essential about Ross. Her purity is neither predictable nor replicable, and so it is of little use to the public good.

We find out later that no one is free of stain, for Garrick's lineage is also unclean. His grandfather had disinherited Garrick's father in a fit of rage, and the father had then suppressed the altered will and kept his family property under false pretenses. A family friend tells Garrick, "it was muddy ground throughout. I never could find a clean path through it" (*Waiting* 98). Garrick is robbed of the fictional purity of his bloodlines by this story and is subsequently obsessed with this dirty blot upon his family history. The legitimacy of his birthright becomes a "festering spot in [his] mind" (*Waiting* 306), an open sore that will not heal.

Though Garrick serves in the army, we do not follow him onto any fields of battle. The war has little meaning for him; Garrick's wound comes from the knowledge of his father's dishonor and his subsequent *loss* of knowledge about himself and the world around him. In perusing the correspondence of alienated kinsmen, "Garrick read page after page, blank of meaning to him, conscious only of a stunning pain in his brain, which no cure, he thought, would ever touch" (*Waiting* 331). Thus his sense of personal security was attached to his faith that he knew his blood and could read others' inheritance; his fall into knowledge makes the world unintelligible, and he imagines himself diseased and unrecognizable.

Garrick's realization that any personal connection, even the most seemingly pure, makes one vulnerable to disease, and his subsequent self-alienation supports the USSC's policy regarding the de-individuation of soldiers. Davis's treatment of dead soldiers further enforces this ethos when Garrick finds a corpse in the ditch by his home. Unable to locate any identifying material on the man, Garrick and Margaret Conrad attempt to read his body. "It is a Northern face, and manly—manly," Confederate Garrick insists (*Waiting* 38). Yet one page later we discover that the man is a Confederate. Garrick then reassesses: "It is an honorable face . . . though I should judge the man to be illiterate and of low birth. It is thoroughly plebian, but full of purpose—observe. I never saw aim or persistent effort so stamped on features" (*Waiting* 39). We later learn that man's name but nothing else about him that would confirm or deny Garrick's interpretation of the man's body. Thus he can remain a representative of his type and a symbol of the logic of blood Garrick initially follows.

Yet Margaret wishes to maintain the myth of the unknown soldier's particularity. "He has an old mother, or a wife maybe, somewhere, who thinks nobody else in the world is like him," she insists (*Waiting* 38). While Garrick attempts to assess the man's valor and situate him in his class, Margaret tries to memorize his face. "There are so many different sorts of people in the world," she observes, adding that she'll memorize his particularity in case she should "'ever find out any of his kinsfolk. I could tell them—' She stopped" (*Waiting* 39). The pause is significant, for what, indeed, could Margaret tell them? Do any kinsfolk exist? In order to re-individuate soldiers, to transform them back from material to men, Margaret manufactures a family that may be nothing but a figment of her imagination. In this way she maintains the myth of his particularity, and ultimately of her own particularity. His body is made to mean, though *what* it means is ultimately irrelevant. Only an anonymous dead body can simultaneously rehabilitate the utility of type and the seriousness of self.

Davis focuses relentless attention on the evacuation of selfhood for white characters, yet she initially insists on the irony of such demands for African American characters, coming so close on the heels of emancipation. The plight of the central African American family makes clear the crucial importance of the rhetoric of bloodties and the political significance of particularity. Early in the novel Nathan is sold away from his enslaved wife, Anny, and son, Tom, and his war story is his lovesick search for them and the promise of identity and emotional legitimacy they hold. When asked if Anny is his wife, Nathan responds, "No, suh; Anny's not dat" (*Waiting* 216). Though Nathan insists, "Tom's my boy, suh," he has no legal claim to him either. The novel reinforces the fact that African Americans had been denied the legitimacy and ontological certainty that fictions of blood promised; Nathan is not limited by his kin and history but by his lack of knowledge and attachment. Though he no longer belongs to his white master, he has no other kinfolk at this point and consequently is illegitimate and indefinite. Almost destroyed by his fruitless search, the narrator claims that for Nathan, "the play's nearly over . . . he is wifeless, homeless, with neither a name nor a country to call his own" (*Waiting* 209). Nathan is defined by what he is not and has not, rather than what he is and has. As they had for Phelps's Mary Cabot, the familial dislocations of the war produce new psychic wounds for Nathan that can only be rehabilitated through the re-membering of his corporeal family. Despite his freedom, Davis suggests that without his family he is still "-less" than a whole person.

Although the recovery of the African American family is posited as a means of rehabilitation in the novel, those intimate ties are still the source of invisible ills, just as they are for the white characters. Perhaps no other character embodies the instability of blood and the disease of attachment more powerfully than John Broderip. As the young enslaved Sap, his mixed racial identification, apparently, was visible and interpretable. In the initial scene of the novel, his "dirty yellow skin" repels the white characters (*Waiting* 7). When we next meet up with Sap he has become the educated and urbane Dr. John Broderip (though we do not initially know the secret). Given the description of Sap on the first pages of the novel, it is hard to believe that his skin color raises no questions. Davis subtly suggests that people see the blood they are looking for. Though Margaret Conrad's blind father discerns that there is a "great deal hid under" Broderip's voice, no one in the novel can visibly discern the supposed "taint" of his black blood. Upon their first meeting, Garrick senses a foreignness about Broderip as well, assuming that he is a "grave Frenchman" (*Waiting* 130). Interestingly, Broderip's mystery is interpreted as a mark of civilization, and not as evidence of racial difference.

Broderip's medical training happens offstage, as does his transformation from black boy to white man. Thus the attainment of whiteness and the acquisition of medical authority are linked; Davis suggests that both systems of knowledge premised on the legibility of bodies are equally unstable. Like Mitchell, who Davis knew intimately and who her war-era surgeon resembles, Davis suggests that medical doctors are merely passing as authoritative figures.[31] Her characterization of Broderip presages Mitchell's fictional alter egos, for Broderip is nervous himself, "as weak as a hysteric, sickly womàn" (*Waiting* 78). Like Mitchell, the bulk of Broderip's war-time practice involves the treatment of lost and lovelorn civilians. Turner J. Lane hospital, the real institution at which Mitchell also practiced, is mentioned in the novel as "Turner's lane," a "roomy, old-fashioned country house in the northern suburb" of "Philadelphia for the cure of nervous diseases produced by wounds" (*Waiting* 369, 364). Broderip's white double and romantic rival, George Markle, is treated there, and he finds that Dr. Broderip is not in attendance at Turner's lane, for some consider him a "quack." Though Davis distinguishes Broderip's Civil War service from Mitchell's in this crucial way, her work echoes his own on malingering in suggesting the quackery of doctors.

Also like Mitchell, Broderip is known for his forceful treatments. He is feared because of his bedside manner; patients whisper about Broderip's "little, hard, cruel face" with a "knife in his hand," terrorizing them. One overhears him turn away a "wretched cripple with a coarse joke about the disease being the only part worth scrutiny, and that the sooner such candles were snuffed out, the better" (*Waiting* 74). His cruelty is his denial of the patients' emotional needs and of their particularity and worth as individuals. Broderip's own callousness surely stems from his hyper-consciousness of his own racial hurts. Though he chooses to pass in white society, Broderip brooks no concealment with his patients: "I have made it a rule to shun all secrecy or deception with patients: as I would a diet of false stimulants. 'Blunt words and sharp knives'" (*Waiting* 88). Broderip acknowledges his emotional cruelty, wielding his words as he does his surgical instruments in efforts to eradicate the disease that makes his own pretence necessary. Yet what does it mean that the surgeon's moodiness and cruelty is allied with a vexed racial identification in this novel? Is Davis "blackening" Mitchell and all other doctors of the era, dramatizing the ubiquitous Africanist presence of which Toni Morrison reminds us?[32] Is she indicting the cruelty of Civil War-era medical practitioners in general?

As in the case of Mitchell's Dr. Ezra Wendell, Broderip's moodiness has dire consequences for those who come under his care. When under the influence of one of his "savage moods," he is needlessly rough with his patients. Davis describes the amputation of a young man's leg: "There was relish, an actual gusto, in his small, colorless face as he cut to-night into this man's flesh. . . . He hacked it cruelly, as if it were his enemy that lay before him, his lips tightly shut, his eyes light in a blaze. Even Hubbard, who was a big bully of a fellow, pulled at his moustache, losing color, growing more subservient to Broderip every moment" (*Waiting* 137). When his assistant can bear the carnage no longer and cajoles Broderip into stopping, he emerges as if "waked from a half sleep." Though most often cruel, Broderip can be kind with his patients when not in the grips of a surgical passion. Indeed, his is the first face young Withers sees upon waking from the ether, and Broderip greets the youth "cheerily" with an "it's all right, young man" (*Waiting* 138). However, such "half sleeps" enable the brutality displayed in this passage. He is an "unconscious" missionary pursuing his work unhindered by emotional attachments. The power in such detachment is evident, as the small man's hacking humbles even a large bully, making the white man "subservient" to the African American. In this passage, Broderip's racial identity is still hidden from the reader (he is markedly "colorless"), and the most disturbing interpretation for racist readers would be the image of an unconscious white boy at the mercy of an armed black man. Clearly, Davis hearkens back to the USSC in presenting disease as an adversary to be defeated. Such strategies distance the patient from the suffering, while firmly situating the enemy within. Given the way that Broderip later succumbs to the dictates of his own "accursed" flesh, this passage suggests that the boy's diseased body, and not the boy per se, is the focus of his cruelty. But can the two be separated? the novel asks. It is this confused logic of flesh, blood and identity that *is* Broderip's true enemy, the source of his alienation. One cannot thoroughly cleanse the body of impurity or disease—racial or not—without exterminating the idiosyncratic spirit that lies within.

Although Broderip easily passes for white in the novel, disrupting the sure footing of racial blood, his emotional attachments weaken him. Broderip claims that no matter "what brain or soul is in [his body], it cannot be done away with" (*Waiting* 147). Like Ross, who knows that intimacy involves the revelation of stains, Broderip knows that bodies accommodate these unsanitary selves: "we all have an ugly, loathsome shell to creep out of, vices and passion left by some accursed old grandfather in our blood" (*Waiting* 148). His racial secret dramatizes most graphically the undeniable claim of family attachments; Davis makes "blackness" stand in for the taint of individualism, the lure of bloodties. Although his race is not discernible on his own body, it is visible in the body of his enslaved brother, Nathan, who Broderip contemplates murdering on a chance encounter in order to keep his secret. To kill Nathan would, in theory, be to cure his disease, not only because Nathan's skin is dark but also because he embodies Broderip's personal history and can lay claim to his emotional life.

Within this logic, the Civil War becomes an inevitability rather than an anomaly. Broderip extends his bodily imagery to the nation-state. When asked if he takes an interest in the war he replies no, for " 'This world is to me only a vast concourse of sound and broken human ware, and I am permitted to tinker therein for a while. That is my only view of life. As for ideas of patriotism, or liberty, or State rights'—with a smile and shrug, 'I leave them to a higher class of physicians. Nations and their laws are sound and unsound, as well as bodies, I presume?' " (*Waiting* 154). Here Broderip imagines the world as a surreal flow of fragmentary human material. His sense of bodies as "broken human ware"—as the only tangible landmarks in an otherwise immaterial world—resonates profoundly with the USSC's own view of the (im)patient bodies with which they also "tinker." The national body is similarly changeable—both "sound and unsound." In linking the national fate to the healthfulness of individual human bodies, writers could justify the metonymic connection between war and disease. "This hyer disease in the country needed bloodlettin'. It don't matter if it was my brother's," Joe Burley claims. Thus some human bodies—any human bodies—must be bled in order to cure the ailing nation.

Broderip's view of the war suggests that he sees all bodies—white and African American—as "broken" at times. In his own case, Broderip's womanly, nervous temperament initially signals the instability of his corporeality, an instability that plagues all of the characters in some form. When he is introduced initially as a renowned white doctor, Davis's characters assume that his effete, nervous behavior is the product of overcivilization. Broderip's penchant for thoroughbred horses, his meticulous good taste, and his hypersensitivity all presumably point to his class identification. However, Margaret's father fathoms in the hidden nature of Broderip's voice, "a feller miserably poor, with an inordinate hungry brain, and the nerves and longings of a woman, and no self-confidence to cover them, going about, stung and bruised at every turn, cut to the quick by every chance word—" (*Waiting* 86). Although his racial identification is easily obscured, the racial hurts he suffers are read as inappropriate, womanly longings that remain uncovered and, then, unrehabilitated. This description resonates with Mitchell's depiction of the hyperaesthetic Dr. Wendell, whose nerves are laid bare and his flesh metaphorically lacerated by criticism. Broderip is described as a young boy as often as he is described as an adult woman: "He is but a boy in size, and has a weak boy's mind in some ways," his benevolent, adopted mother observes (*Waiting* 153). Whereas Broderip's femininity allies him with a neurasthenic fate, his supposed youthfulness firmly places him back in slavery and in recapitulation theory that attributes African Americans' supposed degeneracy to intellectual and psychological immaturity. Yet Broderip also claims that he has been forced "into a brute body" (*Waiting* 147). His fingers at surgery can be both "firm as a steel machine, but tender as a woman's" (*Waiting* 380). He is at once the mechanized black body immune to disease, the deficient, underdeveloped boy's body, and the vulnerable woman's body, diseased by definition.[33] In *Waiting for the Verdict*, Broderip's biracial, bigendered, healing/sick body—a mutable, multidimensional entity—represents the diseased bodies foregrounded by the dislocations of war.

It is, then, a nation where flesh and blood do not hold. Broderip embodies black and white, man and woman, young and old, poverty and wealth, the brutalized and the cultivated. He is everyone, the great concourse of human ware, and then he cannot be any one. As Broderip's race is slowly revealed, he meditates, "'No matter what work or study I begin, the remembrance comes that there is something here' (drawing one finger across his forehead), 'which must one day come to light'" (*Waiting* 146). Here Davis abandons the blood and bodies that had proven so inadequate in explaining her characters' inner lives. This brilliant passage shows that the difference within is not articulable—not found precisely in body or brain. Rather, it is a parenthetical motion—the drawing of one finger across the forehead—that signifies the many differences that are unlocatable even in John Broderip's pliant body. It is not in the body as such, but in its gestures, in the acts of movement, that one can, if not locate, at least track the difference for which explanations of blood are so insufficient.

Broderip may suffer the agonies of his unstable body, but he is tortured most by love. His desire for dull Margaret Conrad makes his voice go "sickly and shrill as that of one of his patients asking for draughts to quench his thirst" (*Waiting* 158). His struggle to win her love is framed in battle terms, allying romance with war and foreshadowing the novel's conclusion: "If she would put one of her cool, strong hands on his throbbing forehead, he could shut his eyes and be content to die, giving up the battle, and owning himself worsted" (*Waiting* 254). Margaret survives the war(s) precisely because she is able to cultivate unconsciousness. Indeed, she finds the petty loves and hates of her compatriots unclean and sickening. "'Why could [people] not keep their paltry pains and joys to themselves?' She turned away from tears, and mourning dresses, and red eyes, disgusted and contemptuous, as from a beggar who showed his sores" (*Waiting* 245). Davis makes visible the psychic disease of individual loves and sorrows here. Broderip is ultimately lovesick because his affection for Margaret evokes a "dreadful consciousness of himself, of his whole self, from the fastidiously clean clothes and skin, into the soul," rather than safe unconsciousness (*Waiting* 243). This painful and sickening sense of self is what the USSC tried to cure. Though Broderip is killed in battle, he really dies of unrequited love and the burning soul sickness it evokes in him.

Broderip's death links black blood, disease, and an excessive sense of self, for it his constant awareness of his "dirty" heredity and his enslaved childhood that forces him to plumb the depths of his soul. The rhetoric of the clean and unclean permeates the end of the novel. "Born below the level of humanity," Broderip tries to convince Margaret that his parents, though African American, were "clean, honest, pious Methodists" and that he has "worked hard to keep [him]self clean" (*Waiting* 400). It is in this pivotal emancipatory moment that "race" became "blackness" in a familiar understanding of color. As one USSC surgeon reported, soldiers remained "dirty, black, and uncomfortable, as not to be recognized by their most intimate friends, until the renovating hands of tender nurses had washed away their blood and dust, and put on them and their beds clean clothes" (*Succinct* 211). Here excessive, dirty blood translates into defamiliarizing blackness, but when that blood is washed away, cleanliness, comfort, and respectability reign again. Only those cleansed of blood's taint are allowed individual recognition. White writers work from the racist premise that white folks are presumably pure underneath, that their bloodlines can be cleansed of taint relatively easily; thus they need not be as obsessed with matters of cleanliness (although as this chapter demonstrates, this belief proves untenable). The former enslaved and anyone whose body harbors even one drop of black blood, however, are inherently dirty in such texts, and thus projects of sanitation must become second nature. Their bodies are endlessly subject to rehabilitation.

Ultimately, Davis disappointingly concludes it is the undeniable claim of his impure, miscegenated blood that urges Broderip to reveal himself to Margaret and renounce his personal intimacies in favor of what Davis argues, despite his mixed racial background, is his rightful national family—the African American race. Davis tells us that in choosing to become African American he had "fought the good fight. . . . The result of it was that he proved his soul to be barred down into an accursed body" (*Waiting* 406). Though earlier in the novel she had suggested that Broderip's mutable body represented the instability of naturalized corporeal categories such as race and gender, Davis ends by arguing that "blackness" trumps all as the source of Broderip's irreducible difference from the white community. The only cure to his lovesickness is Broderip's renunciation of the affections and desires that torture him and make him particular and his acquiescence to the fictions of blood. Broderip abandons the life he had worked so hard to build and that had refuted the biological theories of race. Instead of viewing Broderip's passing as undermining the reality of racial difference, the racial logic of the end of the book insists that Broderip has not been true to his "black" nature. Finally, he is able to "put ease and ambition and woman out of his life, to give life itself for the salvation of a race" (*Waiting* 382). Freed from himself and incorporated into the black community, he can be mythic. Before he dies heroically in battle, he sees himself as a model of Christ, who was also "a childless, wifeless, homeless man, of birth as poor, and skin as dark as his own, who had gone down into the dregs of the people, giving up a man's whole birthright to lead a great reform, to cleanse the souls of imbruted men and women" (*Waiting* 420). Sanitation is the path to salvation for African American men here. And in order to fully cure his own diseased soul, Broderip must die and transcend the "Nature, instinct, blood, what you will" that seals his fate at the end like a "king's hand" (*Waiting* 392).

On the last pages of the novel Davis disregards Broderip's heroic battlefield exploits and focuses, instead, on his death. The dying Broderip testifies that the "blood" that fires his veins "will be troublesome to the last." His friend comforts that the pain his infected blood causes will be gone soon, for "there is no such thing as race yonder" (*Waiting* 464). Davis's novel wonders if such gentle, humanistic myths will suffice on earth in the wake of war. The Civil War is figured as the operation that cuts to the core of unsanitary bodies and reveals the "real" human beings inside: "The knife cut roughly and deep; if some traits and lines which only God had seen before, yawned sudden and black on the surface, it only proved that the chivalric gentleman bore a subtle kinship to us all beneath all difference of blood or color" (*Waiting* 57). Yet even the essential self purportedly buried beneath "blood or color" yawns "black." Such deep penetrations revealed the dark, perpetually racialized stain, the soul sickness that constituted individuality and sentience itself in Civil War texts.

Chapter 4

Experimental Bodies: African American Writers and the Rehabilitation of War Work

> *"Canst thou see the souls around thee*
> *Bravely battling with the wrong,*
> *And not feel thy soul within thee*
> *In the cause of Truth grow strong? . . .*
>
> *"Live for others; work for others;*
> *Sharing, strive to soothe their woe,*
> *Till thy heart, no longer fainting,*
> *With an ardent zeal shall glow . . .*
>
> *"Knowing that to strive and suffer,*
> *With a purpose pure and high,*
> *In a holy cause, is nobler*
> *Than ingloriously to die.*
>
> *—From Charlotte Forten, "The Two Voices"*

As Rebecca Harding Davis's *Waiting for the Verdict* concludes, postbellum white America believed that blackness was a stain that would not out. Despite his education, his wealth, the salubrious climate of freedom, and a body that is inexplicably divested of the visible markers of his racial identity, John Broderip is unable to deny his presumably essential self—the blackness within. Davis's text imagines away the new threat to white cultural hegemony posed by African American military service and by emancipation more broadly. The military machine dehumanized soldiers in order to maintain standardized, disciplined fighting forces. Yet in minimizing difference, martial culture ran the risk of blurring antebellum boundaries of racial distinction. Like many war writers, John William De Forest paid lip service to the liberating potential of the army, asserting that "all distinctions are rubbed out; it is [he] who can fight best, march best, command best" who gets ahead.[1] Given the way that I've argued blackness and individuality are fused in Civil War texts, the possibility of erasing individuality could imply the potential effacement of blackness. Emancipation clearly emerged in an atmosphere receptive to such racial (un)doings.

In its hurry to shut down subversive, humanistic notions—to at least minimally reinvest white Americans with their individuality without divesting African Americans of their racial difference—many white post-bellum Americans reaffirmed their commitment to emerging biological theories of human development, the logic of which assured a preceding and unbreachable racial divide. By the time Darwin's *The Origin of Species* was published in the United States in 1859, the pseudoscience of American polygeny—a discipline premised on the belief that African Americans and other ethnic groups were not members of the same species as Anglo Saxons—was well established. What supposedly distinguished African Americans from white folks was, in part, their susceptibility to a complex of diseases that naturalized their physical and mental inferiority. For example, physician S. A. Cartwright invented two diseases during the antebellum period to explain "aberrant" behaviors. *Dysesthesia* was a disease of inadequate breathing that presumably afflicted African Americans; their physiological inability to expel all of the carbon dioxide from their lungs made them debased, according to Cartwright. *Drapetomania* was a widespread mental disease that filled the sufferer with the desire to run away from slavery.[2] Racist white culture thus meshed undesirable behaviors and the deficiencies of African American bodies, making the former contingent upon the latter. African American soldiers' ethical and competent service initially countered white belief in the ubiquity of such diseases. However, by the time Darwin's *The Descent of Man* and the work of his philosophical colleague, Herbert Spenser, were published in the 1870s, white American thinkers were busily adapting scientific racism to fit the needs of postbellum society. The alienating diseases of the Civil War, which upset antebellum ways of knowing and being, impelled and helped codify this new corporeal logic of race in America.

The fact that African Americans were viewed as inherently and particularly diseased before the war meant that they related, and were related differently, to the corporeal and psychic instabilities magnified by the Civil War. As fate would have it, physical information gathered from the troops by the USSC denied the racial equality that could have resulted from the leveling rhetoric that organization employed. In *Investigation in the Military and Anthropological Statistics of American Soldiers* (1869), USSC director Benjamin Apthorp Gould compiled and categorized physical data gathered from Union soldiers during the war.[3] Detailing everything from age, height, and mean proportions of the body to such characteristics as complexion, head dimensions, and the "pilosity of Negroes,"

Gould shows his readers repeatedly how African American, Indian, and foreign-born soldiers are inherently different from what he ironically calls "Native Americans."[4] Thus Civil War science rewrote colonial history, transforming Anglo-Saxon Americans into the original and proprietary inhabitants of the country, as well as the corporeal norm against which all other races would be measured.

Gould's statistics lent themselves well to the nativist sentiments fitfully quelled by the exemplary Civil War service of European immigrants and African Americans.[5] However, by 1869 Gould attributes the large number of desertions from manufacturing states to the fact that "these cities and towns are crowded with foreigners. The respectable and industrious part of this population did, indeed, produce a mass of faithful troops" (*Investigations* 29). An even more damaging statistic proclaims the "well-known" fact that the heads (read: brains) of Indians and Negroes are much smaller than those of white soldiers (*Investigations* 309). The USSC's findings meshed well with those of contemporary scientists such as J. C. Nott and G. R. Gliddon who in 1868 coordinated the early work of European craniologists with new evolutionary theories, showing Negro skulls as the missing link between the classic Greek and the bestial chimpanzee.[6] In his 1870 work *On the Hypothesis of Evolution: Physical and Metaphysical*, well-known paleontologist, E. D. Cope, "accepted the simian ancestry of humans, endorsed a racial hierarchy defined by 'greater or less approximation to the apes' and speculated about the evolution of humans." Cope also popularized the notion that individuals passed through a series of stages "representing *adult* ancestral forms in their correct order."[7] Thus he provided scientific proof for the long-held belief that the adults of inferior groups were like the children of superior groups.[8]

Gould's investigations continued this scientific project by establishing types of each race, using the statistics gathered during a time of ethnic and racial reconsideration to more firmly entrench distinguishing boundaries. Unfortunately, the large number of African Americans willing to endanger their lives through military service provided Gould with an unprecedented, massive sample of compliant black bodies.[9] The vast congeries authorized sweeping generalizations about ethnicity and race: "It is only when statistical research conducts to the discovery of types, or when the inferences drawn from it may be tested, and confirmed by detection of some systematic subordination to law in their variations, that statistics afford a safe guidance" (*Investigations* 246). Thus the ethnologist could safely and scientifically determine the position of any race relative to others considered in the study. And the USSC could firmly redraw the racial lines they had obscured in their need to manage the soldierly material of the army. Whereas white soldiers were tutored in middle-class virtues and healthful hygiene through the USSC, African American soldiers were firmly inscribed as unteachable and incurable. Apostles of the new biological sciences could proclaim the culture's return to an even more sure-footed hegemony. The numerical force of Gould's statistics vitiated the image of exemplary African American Civil War service. Statistical biology was particularly insidious, for it could acknowledge the accomplishments of extraordinary individuals, while maintaining the degeneracy of the multitudes. Though the end of the war had seemed to promise great rewards for African Americans, the end of the 1860s saw a hurried retreat from wartime racial liberality. According to Stephen J. Gould, the rise of inductive scientific method "imposed the additional burden of intrinsic inferiority upon despised groups, and precluded redemption by conversion or assimilation."[10] Civil War service was eventually used to reinscribe the organic insufficiencies of African Americans.

However, this chapter returns to the turbulent war era, when so-called racial redemption still seemed possible: Civil War writers revealed that many Americans embraced the rupture of corporeal knowledge in general and of racial ideology in particular. Though social constructs that were reliant upon preceding and seemingly natural embodied discourses, racial categories were destabilized by the war's physical and psychological afflictions. The Civil War thus produced a window of opportunity for those hoping to undo bodily truisms that fixed them disadvantageously. Given this opening, there is a strong sense in the war writing of African Americans that the Civil War is particularly historical—that is, a time of both corporeal motility and definite acts. Read back through the reconstruction-era conservatism and racial violence to come, African American Civil War service might seem fated to elicit an immediate backlash. Yet this racist retrenchment was not self-evident during the tempestuous war years, for American racial ideology must have seemed vulnerable given the newly realized instability of corporeality. True, for most white Northerners the Civil War was understood as a battle for the maintenance of the political Union, which would reinforce antebellum knowledge regimes. But for those who had limited access to social or economic privilege, the war was fought not only to quell a rebellious region but also to transform an oppressive antebellum culture. Consequently, social and corporeal change through Civil War service became a therapeutic option for those suffering from social ills imbricated in theories of racial degeneracy.

To this end I consider how two free, literate African American writers explore whether racial rehabilitation could be labored into being through the anomalous corporeal rifts exposed by the Civil War. Charlotte Forten (Grimké) was the daughter of a powerful free family in Philadelphia, a fledgling author and teacher who traveled to the South Carolina Sea Islands to tutor the former enslaved during the Civil War. Forten's fate as an essayist and activist might seem inevitable. Her grandfather, James Forten, was an ardent abolitionist whose diligence, business savvy as a sail maker, and influence with members of Congress brought him fame and wealth. She was daily in the presence of important abolitionists such as William Lloyd Garrison and Harriet Martineau. Her mother died when Forten was quite young, though her paternal aunts, Margaretta, Sarah, and Harriet, were strong female role models. Forten's father, Robert, a racial activist, continued to "impress upon her the importance of scholarship, morality, achievement and selfless dedication to the improvement" of her race. He died serving the Union in a Negro regiment.[11] Some of Forten's written accounts of her life on the Sea Islands were published during the war—notably "Life in the Sea Islands," which appeared in the *Atlantic Monthly* in 1864. However, her more extended and candid journals of the period compel my attention here. Plagued by persistent illness, economic insecurity, and a debilitating sense of responsibility toward the plight of her race, Forten initially finds relief in her Civil War service.

While Forten was performing her Civil War work on the Sea Islands, her guardian and surrogate brother, Charles L. Rémond, was busy drumming up business for a nascent Negro regiment. Among the audience at one recruiting meeting was a talented young writer who was the vice-president of the Colored Citizens of New Bedford, Massachusetts: James Henry Gooding.[12] Gooding, already the veteran of several whaling excursions, became one of the famous 54th Massachusetts's first volunteers. His letters from the front, which began appearing weekly in the *New Bedford Mercury* in March 1863, probe the complicated nature of African American military service, auguring the unpredictable efficacy of Civil War rehabilitation for African Americans.

Forten and Gooding see the war not only as personal cataclysm, as Mary Cabot, George Dedlow, and others had, but also as a rehabilitative opportunity. Although both writers remark upon the physical injuries and psychic wounds sustained through war service, such ills are not the main focus of their texts. Rather, they are most concerned with the Civil War's potential to rectify the economic and political inequalities that were contingent on the presumed deficiencies of the African American race. Explicit descriptions of the individual ills of African Americans are often downplayed to this end, though they are an ever-present subtext to the discussions at hand. Yet the languages of health and history emerging during this period served these writers well as they sought to normalize bodies that were consistently pathologized by the dominant culture. The corporeal instabilities the war engendered both energized public discourse about the "health" of African Americans and provided opportunities for demonstrations of African American fitness. Gooding and Forten are seemingly able to parlay their wartime service into financial remuneration and entrée into "mainstream" society. Ironically, Forten and Gooding exploit the instabilities of an unrehabilitated culture to forge stable selves—in an odd inversion, they claim provisional health through trauma, corporeal wholeness in the midst of partiality. Accustomed to asserting themselves in a climate of personal insecurity and violence, many African Americans seized the dangerous opportunities the war offered, in contrast to those who were just learning to live without safety. Both Forten and Gooding initially remark on their wartime rejuvenation. African Americans' widely publicized labors in the war effort were a therapeutic regimen, seemingly strengthening the sinews of their bodies and cultivating a new thoughtfulness and mental discipline. No longer social phantoms, inconsequential children, lurking degenerates, or unnecessary appendages to the national corps, rehabilitated African American bodies would materialize before the nation's very eyes in the texts of Forten and Gooding.

However, in order to combat scientific racism, Forten and Gooding could not argue that war-era rehabilitation had nurtured new racial attributes. Rather, Civil War service worked like the lens of an eyeglass, bringing into focus a wholesome humanity that had been obscured. Thus, African American writers did not abandon the bodily basis of selfhood, for as Robyn Wiegman remarks, "To imagine ourselves outside such regimes of corporeal visibility is not only at some level unthinkable but also intolerable to our own conceptions of who and what we 'are.' "[13] Although both Forten and Gooding resisted the dominant culture's casual acceptance of their racial afflictions, clearly their vexed self-images were informed by such beliefs. Like their white contemporaries, they longed for corporeal stability. Widely held antebellum explanations of their selves were debilitating, yet they were unable and unwilling to imagine a subjectivity that did not embrace their physicality. In order to solve this dilemma, Gooding and Forten supplant race with gender as the most irreducible mark of bodily difference and measure of subjectivity.[14] Parodying and transforming familiar theories of race, these African American writers imply that gender can operate like a recessive but desirable trait. Gender exists in all bodies but may not be visible on all bodies at all times—and particularly, not visible to all audiences. Forten and Gooding insist that the Civil War activated the gender of many African American bodies *and* that it corrected the gendered perceptions of white America. The Civil War became a stage on which African American men and women offered virtuoso performances of their gender through their nationally significant work. In this way African American Civil War service merged biological and environmental theories of racial rehabilitation.

Many have written of how properly performed gender roles were increasingly invoked as a measure of American citizenship at midcentury and how the Civil War troubled those roles.[15] In March 1863, as the war reached its dark, exhausted midpoint, well-known essayist Gail Hamilton concludes in an *Atlantic Monthly* article, "We shall fail, not because of mechanics and mathematics, but because our manhood and womanhood weighed in the balance are found lacking."[16] Such claims are traditionally used during wartime to mobilize efforts: to be a man during war is to offer one's self up to battle, whereas true women cheerfully exhort their loved ones to the front and reluctantly hold down the fort while the men are away. At the same time, war interrupts social relations and expectations, causing rifts in that gender ideology. Elizabeth Young has explored at length the "disruptive legacies" of the Civil War on women's writing as the war evolved into a "metaphor to represent internal rebellions, conflicts, and fractures"—instabilities that similarly allowed for challenges to cultural hegemony.[17] The adaptability born of a life lived on the margins became a strength during the Civil War, as a myriad of diverse individuals were able to assume the powerful qualities of soldiers, educators, politicians, nurses, lovers, and revolutionaries. Given the relative permeability of gender during the era, Forten and Gooding were freer to test its practicability as a baseline of corporeal fitness, and its potential procurement by people of color.

Finally, this logic of gender allowed Forten and Gooding to account for difference in the African American community—a difference that shifted dramatically and abruptly when slavery was abolished. Gender seems to operate not only as a biological inevitability for them but also as a commodity—skills, knowledge, sentiments, and behaviors that presumably could be cultivated. Given antebellum economics of black bodies, Forten and Gooding were as concerned with the transformation of African Americans from capital to consumers as they were with their movement from pathological and genderless to healthy and engendered beings. Gender and class are inextricably linked in Forten and Gooding's writing; properly performed gender roles became the mark of distinction within the race in postbellum America. I want to emphasize here that I have chosen to study Forten and Gooding because they were *not* enslaved—both were born free, gifted writers who were politically active and were of mixed racial heritage. And their Civil War writings were crucial in formulating postbellum racial politics within the newly constituted African American community as well as in the larger interracial nation. Although the meanings of emancipation were relatively clear for the enslaved (at least initially), they were less clear for those whose lives would not be changed in the same way by universal freedom. Forten and Gooding had already tasted freedom in a racist society and hoped for better treatment after the war. At the same time, they seem to fear that the immediate and profound proliferation of the free African American community would thwart such desires. They want to argue for the humanity of all African Americans, while at the same time maintaining their distinction from the illiterate, uncultivated, and dark-skinned from whom, they now anticipated, they might become indistinguishable in the eyes of white America. In this way their texts nervously prophecy Benjamin Gould's wartime science and its reversion to disabled and disabling type.

And subsequent scholarly treatment of African Americans shows that Forten and Gooding were right to note the postbellum classing of race; people of African descent are often joined together as an indiscriminate underclass in studies of nineteenth-century America, linked by ethnic background and the institution of slavery—whether as lived experience or a reform concern.[18] Although such scholarship often conventionally measures class status by wealth and vocation, Bettye Collier-Thomas and James Turner and E. Franklin Frazier argue that class is historically a much more "nebulous" and dynamic term for African Americans.[19] In the free black communities in which Forten and Gooding operated, ideological commitment, morality, scholarship, and service were prized as highly as wealth.

However, such educational and activist commitments often repudiated middle-class gender roles, which privileged economic achievements that sustained men's patriarchal dominance and women's separation from the public sphere and the world of work. Thus Forten and Gooding also agitate for African Americans' entrance into the domestic circle of the national family and integration into the Northern economy as new laborers and consumers. African American men were battling to maintain their position as defenders of the home and all that it symbolized. As a result, military service proved crucial in subsequent debates about African American citizenship, and the African American soldiers' unequal pay became a particularly important issue for Gooding. Historian Jim Cullen notes that Civil War service anointed African American men as "fighter[s] who leave the home to protect it."[20] Thus the battles being fought by African American troops were for more than emancipation and citizenship: they were battles fought for positions as providers, rather than as slaves, within the domestic matrix. Similarly, war service provided single women such as Forten an opportunity for significant work—work such as teaching which conformed to domestic ideology, but also became publicly meaningful through its association with the war effort. Economic concerns were also pertinent for marginal women such as Forten who were single and largely self-supporting.

As the USSC's work showed, however, even though Civil War service allowed otherwise excluded groups access to the familiar tropes of middle-class manhood and womanhood—and to the new consumer class they conferred—these tropes were also used to exploit African American Civil War service. Gooding's increasing anger and the diminishment of his military corps and Forten's persistent ailments register this cultural malignancy. The lasting effect of the Civil War on civilian society was a potential endlessly deferred, for though African American women might continue as teachers and African American men as soldiers after the war, the Civil War itself was gone. It was *this* war's power as a means of unsettling bodily truths that had allowed for the racial transformations of the era. Eventually, the scientific rhetoric used to account for the Port Royal and Negro regiment "experiments" suggested that the disorder of the Civil War was the temporary laboratory where extraordinary conditions allowed African American men and women to gain nationally significant, but sadly temporary, employment.

Finally, the psychological and corporeal price exacted from African Americans was high, just as it was for their white contemporaries. The epigraph from Forten's poem "The Two Voices" suggests that she wanted to unsettle the association of blackness with self-serving desire, passion, and weakness.[21] However, Civil War service exploited such desires, promising African Americans rehabilitation through dangerous and often deadly service to the very system that pathologized them. As Forten writes, to "strive and suffer" in a "holy cause" is better than "ingloriously to die" (Forten 81, 83, 84). Forten's journals testify to the mental and physical exhaustion that accompanied the expectation of such self-abnegating heroics for many African American Civil War workers. Chillingly, Gooding's correspondence ended abruptly in February 1864, when the editors announced that the vibrant young writer had died. The precipitate conclusion of Gooding's epistolary narrative silently emphasizes the fact that even after emancipation American culture would be built on the backs—or the corpses—of African Americans. Ironically, Gooding implies that those very bodies are payment for potential corporeal stability. But many African Americans had little to lose and much to gain from the Civil War. And so they reconciled themselves to serving in the war for the certain change in American society and in their personal lives that it seemed to promise—for good or ill. I demonstrate that these Civil War participants were not duped victims of war society; rather, they were fully aware of the ironies of their positions.

"Will the Negro Fight?"

The rhetoric of self-sacrifice that Gooding invokes, as well as the economic logic of military service he employs, permeated initial debate and subsequent commentary on what came to be known in the words of historian Dudley Cornish as the "Negro soldier question."[22] Because they were viewed as physically and emotionally unrestrained, African Americans were initially prohibited from serving in the Union army. But as the pace of white enlistments cooled and the death tolls rose, the question "Will the Negro fight?" reverberated through the newspapers of 1862. As one *New York Tribune* pundit editorialized in May 1863, "Loyal whites have generally become willing that [African Americans] should fight, but the great majority have no faith that they will do so." Contemporary stereotypes suggested that African Americans would be unfit for military service, for they would prove "cowardly" in their flight from battle, or "sneaky" in their efforts to avoid combat.[23] In short, they asserted that African American men were not manly enough to face the rigors of the battlefield. More likely, whites feared that long-abused African Americans, once armed, might turn upon their white comrades.

The formation of the Negro regiments in 1863 signaled a hard-fought victory against overt Northern racism. Though war work for the Negro regiments would often be tedious and always rigorous, Gooding insisted on its larger significance. In his first plea for recruits, published in the *New Bedford Mercury* in 1863, an impassioned Gooding testified:

Our people must know that if they are ever to attain to any position in the eyes of the civilized world, they must forego comfort, home, fear, and above all superstition, and fight for it; make up their minds to become something more than hewers of wood and drawers of water all their lives. Consider that on this continent, at least, their race and name will be totally obliterated unless they put forth some effort to *save themselves*. (*Altar* 4)

Gooding sees the war as a fortuitous occasion for demonstrations of the competency and productivity of those traditionally classed as ineffectual and superfluous. Indeed, Gooding asserts that African Americans are irrelevant, even invisible, within the American socioeconomic realm—continued work as laborers will lead, as he says, to "obiterat[ion]," whereas exemplary war work will allow African Americans to "make themselves a people." Whereas white Civil War writers feared the waning sense of selfhood the war inaugurated, Gooding implies that such ontological uncertainties already plagued African Americans: military service would allow for the firm foundation of a self-generated racial identity. In fighting to maintain the Union and to free their enslaved compatriots, African American soldiers would, indeed, "save themselves." Their

uniform-clad and uniformly fit bodies—newly visible to the public—
would represent the additional capabilities of invisible, laboring black
bodies throughout the nation.

Yet Gooding's letters reveal that African Americans were skeptical
about the benefits of their military service. He pleads with his readers to
offer themselves up to the nascent Negro regiment, not only for the
good of the race but also for their own satisfaction. In March 1863, he
flatters his fellow New Bedfordians: "The New Bedford men stand A No.
1 in military bearing, cleanliness and morality," implicitly endorsing and
promulgating the sanitary standards the USSC institutionalized (*Altar*
5). And yet Gooding's editor, Virginia Matzke Adams, notes that 439
men—only half of a regiment—had signed up after two months of
intense recruiting.[24] In his efforts to convince African Americans of the
benign employment waiting for them in the army, Gooding insists that
his superior officer, Captain Grace, has studied the colored man's
"peculiar modes of thought, action and disposition" and that he will go
to great lengths to "assist or benefit an inferior." Though Grace exem-
plifies "military discipline," he is also distinguished by his "kindness"
(*Altar* 6). The soothing tone of this epistle suggests that Gooding's contemporaries feared abuse and mistreatment in the army—another form
of enslavement. He tries to convince his readers that Captain Grace
earns, rather than compels, the "veneration" and "cheerful obedience"
of his company (*Altar* 6). Yet Gooding's rhetorical strategies make clear
his audience's apprehension. For example, he is surely tongue-in-cheek
when he writes of how the "boys" of Co. B became a little "pugnacious"
for their "bounty" but were quieted "wonderfully" by threats of the
guard house, "wearing patent bracelets, and sundry other terrors"—
punishments that clearly mimic those of slavery (*Altar* 10). Gooding
finds the quieting of these men reassuring, for he argues initially that
pay was incidental—what really mattered was that African American
men were given the opportunity to prove themselves men. Yet unequal
pay was the injustice that eventually aroused Gooding's ire.

Still, Gooding viewed camp life as a great means of rehabilitation, particularly for those men, unlike himself, who did not yet "comprehend
the future benefits of enlisting" (*Altar* 6). Gooding was often conde-
scending toward those he perceived as less cultivated than himself. For
example, he finds a "source of amusement" in watching the "odd
capers" and listening to the "ludicrous speech" "peculiar to some of
our class of people" (*Altar* 6). Interestingly, he invokes race as a class
identity ("our class of people"), but also undermines racial singularity
by emphasizing his difference from other African American men. His
own biases confirm one scholar's contention that members of the African American press were often "representative of the portion of the

community which was articulate and accumulating property and becoming upwardly mobile."[25] Gooding feels that military service will homogenize the race by bringing all up to a higher standard of comportment and discipline. Like the USSC advocates, Gooding is happy that soldiers are tutored not only in military matters but also in spiritual growth, personal hygiene, and so on. In this way the inner character would be reformed as well as the outer man. When observing the great reviews, Gooding's heart swells when he "looks upon those stout and brawny men, fully equipped with Uncle Sam's accoutrements upon them[; he] feel[s] that these noble men are practically refuting the base assertions reiterated by copperheads and traitors that the black race are incapable of patriotism, valor or ambition" (*Altar* 9). Gooding reflects the fact that a crucial part of the army experience for black men was literal rehabilitation—that is, the reclothing of the men in the national uniform and their outfitting with rifles. Armed with "Uncle Sam's accoutrements upon them," they are made over into men. Gooding implies their uniform(ed) bodies redress racial stereotypes.

The Negro regiments were perhaps the most visible, widely publicized, and highly scrutinized "experiment" of the war. One antislavery reporter declared in 1863 that the Negro was "the observed of all observed; the talked of by all talkers; the thought of by all thinkers; and questioned by all questioners."[26] Gooding reports that everyone from local civilians to legislators and statesmen flocked to watch the troops at their drills and inspect their quarters. When they went on "grand review . . . the crowd was so great that the officers would allow no carriages within the lines" (*Altar* 17). Military service served as a provisional laboratory; Gooding claims that a favorable response to the rigors of martial training and the trials of battle would produce observable, measurable results. "If the colored man proves to be as good a soldier as it is confidently expected he will, there is a permanent field of employment opened to him, with all the chances of promotion in his favor" (*Altar* 4). The Civil War was a crucial test case: if African American men rose to the challenge of war and proved their manhood, as Gooding so confidently expected that they would, new worlds of advancement would be open to them. Although the desire of Massachusetts's abolitionist Governor Andrews to create a "*model* regiment" in this regard is laudable, he also invokes the linguistic architecture upon which more negative connotations were eventually built. Andrews surely meant to compliment his regiment, implying that they were worthy of imitation. However, "model" regiments might also be understood as small-scale, preliminary, and disposable prototypes of the "real" armies. Terms such as "model" and "experiment" suggest the impermanence of African

American accomplishments; the Negro troops are framed as passive, albeit eager, objects of observation and study.

The experience of soldiering for the Negro troops themselves continued to be expressed through two dominant discourses: gender and economics. On the one hand, Gooding clearly understood the economic basis of racism and slavery. Appeals to African American patriotism were fraught, for even free blacks were not granted full citizenship. Thus Gooding does not argue that African Americans should fight to maintain the Union; rather, he urges African American men to fight for a new role in the American economy. The basic trajectory of uplift he posits is not just from slave or second-class citizen to soldier-citizen but also from producer to consumer. He argues for the viability of the freedmen based on their potential purchasing power: "The looms of New England will have employment weaving for these people, for their money will be as good to the manufacturers as that paid by others; and instead of emancipation being a losing operation, it will prove as it already begins to do, a commercial success" (*Altar* 111). Gooding insists that the "future benefits" of enlistment must be pecuniary and salutary. The dignity attained in carrying a musket will raise African American men out of the degradation of "shaving a man's face, or waiting on somebody's table," tasks that keep African Americans as perpetual "appendages" to national economic and social life (*Altar* 4). In making African Americans into a subordinate and nonessential part of the national body, Gooding implies that they are inconsequential to the maintenance of that body and that "amputation" of the race was a possible outcome of emancipation. He uses economic rhetoric in order to fuse the supposed "appendage"—the African American race—to the main body of the nation, transforming emancipation from a "losing operation" (a phrase that connotes both an unsuccessful business venture *and* amputation) into a "commercial success."

Gooding's authorial body fluctuated during the run of his letters, sometimes highlighted by the editors, and at other times cloaked. The editors at the *New Bedford Mercury* clearly nurtured abolitionist sympathies. For the first six months of their publication, Gooding's epistolary efforts to recruit African American soldiers appeared prominently at or near the top of an inside page of the paper and were signed simply with Gooding's initials—JHG. Oddly, after six months of this practice the editors were apparently compelled to append an attestation to his letters: "Our correspondent JHG, is a member of Co. C., of the 54th Massachusetts regiment. He is a colored man, belonging to this city and his letters are printed by us, *verbatim et literatiim,* as we receive them. He is a truthful and intelligent correspondent, and a good soldier" (*Altar* 43). His race, city of residence, and character would presumably influence the way readers responded to his letters. Although it was relatively clear before this announcement that Gooding was a man of color, his subtle shifts between "our" and "them" in describing his relationship to the members of the regiment made his body waver. He speaks of "our race," but then refers to the men as if he is apart from them: "The men were all supplied with uniforms, and now they are looking quite like soldiers" (*Altar* 5). Readers might have wondered if he was among those men. Gooding surely found himself negotiating many audiences through the venue of the white-owned *Mercury*: sympathetic white abolitionists who ran and read the paper, potentially hostile white readers, and black community members back home who also subscribed. And his relationship to those varied audiences might also have influenced the way he represented his identification with the regiment. Gooding's voice initially mediates among many constituencies; the Civil War sanctions his mutable and yet commanding textual presence.

The editors attempt to make Gooding's racial and class status unambiguous and static by making his body, his profession, and his character visible to readers. His authority is taken away to some extent as his editors reinscribe his body and his words in racist paradigms; their characterization of Gooding as a "truthful and intelligent correspondent" merely served to remind readers that they were to assume his colored body made him false. Not long after the attestation, in September 1863, Gooding began to use the pseudonym "Monitor," no doubt, according to Adams, in response to orders that prohibited soldiers from releasing military information to the public (*Altar* xxxiv). But why Monitor? Who was Gooding monitoring? Certainly he served as a watchdog for the treatment of the regiment, monitoring their image in the popular imagination. Injustice, subtly pleaded, and military achievements, loudly proclaimed, were immediately brought to the attention of a wide and sympathetic audience. Monitors were also armored battleships; in invoking their names Gooding allied himself with their modern power and their impregnability. However, although the "monitors and iron boats were expected to revolutionize naval warfare," Gooding explains, they had done nothing as far as he could tell except "blow off steam." One comrade jokes that the warships are "having a dress parade"; by extension, Gooding implies that his regiment, and his own correspondence, serve as liberal window dressing of oppressive army service (*Altar* 60). But ultimately Gooding's text is self-monitoring, gaging how well his own efforts, and those of his fellow soldiers, measure up to the standard of manhood.

While Gooding's regiment did get to fight in key military episodes—notably in the infamous assault upon Fort Wagner—the troops were most often employed at the physical labor Gooding denigrated. Soon after the battle at Fort Wagner they were "introduced to Messrs. Shovel and Spade, a firm largely interested in building rifle pits, breastworks and batteries" (*Altar* 47). And the regiment was eventually decimated in undramatic ways: sniper shot, infection, and disease wiped out the men as they persevered in their unmanly labors. He begins one letter, "There is nothing to record the past week, other than the (insignificant?) death of a dozen pickets, or as many more laborers in trenches" (*Altar* 55). Though Gooding insists that a man killed in this way "dies none the less gloriously" than those cut down in the heat of battle, he clearly feels that African Americans must die fighting to earn their claim upon the national body and their new place in the American economy. In September 1863, Gooding wrote an audacious letter to President Lincoln descrying the unequal pay of the colored troops and demanding of the commander-in-chief, "Now the main question is, Are we *Soldiers*, or are we *Labourers?*" (*Altar* 119). Gooding invokes the bodies of his dead comrades to make his case for the former: "Let their dusk forms rise up, out [of] the mires of James Island, and give the answer. Let the rich mould around Wagner's parapets be upturned, and there will be found an eloquent answer. Obedient and patient and Solid as a wall are they" (*Altar* 119). Here Gooding reconstitutes the decomposed bodies of the men who have died in manly warfare, insisting that only their bodies can offer the "eloquent answer" to the question of whether or not manhood inheres in African American bodies. In this way, Gooding combats the corporeal logic of race by substituting a more compelling logic of gender. Gooding makes the moldering bodies as "Solid as a wall"—a concrete foundation for postbellum African American identity.

The pivotal issue of the soldiers' unequal pay conflated African American manhood, labor, and money and lent materiality to otherwise nebulous ontological matters. According to most accounts, manhood was identified as the primary result of the 54th's heroic assault upon Fort Wagner. Gooding transcribes Governor Andrews's comments to the regiment: "Today we recognize the right of every man in this Commonwealth to be a MAN and a citizen. We see before us a band of as noble men as ever came together for a great and glorious cause; they go not for themselves alone, but they go to vindicate a foul aspersion that they were not men" (*Altar* 21). But what it means to be a "MAN" is never clear-cut. Given the nature of midcentury capitalism, and particularly the way that African Americans were perceived as capital under slavery, the issue of the soldiers' salaries provided an apt forum for this debate. Negro troops were still paid $10 per month ($7 after a fee had been automatically subtracted to cover the cost of their uniforms) for every white soldier's $13. Thus manhood was comprised of more than mere brute strength or courage. In Gooding's world, manhood is a matter of material worth, in this case, of African American labor—and life—being worth as much as that of white men. "If the nation can ill afford to pay us, we are men and will do our duty while we are here without a murmur, as we have done always, before and since that day we offered to sell our manhood for ten dollars per month," Gooding concedes. However, he continues, "Too many of our comrades' bones lie bleaching near the walls of Fort Wagner to subtract even one *cent* from our hard earned pay" (*Altar* 49). Their military service unequivocally affirmed their gendered identification—indeed, Gooding seems to believe that a sort of corporeal bargain was struck through military service, where the dead bodies of African American soldiers purchased manhood for those who survived. Thus the economic logic of manhood required that the material signifier of manhood—here the arbitrary sum of $13—be awarded to African American soldiers in order to confirm their gender. As Gooding later makes explicit, "A soldier's pay is $13 per month . . . to say even, we were *not* soldiers and pay us $20 would be injustice, for it would rob a whole race of their title to manhood" (*Altar* 83). In a shocking parody of the situation, Gooding reports that during Thanksgiving Day festivities members of his regiment tied a pair of new pantaloons to the top of a greased pole with $13 in the pocket. Climbing the greased pole makes them look "laughable indeed," as ridiculous as they feel when they are denied the $13 issued to white soldiers (*Altar* 85).

The question "Will the Negro fight?" was answered emphatically by the regiment's well-known accomplishments as brave combatants, loyal comrades, and tireless laborers. As Governor Andrews initially predicted, the success of the Massachusetts 54th went "far to elevate or to depress the estimation in which the character of the Colored Americans would be held throughout the World" (*Altar* 106). Their efforts were rewarded with enfranchisement, and, eventually, some back pay. However, the results of this grand experiment were also used to ensure African Americans' continuing degradation. For example, favorably impressed legislators had remarked upon the "efficiency, discipline and cleanliness of the men" (*Altar* 15). Such pronouncements reinscribed stereotypical characteristics that, it was argued, made African Americans such good laborers and domestics. By the end of the war, Gooding seems incensed that African American military service is not viewed in the same vein as that of white soldiers: "It is all very well to pat a battle-scarred soldier on the back, and say 'you're a brick, old chap'; but people stroke a dog, or play with a monkey on the same principle!" he seethes (*Altar* 105). This last characterization of African American soldiers as trick monkeys is particularly troubling given the new polygeny that linked African Americans to apes in the great chain of human evolution.

But military service was more than humiliating—it was life threatening. The grand reviews of Gooding's early letters are eventually upstaged by images that represent the astronomical mortality rates of the Negro regiments. Gooding reports that while one troop is on review, "the stretchers are borne along from the front, dripping with blood" (*Altar* 80). Further, army life is typified by blind obedience and paternalistic control; it is no democracy. After nearly a year of service Gooding admits that the army is no longer a great opportunity for career advancement. Now, the army is enslaving them: their labor is stolen from them; and their efforts to return home to help support their families, or to peacefully protest their unequal pay, result in execution. More than half of those subjected to military execution during the war were African American; according to Hondon Hargrove, significantly, the first African American executed was charged with leading a strike.[27] Gooding describes one conscript who was "escaping" to the enemy lines; his arrest and subsequent execution is an elaborate ceremony, witnessed by the whole troop just as whippings had been performed on slave plantations (*Altar* 92). Finally, the lower pay given to Negro troops for the same work as white soldiers is the model upon which subsequent economic relationships were based. Though the army was not slavery, certainly it did not prove African Americans' fitness for self-government or capitalism. Indeed, postbellum reformers might have noted the similarity between prison life and the soldier's plight; African Americans did so well in the army because they needed structure, discipline, and constant surveillance. Thus their exemplary war service could have been seen as supporting postbellum efforts to criminalize African Americans and transfer them from "the plantation to the penitentiary," as H. Bruce Franklin argues; the crucial pivot of this relocation was the Civil War.[28] Ultimately, exemplary Civil War service was used to undercut continued movement toward racial equality. Though the audacious assertion of both living and dead corporeal selves into the altered public arena garnered African American male enfranchisement (if only in theory), it did not alter scientific theories that reduced African Americans to their diseased corps.

"Genius and Beauty and Deathless Fame"

Charlotte Forten's early life was imbued with a constant awareness of her corporeal difference. The bulk of her remarkable journals span her life from the age of sixteen—when she left her family in Philadelphia to attend racially integrated schools in Salem, Massachusetts—to the age of twenty-six—when she was forced by ill health to retire from her Civil War service on the South Carolina Sea Islands. In an effort to prove the fitness of African Americans for freedom, the Port Royal "experiment" in which she engaged was begun by abolitionists as soon as the Sea Islands were captured by Union troops. The island's isolated inhabitants were considered primitive by abolitionists and slaveholders alike, mainly because their English, which was interspersed with remnants of African Gullah, was barely intelligible to English-speakers from the mainland. Bonny Vaught guesses that they were perhaps the first African Americans Forten had encountered whose skin color had not been diluted by interracial relationships with whites; that "darkness" also was perceived as a barrier to their educability. Consequently, the islands were regarded as a severe test of abolitionist hopes that the enslaved could be turned into responsible free citizens.[29]

Scant attention has been paid to the fact that the Sea Island inhabitants were as foreign to Forten as they were to her white contemporaries. Her presence on the Sea Islands was also something of an experiment, for she was the only African American teacher in the area for nearly the whole war. By bringing her into intimate, continuous contact with white men and with the former enslaved, the war brought Forten face to face with the specters of class, racial, and gender identification that haunt her early journal entries. Forten's race, despite her supposedly middle-class status, affected her relationships with the other teachers and the army officers—all of whom were white—and with her students and the Negro soldiers—most of whom were former slaves. Whereas white Civil War workers such as Louisa May Alcott railed against the constraints of middle-class womanhood in their own wartime confrontations, Forten derives power from her fragility, her genteel manners, her sexual desirability—even her chronic ill health, which resisted the labor to which so many African Americans were pressed.[30]

Only recently have scholars begun to acknowledge the ways in which Forten's wartime travels in the South cogently highlighted the tensions between middle-class gender performance, racial activism, and financial pressures for a free woman of color. Ray Allen Billington's extensive and selective editing of the first—and for many years the only—published edition of her journals (1953) actually hindered efforts to study Forten.[31] In particular, Billington's seminal characterization of her as a passive observer to the "real" war, untouched by the people and events around her, historically has framed discussion about Forten's Civil War experience. In Billington's view, Forten merely records others' Civil War actions: "Charlotte Forten witnessed these stirring events from the comparative safety of Port Royal. She cheered the Negro troops [and] suffered while awaiting news," he explains.[32] Fortunately, the Schomburg Library of Nineteenth-Century Black Women Writers published Forten's journals in their entirety in 1988. Yet Forten's journals still have remained relatively obscure, overshadowed perhaps by the common misperception that she was economically privileged and somehow, then, unrepresentative of African American women of the period. Historian Emma Jones Lapsansky hyperbolizes, "Pampered and protected from the harsh realities of fending for themselves, [the Forten women] drank greedily from the Forten wells of privilege, always assuaging the thirst with a clear sense of *noblesse oblige*." Even Forten's most recent and discerning critic, Carla Peterson, contends that Forten's "elite status" "singles her out as remarkable"; thus Forten is distinguished not only from the extraordinary African American women lecturers, travelers, and writers who people Peterson's study but also from the mass of African American men and women.[33] One could argue that as a member of the free black intelligentsia, encouraged in intellectual pursuits by family and friends, Forten shares more in common with young white intellectuals than with her enslaved contemporaries. Be that as it may, I argue that though she was a member of a relatively privileged community, Forten's solitary, daily economic struggles complicate the notion of her apparent elitism.

Forten's story has been eclipsed by contemporaneous slave narratives, the ultimate American success stories. Henry Louis Gates notes that this critical preference for slave narratives dates back at least to 1846 and Theodore Parker's comments about their "originality [and] peculiarly American quality."[34] For example, dramatic, heroic, and unambiguous in its indictment of white America, Harriet Jacobs's *Incidents in the Life of a Slave Girl* (1861) is in many ways more compelling than Forten's journals. Obviously, Forten's comparatively circumscribed experiences do not compare to the horrors that millions of her enslaved compatriots endured. In addition, her sometimes melodramatic and meandering personal musings have not made easy reading for some. Joanne Braxton writes of being put off initially by Forten's "romantic language, as well as her class pretensions."[35] Forten's journals are sometimes thorny territory, for she reveals herself as an unapologetic assimilationist who wrote derisively of her own race and fawned over the most trivial accomplishments of white abolitionists. But the raw, honest tensions in Forten's journals—caused by her travels to a new region, a new job, and the quickly evolving status of African Americans—make them, perhaps, more insightful. Forten gives us an extremely nuanced picture of her growing class-consciousness, which registered most cogently at the crucial moment of emancipation. The way that Forten, her newly freed African American students, and her white colleagues negotiated power and authority in war-era classrooms revealed new and momentarily fluid social strata that quickly settled into the familiar striations of postbellum American society. Though clearly problematic, Forten's insistence on difference within the African American community resisted reductive racial formulations and the singular and immutable character of black-ness.

Forten's own words counter academic versions of her life that empha-size her stellar connections and privilege and describe her interchange-ably as "elite" and "middle-class." The wealth her grandfather had amassed had deteriorated by the time of Forten's birth. The family's waning fortunes trickled down through the generations, impeding her father's activism and leaving Forten constantly on the brink of financial ruin. Forten became economically independent in 1855 as an eighteen-year-old student, when her already emotionally distant father moved to Canada with Forten's step-family and stopped sending her money. In 1856 she writes anxiously, "Still no news from Canada. I have heard from father but once since he removed thither" (Forten 150). She immediately adds that her "indebtedness" to her landlady weighs upon her, and finally vents, "All my day dreams of independence and useful-ness, seem to have been dissipated one by one. And harder and sterner become the realities of life" (Forten 150). Her father finally wrote in 1857 that he was "*utterly unable*" to help Charlotte financially (Forten 272), forcing her officially into the ranks of the working classes. Forten's economic woes were compounded by her propensity for headaches and weakness, which rendered her incapable of working for periods of time and left her, to her shame, reliant on relatives for food and shelter. In announcing her determination in 1858 to leave a teaching position in Salem after a bout of illness, she vows that she should "ten thousand times rather die" than be "miserably dependent" on others for eco-nomic sustenance (Forten 290).

Thus Forten's class/gender identification was remarkably vexed. She was clearly not of the slave or laboring classes; her fine education and well-connected associates distinguished her from those of her economic rank and kept her from the manual labor her delicate health forbade. Nor was she a lady of leisure. After a couple of odd jobs—weaving hair in an aunt's store, for example—Forten had reluctantly settled into a career as an educator. Her father had pushed her in this direction, per-haps motivated as much by the realization that his daughter would need to support herself as he was by the belief that teaching would give her some practical skill with which she could aid her race. As early as 1854 Forten pledges, "I will spare no effort to become what [Father] desires that I should be; to prepare myself well for the responsible duties of a teacher, and to live for the good that I can do my oppressed and suffer-ing fellow-creatures" (Forten 105).

Forten's ideological commitments also inflected her gender identifi-cation. Young African American women of Forten's class were expected not only to be "true women" but also to be informed and involved in public affairs.[36] It seems clear from many contemporary accounts of her behavior that Forten strove above all to be a "lady." Family friend John Greenleaf Whittier wrote of her as a "young lady of exquisite refinement, quiet culture and ladylike and engaging manners and personal appearance."[37] Such aspirations were painfully at odds with communal expectations that she also be, in Peterson's terms, a "doer of the word." Forten's ladylike behavior necessarily combated imputations that African American women were naturally immoral and promiscuous. Thus the pleasure achieved through passion and personal intimacy were traded for the rigors of an intellectual and high-minded life. At the age of twenty-one Forten writes:

I am *lonely* tonight. I long for one earnest sympathizing soul to be in close communion with my own. I long for the pressure of a loving hand in mine, the touch of loving lips upon my aching brow. I long to lay my weary head upon an earnest heart, which beats for me,—to which *I* am dearer far than all the world beside. There is none, for me, and never will be. (Forten 344)

Her belief that she must "sacrifice rather than indulge the self" to the "*stern performance of duty*" was an expectation Forten found burdensome (Forten 137). Her youthful journal entries directly respond to racial stereotypes; she repeatedly spurns her own desires and belittles her physical beauty, repressing her sexuality in efforts to disassociate herself from the stigmatization of African American bodies.

Forten's earliest antebellum entries reveal a young woman sickened by the high expectations placed upon her—by others, but most important, by herself. Despite the fact that by the age of twenty-one she had read hundreds of books, left home to study in an integrated school system, and become the first African American teacher in Salem, she claims she has "only a *wasted life* to look back upon," one riddled with "intellectual defects . . . want of energy, perseverance and application," and a "fretful and despondent disposition" (Forten 316). Forten's twenty-first birthday journal entry reveals that she is a deeply unhappy, even suicidal, young woman who is so "weary of life" she would "gladly lay me down and rest in the quiet grave" (Forten 344). The entry continues as an extended meditation on the "sorrow, shame and self-contempt" her short life to date evokes in her. Finally, she writes of how she wishes to "reform. . . . But how to begin! Hav'nt the least spark of order or method in my composition, and fear I'm wholly incapable of forming any regular plan of improvement" (Forten 315). Forten does not consider the difficult circumstances of her life as an impediment but, rather, excoriates her own irascible and defective nature. But Forten's desire to be in absolute control of her behavior and of others' perceptions of her certainly derived from common beliefs in African Americans' inability to rehabilitate themselves; after all, such cant was used to justify the "benevolent paternalism" underpinning the Southern way of life at midcentury.[38]

Central to her disappointment was the belief that her lack of discipline had precluded her from success as it was defined in the abolitionist community: she had not become an "Anti-Slavery lecturer" (Forten 91). Repeatedly, Forten expresses her discomfort with the public modes of expression she desperately desires to master. Early in her diary at age sixteen she complains that "reading one's composition before strangers is a trying task" (91). She adds that as she grows older, the "inspiration of the subject" will help her to overcome her discomfort. Yet ten years later on her great mission to the Sea Islands she still laments, "I do not know how to talk. Words always fail me when I want them most. The more I feel the more impossible it is for me to speak" (Forten 433). Brenda Stevenson supposes that Forten's negative self-esteem resulted from a subconscious inculcation of popular views of African American inferiority. I would add that Forten's double identification as a middle-class woman and as an ardent abolitionist leaves her uncomfortably tongue-tied. Public speaking was inappropriate feminine behavior. But her discomfort with public speaking seems infinitely more trying than the discomfort of most white women, for she desperately wants to contribute to the abolitionist cause.

Forten's audience came to both her speaking and writing with a prohibitive set of expectations. Frances Smith Foster remarks:

[African American women] knew that their very acts of writing tested social attitudes toward their intelligence and their historical situation. As black women they knew that their gender and their race infused their words with connotations which were complex, complicated, and difficult to control. In transgressing social conventions, they faced condemnation as "unnatural" beings.[39]

Public speaking was an even more precarious forum, for the speaker herself was presented as text to the audience. Interlocutors such as Sojourner Truth had exploited their cultural marginality in a manner that was surely repugnant to the refined Forten. She would have never appealed to her audience with "folksy" language or used her body as Truth had done so audaciously. For example, at an 1858 antislavery meeting, Truth was challenged to strip to the waist in order to prove that she was a woman. Apparently, Truth calmly complied, informing her audience "that her breasts had suckled many a white babe, to the exclusion of her own offspring" and asking them "if they, too wished to suck!"[40] The stereotypes associated with African American women's bodies were enough to put off many young women, especially those such as Forten who were of mixed heritage (considered exotic seductresses or "Jezebels"), and especially one such as Forten who repeatedly denied herself pleasure and praise in efforts to disassociate herself from the pathology of African American bodies.[41] Still, only public acclaim and recognition could give her the approval she felt she must have in order to be accepted both by the African American community and the white abolitionist world in which she functioned. Ultimately, Forten aspired to be something she could not be: a disembodied, de-gendered, "big voice." Whereas Gooding's soldiers let their bodies do the talking, Forten longs for a weighty effect sans the drag of the corporeal.

In 1863 Forten embraced Civil War service for the break it offered from this alienating, stultifying life. On a pragmatic level, work in the South, with its stipend and sunny climate, allowed Forten to escape the endless cycle of intense teaching and incapacitating illness to which she had fallen prey in the North. Though Forten had deep ideological commitments before the war, she could find no clear-cut, economically viable means of contributing to her causes. During the Civil War Forten was freer to craft her own definition of African American womanhood, one that fulfilled community expectations that she be moral and visibly active, while also permitting her liberating personal experiences. Forten articulates that complex of often contradictory ambitions precisely as the attainment of "genius and beauty and deathless fame" (Forten 331). Most African American women who worked near the front lines washed clothes, cooked, or nursed; they were classed only as "laundresses" by the government and denied compensation for their labors. Forten procured an official paid position. But primarily her war work was attractive because it gave political force to work traditionally performed by women in pseudodomestic settings, such as teaching.

Forten's selfless dedication to her race was, at best, a burdensome ideal and, at worst, a pathological one. Her Civil War service offered a therapeutic response to her myriad and interrelated ills. Ironically, it was during her stint as a teacher on the Sea Islands that she was able to find personal fulfillment and to keep the depressions and physical ailments at bay. Forten pauses shortly before her departure—here, her twenty-fifth birthday—to take stock of her life and to assess the potential of the Port Royal experiment for both what she can contribute and what it can do for her. Forten writes, "The accomplishments, the society, the delights of travel which I have dreamed of and longed for all of my life, I am now convinced can never be mine." Yet she clearly sees the potential of Sea Island service, hesitantly pledging, "If I can go to Port Royal I will try to forget these desires. I will pray that God in his goodness will

make me noble enough to find my highest happiness in doing my duty"
(Forten 376). Though she is still subdued, this birthday entry is quite
different than that of the despondent twenty-one-year-old Forten. There
is hope based on the Civil War opportunity that she may yet accomplish
something worthwhile.

As it turns out, Port Royal provided all of the travel, adventure, and
romance for which she had longed. Her early journal entries had imagined foreign excursions as a means of achieving self-fulfillment. Thus a
brief look at Forten's youthful passion for travel literature is in order, for
it presages the way that she eventually framed her Civil War adventures
in the exotic South. Rome, Italy, emerges in both pre- and postbellum
journal entries as the fictitious, geographical location of liberating experience. European travel was an enthusiasm shared by many of her mid-
nineteenth-century contemporaries—particularly those of the upper
classes and those with a scholarly bent for whom a European tour was *de
rigueur*. Writers ranging from Washington Irving to Harriet Beecher
Stowe wrote travelogues detailing their Italian excursions.[42] According
to critic Leonardo Buonomo, although popular England offered the
"pleasure of a familiar past" to American travelers, Italy was both
"homeland of the arts" and the possessor of "the irresistible charm of
the exotic."[43] For nineteenth-century women writers Margaret Fuller
and Julia Ward Howe, Rome "represented a unique opportunity for free
conduct and association, for unprecedented independence." Reading
travelogues became a form of travel itself for Forten, a fantastic escape
from the harsh realities of daily life. She writes of checking out *Travels
in Europe* from the library, though she was "determined *not* to take a
book of travels, for already the foreign fever burns high. But on opening
the book, the magical names of places and people fascinated me, and I
could not resist temptation" (Forten 237). Daydreams of European
travel were forbidden self-indulgences.

In her antebellum journals Forten repeatedly invokes Rome as a
totemic place "sacred to genius and beauty and deathless fame" (Forten
331). Psychologically, Rome symbolized both the far-ranging celebrity
and the intimate relationships she craved; in Rome she would have the
genius of articulation, the fame that such a skill would bring her, and
the beauty to attract admiration and love. On her twenty-first birthday
Forten laments that she has not realized the "cherished all absorbing
dream of my heart" in failing to visit Rome (Forten 331). Geographi-
cally, a trip to Rome would have meant that Forten's sphere of influence
as an exemplar of African American intellectual potential had exceeded
the narrow confines of New England. As it had for Fuller and Howe,
Rome signaled a liberating spirit for Forten, allowing her to indulge her
passions rather than repress them in the name of duty. However, Roman

indulgences are initially out of Forten's reach. She writes of how Miss Whittier shows a gathering of abolitionist luminaries a picture of an "Italian girl" and then comments upon the striking likeness it bears to Forten. Forten protests, "I utterly failed to see it: *I* thought the Italian girl very pretty, and I know myself to be the very opposite" (Forten 373).

Yet Forten may include this passage to suggest that she has the potential to be Roman. Unable to travel abroad, Forten transformed South Carolina into her foreign reality. Forten makes the connection explicit, noting during a stroll at daybreak, "'Twas a lovely, dreamy kind of morning. . . . I think the air to-day must be like that of Italy"; she repeatedly comments upon the "soft, Italian air" (Forten 474), which creates an atmosphere conducive to wartime romance. The male protagonist in this liaison was Dr. Seth Rogers, the surgeon attached to the First South Carolina Volunteers stationed near Forten's school. Forten already knew Rogers (and his wife), having visited his clinic in Worcester, Massachusetts, where she had gone for relief of her chronic respiratory ailments. It is significant that her doctor effects the cure to her emotional ills as well. Dr. R., as she calls him in her journals, comes often to visit Forten at her residence. Many journal entries are devoted to rich narratives of twilight rides with Dr. R.:

He came to dine with us, and then we—just he and I—had the loveliest horseback ride. . . . Dr. R. broke off long sprays and twined them around me. I felt grand as a queen . . . Dear A. I can give you no idea of the ride homeward. I know only that it was the most delightful ride I ever had in my life. . . . How wild and unreal it all seemed and what happiness it was, as we rode slowly along to listen to the conversation of the dear friend . . . There is a magnetism about him impossible to resist. (Forten 454)

Though Forten never explicitly admits to more than a dear friendship with Dr. R., it doesn't seem too much of a stretch to detect a romantic feeling in her journal. With Dr. R. Forten felt special, physically "twined" with attention and affection. Her self-entitlement as a "queen" suggests that she had secured the respect befitting a lady, and not merely the salacious attentions of a man intent solely upon seduction. Whereas African American manhood is measured in economic capital, African American womanhood is gauged in part by male attention.

The relaxed social mores of wartime allowed her to spurn the intellectual and to indulge in the sensory experiences that were repressed in the abolitionist community. Forten emphasizes the sense of physical well-being she enjoys in the Southern climate; perhaps for the first time in her life Forten feels free from probing, censoring eyes.[44] In this provisional community she could "*luxuriate*" in a ride through the lush countryside and in the intoxicating presence of a handsome, attentive man (Forten 474). The intensity of her new feelings is almost beyond words, "'too much, too much.'" And Dr. R. is not the only man who courts Forten, for she confesses that a "report says that [Mr. Thorpe, another neighbor] likes me" (Forten 484). Though she denies such rumors, reasoning that Mr. Thorpe could never love one of the "prescribed [*sic*] race," still she goes on a nighttime ride through the woods with him. "Often in such perfect darkness we c'ld see nothing," she confides to her journal, adding "—how strange and wild! I liked it!" (Forten 484). Forten's oblique journal entry could telegraph a sexual indiscretion. Yet the blinding darkness of night might also be read metaphorically as Mr. Thorpe's disinclination to see race—the darkness of the Sea Islands is freeing.

Not only are her romantic liaisons associated with tender affection and attention, the whole Sea Island experience is characterized by a liberating, enlivening wildness and danger; it brings out the adventurous spirit in Forten, who had always been so timid, so proscribed. As she describes it, her life is a "strange wild dream" and she is the "fearless" protagonist (Forten 393). The liberation begins immediately on the boat trip from New England to South Carolina. Forten relates how she and her companion, who are seasick, decide to sleep on deck. After being entertained by the fine singing of two young men from Hilton Head, they "pass the rest of the night in the society of the Ocean alone. How wild and strange it seemed there on deck in the dark night, only the dim outlines of the sea and sky to be seen, only the roaring of the waves to be heard. I enjoyed it much. The thought that we were far, far, away from land was a pleasant one to me (Forten 382–83). Wooed by strange men, braced by ocean air, freed from the land and all that society entailed for her, the ocean trip becomes a liminal space where convention is suspended, and so too are the strict expectations Forten seems constantly to place upon herself. The Civil War created these new spaces where the "roaring of waves" drowned out the voices of self-censorship and the "dark night" obscured difference. When a storm blows in, many of the passengers are alarmed, but Forten "felt no fear" and is glad that she has experienced a "veritable storm at sea" (Forten 385). Forten's "storm at sea," like the volcanic eruptions her contemporaries endured, altered her world. She is not wounded but, rather, rehabilitated by her service. Though she is close enough to hear artillery on the Sea Islands, she writes, "I have never felt the least fear since I have been here. Though not particularly brave at home, it seems if I *cannot* know fear *here*" (Forten 461). Her bravado is particularly ironic, as her life on mainland New England was characterized by constant anxiety and physical ills.

Forten's Civil War service also cures the vocational disease that had plagued her in the North. Her inability to fulfill her commitment to the abolition cause is heroically remedied through her missionary work; on the Sea Islands she is an exemplary activist. For example, she successfully fulfills her goal of becoming a visible abolitionist by teaching the former enslaved about an exceptional African, Touissant L'Overture: "It is well that they sh'ld know what one of their own color c'ld do for his race. I long to inspire them with courage and ambition (of a noble sort), and high purposes" (Forten 397–98). Such observations are often accompanied with proclamations of her good health. On this day she proclaims, "I forgot that I was almost ill to-day" while sauntering through the woods before class (Forten 397).

Clearly her war years were the happiest of her young adulthood, full of new places and people, romance, adventure, and satisfying work; she writes, "I have never felt more hopeful, more cheerful, than I do now" (Forten 394). Yet they were also quite dangerous years; not only were the battlefields perilous, so, too were the relationships in which Forten engaged. It is not surprising that the lonely Forten would develop a romance with one of the equally lonely white men with whom she came into constant contact and with whom she shared common interests. As Dorothy Sterling comments, "Although the black teachers had the black community to reach out to, the cultural gap between educated women and ex-slaves was not easily bridged."[45] Yet the fact that Forten is African American—the only educated, Northern African American woman in the area—brings a new set of concerns to her relationships. Common knowledge about the sexual vulnerability of African American women serves as a subtext to the narrative; reputed to be women of easy virtue, they always had to be on guard against rape.[46] Forten's singular position on the Sea Islands was particularly problematic: one wonders if Dr. R. would have been so free with Forten if she had been white, or if he would have been as eager to engage in flirtation if she had been unconnected or uncultivated. Dr. R. and Colonel Thomas Wentworth Higginson claimed Forten as the "Daughter of the Regiment," though this was an honor more appropriately conferred upon the wife or daughter of an enlisted man.[47] The gesture was apparently benign, yet it announced Forten's intimacy with those to whom she was not otherwise related.

Significantly, Forten's special title allows Higginson and Dr. R. to request her company when the regiment is slated to move to Florida.[48] Forten disavows feeling any fear of the moral risks she runs, ingenuously joining in the general condemnation of some anonymous women who have been acting inappropriately while in the South. Even as she is in the thick of her affair with Dr. R., Forten writes that there "have been of late very scandalous reports of some of the ladies down here, so of course as usual, *all* must suffer to some extent" (Forten 484). The rumors keep Forten from traveling to the front with Dr. R. and his regiment. Forten is crushed, not only because the request for her presence attested to her "usefulness" in the war cause but also because she would have "enjoy[ed] the 'spice' of danger" at being closer to the Rebels (Forten 464). Yet the dangers associated with her adulterous flirtation, I would argue, were more imminent than any Rebel gunshot.

Forten's relationships with the former enslaved and Negro troops were equally complicated. Her journey from the predominantly European, alienating North to the warm "folk-life" of the South neatly fits within Robert Stepto's definition of an "immersion narrative," which is "fundamentally an expression of a ritualized journey into a symbolic South, in which the protagonist seeks those aspects of tribal literacy that ameliorate, if not obliterate, the conditions imposed by solitude."[49] Forten's trip to the South was clearly an effort to rediscover her racial identity, to work for and connect with her people. Ultimately, however, she must remain outside the community of the former enslaved as a "sympathetic but patronizing ethnographic observer."[50] Her response to an Oliver Wendell Holmes poem, "Anis," tells of Forten's psychic maneuvers through this racial hegemony. She describes the story as a "touching one, that of a poor forsaken colored child in one of the hospitals (I believe) of Mass. who had a disease so disgusting and malignant that no one could be found to nurse her, until a fair and noble young girl of high position, offered her services, and went and kindly and carefully nursed the poor child until she recovered" (Forten 346). As Forten summarizes the story, the child's race, and consequently her own, is pathologized, requiring the "healing" attentions of a stereotypical ministering angel. The position of a white woman of means reading this story is unambiguous. But where is Forten in the story? Is she the noble nurse or the child with the "malignant" disease/race who needs to be nursed?

Forten became increasingly aware of this dilemma as she moved from North to South, from peace to war. As Frances Smith Foster explains, Northern readers—including white abolitionists—would have expected, even required her to intimately associate her fate with that of the former enslaved. "Because American racism consistently associated African Americans with slavery, making little distinction between middle-class, free northern women and the most oppressed and brutalized slaves of the rural South, it allowed, even imposed upon, virtually every African American woman writer the authority of slave experience."[51] Obviously, Forten was a constant target of racial prejudice. She relates how a navy officer will not sit at a table with her on the boat ride South but expresses her resolve not to be "wounded" by him. "The name of his kindred is Legion," she goes on, "but I defy and despise them all. I hope as I grow older I get a little more philosophy. Such things do not wound me as deeply as of yore" (Forten 370). But slave experience was as foreign to her as to any of her white contemporaries. Once on the Sea Islands, Forten tells of an old former slave, Scipio, who rejoices that he " 'Don't hab me feelins hurt now. Used to hab me feelins hurt all de time.' " She rejoices with "him that he and many like him no longer have their 'feelins hurt' " (Forten 408). Though her own journal is full of slights and disappointments, Forten suggests throughout that she feels differently than the former enslaved and that Scipio's Civil War liberation is appreciably different than her own.

Race is initially a monolithic category in Forten's thinking that seems at once never to be a consideration and always to be a consideration in her writing,. It is rarely mentioned except in abstract rhetorical commonplaces in her youthful entries. At the very beginning she passionately proclaims that the recent outcome of Henry Burns's trial "shall be a fresh incentive to more earnest study, to aid me in fitting myself for laboring in a holy cause, for enabling me to do much towards changing the condition of my oppressed and suffering people" (Forten 67). As Peterson too has noted, Forten's youthful entries consistently use possessive pronouns in referencing enslaved peoples: that is, "my people," "we" or "us," and "we are indeed a wretched people" (Forten 183). However, after arriving on the Sea Islands her rhetoric quickly shifts to distancing pronouns: "them" and "they."[52] Forten never reflects on her own racial identification as a "mulatta," though she calls the former enslaved "Negroes" when she arrives in South Carolina (a term she had not used to describe her Northern companions) and remarks on how "few mulattos there are here. Indeed in our school, with one or two exceptions, the children are all black" (Forten 398). She even begins to associate character with color; one soldier is described as having a "good, honest face," "although it is black" (Forten 496–97). Forten rarely identified with the former enslaved she finally encountered, nor did she seem to fully associate their educability with her personal vindication as a woman of color. She wanted to speak for the race but to be exempt from the class identification assigned by white culture to anyone of African descent.

In comparing Forten's version of her arrival at her new home with that of her school's white administrator and in-house physician, Laura Towne's, we can see that both whites and African Americans observed Forten's anomalous yet pivotal position.[53] Forten writes only that the "negroes on the place are very kind and polite. I think I shall get on amicably with them" (Forten 391). Towne tells of how the servants assigned to care for her initially refused to serve Forten and derisively labeled her "dat brown gal." The reaction of the former enslaved servants, though secondhand, suggests that they were fully aware that class formation hinged not only on the white-black color line; they initially resisted class distinctions within the race. However, Higginson explains that the servants were won over by Forten's piano playing, apparently assured that even though she too was "colored," she had the power to aid their emancipation and education. Significantly, it is not just literacy, but the refinement of a specifically gendered and class-marked skill—piano playing—which, according to Higginson, convinces the servants of her superiority.[54] Forten's body becomes visibly engendered here, and consequently she is transformed from merely a colored body—a "brown gal"—to a subject invested with inner depth and accorded privacy and respect.

For Forten, too, the material *realities* of slave life as opposed to racial prejudice filtered through her own life, began to register when she was in the Sea Islands. In a letter to abolitionist Garrison, which was eventually published in *The Liberator,* Forten writes that sometimes her life and work in South Carolina seems like "a strange wild dream. But when I see the people at work in the cotton fields, and visit their 'quarters,' and listen to their strange songs, it becomes more real to me."[55] The surreal, carefree quality of her Civil War experience is grounded by her exposure to the former enslaved. Carla Peterson and Nellie Y. McKay contend that Forten's Civil War experience gave her a "usable past," a "*lieux de mémoire*" that allowed her to locate and unravel the complexities of her racial identity.[56] She encounters people working in fields instead of going to school and lectures as she had done; she visits the primitive living quarters and writes of the incipient illnesses that accompany poverty. Forten is uniquely positioned to reflect on the reality of slavery and the changes wrought by emancipation as slavery passes into history right before her eyes on January 1, 1864. Indeed, she is unable to give a "regular chronicle of the day" for it elapsed like a "brilliant dream" (Forten 429). The corporeal transformations taking place—changes that would undoubtedly affect Forten's life as well as those of the enslaved—were so dazzling and fantastic that they were unaccountable. Emancipation was clearly the historical core of Forten's turbulent Civil War service. However, like the eye of the storm, the moment of corporeal transformation lacked the substance necessary to make it discernible.

The Civil War relationships forged between women such as Forten and the former enslaved were crucial in shaping subsequent patterns of class differentiation within the African American community. No longer separated by enslavement after emancipation, new criteria emerged to distinguish African Americans from each other. Often excluded from the economic opportunities of the postbellum period and effectively disenfranchised by Jim Crow laws, many African Americans embraced education as a means of measuring racial progress. W. E. B. Du Bois observed that in the years following the war

a new vision began gradually to replace the dream of political power. . . . It was the ideal of "book-learning"; the curiosity, born of compulsory ignorance, to know and test the power of the cabalistic letters of the white man, the longing to know. Here at last seemed to have been discovered the mountainpath to Canaan; longer than the highway of Emancipation and law, steep and rugged, but straight, leading to heights high enough to overlook life.[57]

Forten's travel to the South to lead her more unfortunate compatriots on this rugged path was clearly altruistic; at the same time, the hierarchical nature of those associations reinforced a boundary that she was unable to bridge. Those African Americans such as Forten who already had an education and had inculcated Northern behaviors and values attained a status comparable to that conferred by "old money" in an economic class paradigm. Advertisements for Northern missionaries appealed explicitly to such superior sentiments: "Philanthropic people of the North" were exhorted to "aid the poverty-stricken and illiterate refugees."[58] And the teachers were responsible for more than reading, writing, and arithmetic: they taught the former enslaved middle-class notions of personal hygiene and cleanliness, the proper way to dress and speak, and probity. Like other schoolmarms, Forten taught children by day and adults at night, organized Sabbath schools, and even visited her pupils' homes.[59] Such wholesale instruction laid the groundwork for postbellum efforts to uplift the "untalented" ninety percent of African Americans. For example, Booker T. Washington's "gospel of the toothbrush" was used to indoctrinate students at Hampton and Tuskegee Institutes. "The matter of having meals at regular hours, of eating on a tablecloth, using a napkin, the use of the bathtub and of the toothbrush, as well as the use of sheets upon the bed" were integral parts of the curriculum.[60] In 1892, Forten's great friend Anna Julia Cooper (who transcribed Forten's journals after her death) insisted still that "there exists a quiet, self-respecting, dignified class of easy life and manners . . . of cultivated tastes and habits, and with no more in common with [the colored working classes] than the accident of complexion."[61] Though members of the African American middle and upper classes worked diligently to uplift uneducated, poverty-stricken members of their race, for a variety of political, social, economic, and psychological reasons, many felt compelled to maintain their class status.

Eventually, Forten's position in the Sea Island experiment took its toll on her. Her delicate health, which had initially driven her to seek employment in the South, gave way under the strain of teaching and her anomalous position in Sea Island society. First and foremost, teaching was hard work, and as Sterling reminds us, "The schoolmarms were not superwomen. The stress of teaching in an unfamiliar and often hostile environment and the heavy emotional investment in their pupils brought on headaches, neurasthenia, and mental breakdown."[62] Further, the teachers did not have clear positions of authority; as an employee of a religious/missionary organization and as an African American woman, Forten was under the supervision of white male missionaries, Union officers, and the white women with whom she taught.[63] After her first teaching experience she confides to her journal, "To you and you only friend beloved, will I acknowledge that it was *not* a very pleasant one. . . . I fancied Miss Towne looked annoyed" when the young children were restless (Forten 394). And there are other moments where she feels that she is under disapproving surveillance. Forten even assumed the rhetoric of war in describing her daily teaching activities: "A hard day at school. This constant *warfare* is *crushing* me. I am desperate tonight" (Forten 257). Though unshaken by approaching military engagements, Forten's personal battles exacted a high price.

I believe, finally, that Forten's illnesses expressed an ontological crisis precipitated by her Civil War service.[64] A close examination of her journals reveals that her bouts of illness seem to correspond with feelings of alienation, stress, and shame.[65] For example, the minute she is turned away from the opportunity to go to Florida with the colored regiment and her beloved Dr. R., Forten is "very unwell with the worst cold I've had. It *stupefies* me. . . . Drearily, drearily the days drag on. Can do nothing but knit, and that grows wearisome" (Forten 466–67). Her reference to being "stupefied" and to being engaged only in the action of "knitting" suggests a mental torpor and physical expense of anxious energy that infects Forten's mental well-being and her body. I point this out not to argue for Forten's hypochondria but to suggest how thoroughly the paralyzing oscillations of war-era identity politics are associated in Forten's psychopathology. Forten's class inflected her illness in unique ways. Her physical weakness allied African American women—who were by definition laborers and thus not susceptible to disease—with the delicate constitutions that increasingly signified the privilege of middle-class white women. At the same time, her susceptibility to disease confirmed the common belief that "mulattos" were a degenerate, sterile, and ultimately doomed mixture of two distinct races. As Diane Price Herndl remarks, women such as Forten walked a narrow line: if they were seen as invalid, "the dominant culture could interpret this as evidence of their unfitness for freedom." Yet if she evinced no weakness, Forten could have fueled "the ideology that black women's bodies were fundamentally different and indestructible."[66] Her illnesses are not caused solely by war but are generated by the persistent corporeal instability her war-era rehabilitations both express and resist.

During her frequent bouts with depression Forten expressed her horror at an eroding sense of reality. In an 1867 letter to her friend Lucy Chase, Forten writes of her wartime employments: "Often, I was haunted by the fear of insanity, & indeed, I think I should have become insane had I continued to teach. Oh, if one could only be well! I am disgusted with myself."[67] These confessions echo her adolescent journal entries, where she wrote of how feeling like an outcast might drive her to insanity (Forten 183). Thus I am inclined toward Ann Folwell Stanford's claim that "health" for women such as Forten "caught in its own complicated webs of oppression and hegemony is an impossible dream."[68] As she closes her wartime journals Forten writes, "The Southern dream is over for a time. The real life of the Northland begins again—Farewell!" (Forten 502). Thus despite—perhaps because of—its dangers and upheavals, the "dream" of the Civil War had provided the solidity Forten craved. Forten feared, I believe, that such a time of opportunity would never come again. As Wendell Phillips warned increasingly complacent former abolitionists in 1869, "Our *day* is fast slipping away. Once let public thought float off from the great issue of the war, and it will take perhaps more than a generation to bring it back again."[69] Though Forten became so ill while teaching that she was sent home to recuperate, she was eager for reassignment. She writes that she is only on "furlough" on the uneventful sea voyage back to Pennsylvania, lamenting that the "sea is unusually calm. . . . Am rather sorry that nothing has occurred. Think I sh'ld like a storm" (Forten 501). There would never be another "storm" quite like the Civil War.

Ultimately, African Americans were subject to the same feelings of corporeal dissolution as their white compatriots and remained dissolute and nebulous in the white gaze as the war ended. As one commentator observed of defeated rebels viewing a jubilant black regiment in May 1865, "[The rebels] look back at these magic lords, swaggering on in their exultant conquest, and seem to be musing as to whether they are actually in another world, or whether this one is turned upside down."[70] These African American men are not solid, but otherworldly and spectral, to the white rebels; they are visible only in the backward glance, signifying the passage of the Civil War and its opportunities.

Chapter 5

Soldiers' Bodies: Historical Fictions and the Sickness of Battle

> Wars are largely the result of unbridled passions, . . . organized mobs, they tell us. We are not without that seed in our fair land to-day.
>
> —Mary A. Gardner Holland, *Our Army Nurses: Interesting Sketches, Addresses, and Photographs of Nearly One Hundred of the Noble Women Who Served in Hospitals and on Battlefields during Our Civil War*

In 1892 and 1893 S. Weir Mitchell and his son, Dr. John K. Mitchell, began a follow-up study of some of the elder Mitchell's very first Civil War patients. They wrote to those Turner J. Lane patients who had lost limbs, pursuing a "matter" that they claimed had "never been investigated." The questionnaire accompanying their letter focused primarily on the patients' abilities to feel: "How are you as to the sensation of touch in the parts injured? How do you feel heat and cold? How strongly do you feel a touch and do you feel it as a pinch or a prick?" the doctors wanted to know. "How much movement have you in the part injured, and what powers have you lost and regained?" they continued.[1] And finally, "Has the loss of your member altered your general health?" A few of the respondents proudly claimed that their lives had been unimpaired by their injuries. But most—the majority—noted alarming, life-altering changes that extended beyond their physical injuries. Almost all claimed that they had become "more irritable," "cranky," "quick tempered," and "nervous" since their injuries. Frank Mark of St. Louis, Missouri, became "excited on slight provocation." A desperate L. S. Benton of Wilmington, Deleware, wrote an unsolicited letter to Mitchell begging help for his "greatest trouble . . . nervousness and Insomnia, from which [he had] suffered extremely for the past seventeen years." Almost all felt pain where there should be none—in their invisible, phantom limbs; one man notes that the fingers of his amputated hand "remain closed all the time the same as they were when I left the hospital."

Another writes poignantly, "I was 24 years old when I lost my arm, and am now 67. Almost two-thirds of my life has passed without thought of the possible use of my right arm, and yet never have I dreamt once, that I was not without two arms."[2] Again and again, veterans suffering from a variety of nervous disorders begged the doctors to send them "what they think are the causes of so much suffering," to assuage the physical pain and mental disquiet that had given them no peace since the war.

The enduring diseases of the Civil War not only served as measures of postbellum health but also became deeply embedded in turn-of-the-century understandings of the Civil War, American militarism in general, and modern selfhood. Though neurasthenia has often been understood as a disease that was limited to white, upper-class Northerners, scholars have recently noted that "Americans of all social classes and a variety of occupations were diagnosed as neurasthenic and treated by rural, urban, and small-town physicians . . . across the country."[3] Once dismissed from the battlefield, S. Weir Mitchell's patients had settled all over the nation. Even those who sustained no visible scars during the war nursed some illness for, as Mitchell maintained, disease and the experience of war were interchangeable. Consequently, late-century male nervousness was often expressed through the trope of the Civil War. As Tom Lutz explains, battle, like nervousness, is both a "topos and a painful emotional reality." T. J. Jackson Lears, too, writes of how martial violence was used as a means of "personal regeneration" by discontinuous, "weightless" modern Americans.[4] It became commonplace for neurasthenic treatments for men to mirror Civil War boot camps. Ironically, in such reckonings the Civil War was both the source of disease and the contemporaneous site of rehabilitation.

However, wartime service is reconstructed in the historical fiction under consideration here not as therapy but as the occasion for an attack of the nerves. I contend that by the century's end the "red sickness of battle," as Stephen Crane phrases it, was endemic to contemporaneous expressions of white masculinity in particular and modern life in general. Ambrose Bierce's short story "An Occurrence at Owl Creek Bridge" (1892) powerfully links the physical symptoms that signal this modern sense of psychic dislocation to the Civil War.[5] In the story, we are privy to the dying thoughts of well-to-do planter, Peyton Farquhar. As the Southerner is executed by stony-faced Union troops, Peyton explains that "something in the awful disturbance of his organic system" had made his physical senses "preternaturally keen and alert" ("An Occurrence" 49). The ticking of his watch "hurt his ear like the thrust of a knife"; the troops on the shore are "grotesque and horrible, their forms gigantic"; the bullets the regiment rains upon him move in slow motion ("An Occurrence" 47, 50, 51). Finally, even time becomes relative; we learn that Peyton experiences as days the few seconds it takes for his neck to snap in the noose. Ultimately, he is no longer corporeal, but sensate motion, "circular horizontal streaks of color" "whirled on with a velocity of advance and gyration" ("An Occurrence" 51). Peyton roams through a land reminiscent of the Garden of Eden, only to end up in a modern wasteland—an "untraveled land" with no "human habitation" where the stars overhead are "unfamiliar," and he hears only "whispers in an unknown tongue" wafting in the wind ("An Occurrence" 52).

Bierce's modernist relativity echoes Mitchell's excursions with George Dedlow; his afterlife is the uncanny antithesis of Elizabeth Stuart Phelps's cozy, corporeal heaven. Such turn-of-the-century fiction insists that the Civil War is not a sign of "personal regeneration," as Lears argues. There is no redemption in Peyton's disorienting and existential death, nor in the actions of his ambivalent, almost inhuman executioners. In his *Devil's Dictionary* Bierce defined history as "an account mostly false, of events mostly unimportant, which are brought about by rulers mostly knaves, and soldiers mostly fools."[6] Bierce is painfully aware of the unreliably singular and corporeal perception associated with the war's events. Neither histories nor historical fictions, both of which sought to pin down what remained surreal and ephemeral, were sufficient to account for the actions of "knaves" and "fools." Postbellum Americans were too lacking in sense to perceive the important and the true.

What is disclosed in Civil War historical fiction of the Progressive Era is degraded white manhood. As Gail Bederman has argued, white men's race became a "palpable fact" and a "manly ideal" as they worked to maintain their privilege at the turn of the century.[7] Bederman goes on to explain that bodily strength became a metonym for social authority. In Crane's *The Red Badge of Courage* (1895) and Paul Laurence Dunbar's *The Fanatics* (1901), corporeal authority derives not from a disciplined, well-toned body but from hysterical, fever-induced bursts of strength; white men are defined by self-indulgence, vacillation, and violent prejudices. Although neurasthenia has been understood as a woman's disease or as universally effeminate at the very least, social historians Francis Gosling and Joyce Ray find that men were more frequent topics of medical discussions of the disease than women at the end of the nineteenth century.[8] The still-recent Civil War experience explained the paradox of white masculinity, wherein white men were at once enervated and weak, and decisively violent.

In pathologizing war and explaining Civil War hysteria as a culturally induced, temporary illness that was cured upon the cessation of hostilities, turn-of-the-century consensual writers exculpated American men of their wartime offenses. But the war's disturbing legacy had not disappeared: it remained sealed inside veterans, hidden metaphorically

under smooth, pink scar tissue. Thus Crane's Henry Fleming notes at
the end of *The Red Badge of Courage* that "scars faded as flowers" as he
trudges from the battlefield.[9] Crane biographer Christopher Benfey is
correct to note that Henry's emergence is figured here as his "recovery
from disease."[10] Many critics take Crane's narrative closure at face value.
In doing so they follow a long tradition of disregarding the potential
effects of Civil War service, for an otherwise loquacious horde of turn-
of-the-century historians and memoirists also maintained a contemporaneous silence about the barbarity of Civil War combat and the compromised health of the veterans. Historian Gerald Linderman claims that
Civil War soldiers saw no reason to keep the horror of combat alive,
"curing" themselves by saying what would "cause the least discomfort
to themselves and others—little or nothing." In *The Unwritten War*, Daniel Aaron agrees, finding that "men of culture" felt it necessary to cen-
sor their accounts of war so as not to upset their delicate readers.[11]
According to Linderman, the "quiescent years," characterized by the
virtual silence of veterans and authors about the war, lasted until at least
1880.

As the century drew to a close, interest in the war grew keen, resulting
in an avalanche of publications. Consensual politics permeated both
popular history and the new academic history that increasingly superin-
tended representations of the Civil War. For example, from 1884 to 1887
Century Magazine published a series on the Civil War called "The Century War Series." The endeavor proved so popular that it boosted the
magazine's circulation by one hundred thousand and prompted them
to issue a condensed, bound version of the series in 1894 as *Battles and
Leaders of the Civil War*. Crane is said to have used this work as a point of
reference for his fiction. Lavishly illustrated, the text brought together
the writings of such wartime luminaries as Union Generals Ulysses S.
Grant and William T. Sherman and Confederate Generals G. T. Beaure-
gard and Joseph E. Johnston, presenting dual coverage of the significant
battles of the war. It drew upon the prowess of professional historian
Warren Lee Goss and the sensitivity of Walt Whitman. "The good temper and the unpartisan character of the articles have been an important
means of bringing about a better understanding between the soldiers
who were opposed in the War for the Union, and indeed between all
the people of the North and the South," according to the book's editors.[12] For example, an essay detailing the events of Antietam, the bloodiest battle of the war, is graced by an illustration entitled, "Between the
Lines during a Truce," which depicts a Yank and a Reb intimately sharing a match as they stand among a field of corpses (*Battles and Leaders*
155) (Fig. 3). Another illustration portrays a "Confederate Camp-
Servant on the March"—a caricatured African American man clown-

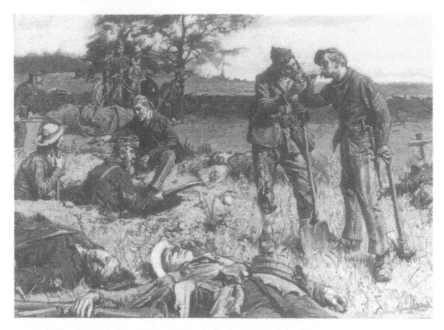

Figure 3. "Between the Lines During a Truce." From *Battles and Leaders of the Civil War: Being for the Most Part Contributions by Union and Confederate Officers, Condensed and Arranged for Popular Reading*, ed. Robert Underwood and Clarence Clough Buel (New York: Century Company, 1894).

ishly draped with camping gear (*Battles and Leaders* 131) (Fig. 4). This visual imagery reinforced the regional camaraderie and racism that undergirded turn-of-the-century history. As David Blight eloquently argues, reconciliation was largely founded on the shared racist sentiments of whites from both North and South.[13]

The posthumous publication of General Ulysses S. Grant's popular memoirs in 1885 could be interpreted as inaugurating this era of cultural reconciliation. Bound in handsome brown leather and embossed with golden seals, the "thick pair of volumes used to stand like a solid attestation of the victory of the Union forces on the shelves of every pro-Union home," according to critic Edmund Wilson.[14] The memoirs went through at least three editions, earning nearly one-half million dollars for Grant's estate. Their physical heft and opulence suggested stolidity and comfort to Gilded Age Americans. The engravings of Grant, graced by a personal inscription that reads, "These volumes are dedicated to the American soldier and sailor," made the books familiar, even familial. Finally, the fact that Grant was dying from throat cancer as he wrote the memoir, succumbing to the disease a week after he finished, lent them

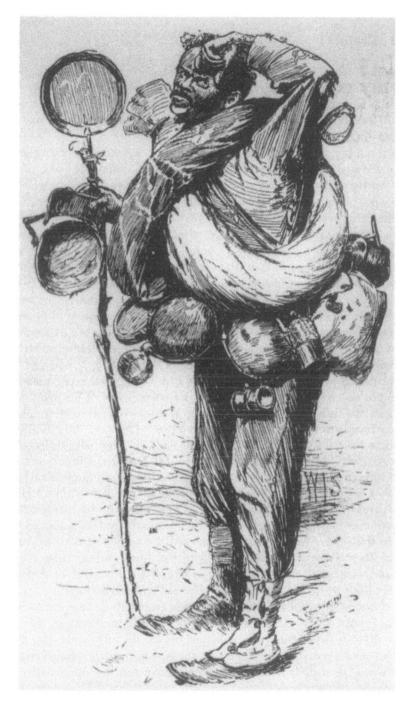

Figure 4. "Confederate Camp-Servant on the March." From *Battles and Leaders of the Civil War: Being for the Most Part Contributions by Union and Confederate Officers, Condensed and Arranged for Popular Reading*, ed. Robert Underwood and Clarence Clough Buel (New York: Century Company, 1894).

an aura of truth and prophecy. Though Grant's cancer was not explicitly linked to his Civil War service, the absent presence of this dying veteran's body served as a powerful textual undercurrent. The once-reviled Grant was transformed by his illness and his association with the war into a conciliatory symbol.

It is a sober, reflective Grant who pronounces slavery the cause of the "great War of the Rebellion against the United States." However, it was not Northerners' abhorrence of the system that prompted the conflict. "The people of the North had no particular quarrel with slavery," Grant insists.[15] Rather, it was the South's efforts to foist the maintenance of their "peculiar institution" upon Northerners that spurred the violence. Yet the former president proves himself no champion of racial equality when he maintains only that because African Americans were "brought to our shores by compulsion," they have "as good a right to remain here as any other class of citizens." More positive are the nationalizing results of the war and Reconstruction era. The war "begot a spirit of independence and enterprise," Grant praises, which has resulted in exploration, travel, industry, and a "commingling of the people" connected by the completed transnational railroad system (*Memoirs* 588–89). Grant thus cements regional reconciliation, poignantly writing that even though he "cannot stay to be a living witness to the correctness of his prophecy," he sees this time as the "eve of a new era, when there is to be great harmony between the Federal and Confederate" (*Memoirs* 590). Frederick Douglass decried the "mawkish sentimentality" that stimulated these dangerous alliances as early as 1871, sensing perhaps that white rapprochement would be forged in large part through shared racism.[16] Here, a national hero gives his deathbed blessing to the "commingling" of discrete white bodies into a national mix; however, he surely did not mean to condone miscegenation, for he clearly endorses the ambivalence that many Northerners felt toward the plight of African Americans. They were a people apart from the burgeoning white nation, characterized still by the circumstances of their arrival in America, rather than by their Civil War service or subsequent actions.

Academic historians too saw themselves engaged in the great national task of rapprochement. In reminding readers of the brutality they had once loosed upon each other, historians would only stoke the dying embers of sectionalism. Indeed, as Peter Novick argues, eliminating sectionalism from their histories also demonstrated the impartiality and objectivity historians were working hard to establish.[17] Thus representations of the Civil War became inextricable from the foundation of the American historical project. In his immensely popular, seven-volume *History of the United States from the Compromise of 1850 to the Final Restoration of Home Rule at the South in 1877*, Harvard-affiliated James Ford Rhodes created a consensual "usable past" for the middle-class readers who ostensibly bought his books.[18] In praising the antebellum Republicans as a "pure," "disinterested," and "intelligent body of men banded together for a noble political object," while at the same time referring to Southerners as characterized by "good breeding, refined manners, and dignified deportment," Rhodes placated readers from both regions, while emphasizing the reasonable and magnanimous nature of Anglo-Saxon men across the country.[19] The similar racial "pur[ity]" and "breeding" of white men from North and South—and, by association, the reliability of the white historians themselves—became the biological basis of historical truth in the period. Rhodes's work was praised widely and led to his election as president of the American Historical Association. Amazingly, one of his few detractors, respected Columbia history professor John W. Burgess, critiqued the text for its abolitionist bias, arguing that more "impartial" work remained to be done on the "true" relations between "the highly civilized white race and the deeply barbarous negro race."[20]

In their explorations of turn-of-the-century Civil War culture, contemporary scholars too have focused primarily on the "romance of reunion"—a highly sentimentalized narrative of sectional conciliation, often dramatized through cross-regional marriage. Most recently, Nina Silber argues that this stock narrative allowed the still disparate regions to forge financial reconciliation, while enabling Northerners to come to terms with a "victory that necessarily entailed the defeat of fellow Americans."[21] In the fiction I cover in this chapter, this "romance of reunion" is supplanted by the "sickness of battle." Crane's and Dunbar's novels formulate a different consensus than that of contemporary historians, showing that white men were linked by their degenerate natures. Thus Crane's *The Red Badge of Courage* dramatizes how American culture cultivates the murderous impulses of its citizens by incorporating individuals into a monstrous mob. And in *The Fanatics*, Dunbar reveals that the virulent violence that white men had trained on each other during the Civil War had persisted and mutated into organized, racist violence. Crane and Dunbar propose that the culture's inability to suppress the pain of war or to forget its inhumanity exacerbates the battle sickness; the shame and violence that lurk beneath deceivingly smooth scar tissue, like the barely leashed irritability of Mitchell's suffering veterans, can—and must—erupt. Once exposed, the sickness becomes hysterically contagious, spread by impassioned narrative. Although I agree with Lutz's contention that American nervousness lent itself to an increasingly pluralistic society, addressing the fears of those "experiencing the disorienting effects of cultural and social change," these historical novelists read the persistence of Civil War nervousness as a frightening sign of stability.

The conflation of neurasthenic and martial discourses produced the image of worn-out, enervated men who were encouraged to challenge the inertia of their illnesses by replicating the rigors of war in sporting competitions and rough-riding vacations. Yet locating this discursive conjunction in the equally ubiquitous representations of the "real" war—the Civil War—reminds us that white, male nervousness was *not* ineffective, but potentially destructive.

Ultimately, these authors' clear and consistent references to neurasthenia and hysteria invite comparisons between the Civil War and contemporaneous theories of race suicide, for the disease's place in theories of evolutionary degeneracy and eugenics was commonplace. The internecine rhetoric of the Civil War did not accommodate turn-of-the-century military endeavors well: the Civil War was not an imperial pursuit, nor did it conform to dominant narratives allying war and illness—developed most clearly in Theodore Roosevelt's writings—wherein effeminate sickness could be vanquished symbolically through the militaristic discipline of dark-skinned races.[22] Thus the Civil War could be read as the occasion for incipient race suicide, rather than the fondly remembered proving ground of nationalism. Crane and Dunbar reveal what the whitewashed stories of reconciling veterans that saturated the popular press sought to obfuscate: the Civil War was all about white men killing other white men.

Given turn-of-the-century America's fascination with neurasthenia and degeneracy, it seems reasonable that young novelists were attracted to the Civil War and conflated its battlefields with the struggles of disease. Indeed, both Crane and Dunbar were plagued by poor health throughout their lives, and both succumbed to disease at very young ages. Benfey writes of Crane that "illness, ill-defined and undiagnosed, in a characteristically nineteenth-century way," punctuated Crane's whole life, starting with his childhood "sickliness," continuing through his bout with "Cuban fever" during the Spanish-American war, and ending finally with tuberculosis.[23] Dunbar, too, was a frail child; his chronic illnesses, ranging from pneumonia to the tuberculosis that also took his life, were exacerbated by his alcohol abuse (ironically, the prescription for his disease). Yet a quick perusal of this period reveals that they were not atypical. Ill-defined and incurable ills, and a microscopic and genetic fascination with the human body, permeate the literature and science of the period. Neurasthenic imagery finally yokes the American Civil War and turn-of-the-century eugenics; America's internecine warfare endangered the fate of the whole white race.

The Red Sickness of Battle

Mitchell, of course, continued to evince great interest in the Civil War, displaying at least a passing familiarity with Crane's *The Red Badge of*

Courage. Exploring the nature of battlefield heroics, Mitchell apparently asked Civil War veteran General Smith to detail the "conduct of battle" for him. Smith complied, writing to Mitchell, "It is an almost universal rule that, through the nerves I suppose, the brain is excited to unwonted action." According to the bellicose Smith, fine yet phlegmatic soldiers could be "great" with "more of nerves." Finally, he labels Crane's Henry Fleming a "philosophical private" who is made nervous, not nerved, by his fear.[24] Thus Smith carefully tries to distinguish the unusual behaviors of battle from those of daily life, nervousness from nerve—distinctions that are tenuous at best given their reliance on moral judgments about the appropriateness of one's heightened state under the unsettling conditions of combat. What is most striking is the way that Crane's fictional protagonist is woven into the fabric of General Smith's factual musings on the "various phases of courage under fire."

Since its initial publication in 1895, Crane's impressionistic *The Red Badge of Courage* has been heralded as the most accurate portrayal of Civil War experience. Contemporaneous critics were the first to marvel at young Crane's ability to re-create the psychological reality of war. How could a young man who was not even born during the Civil War and had never been in any other military conflicts know so intimately what happened during battle? they wondered. The *New York Times* reviewer noted that Crane's work eerily echoed the recent autobiographical accounts of the war and praised Crane for "defying every accepted tradition of martial glory . . . [for] war, as he depicts it, is a mean, nasty, horrible thing."[25] George Wyndham, one of Crane's most ardent admirers, found Crane's work even more compelling than the memoirs and diaries published contemporaneously by actual veterans.[26] Apparently, firsthand evidence was irrelevant to these Crane critics; more important to them, he captured how the men of 1895 remembered and filtered their war experiences through their turn-of-the-century realities.

Contemporary critics have speculated that Crane's intense experiences on the football gridiron gave him insight into the mental and emotional rigors of battle. I argue that it is Crane's understanding of the psychology of illness, rather than his athletic prowess, that generated his uncanny representation of Civil War battle. One of Crane's few turn-of-the-century detractors, Alexander C. McClurg, angrily charged that the text was the product of a "diseased imagination" because it denied the heroic myths of the Civil War.[27] Crane reveals that it is precisely such disease that is at the heart of Civil War battle and white masculinity. Lured by heroic myths of the nobility to be achieved on the battlefield, Crane's protagonist, Henry Fleming, joins the Union army over his mother's protests. As the novel proceeds we learn less about Henry's battlefield exploits and more about the insidious infections that compel him and his comrades to kill other men. Henry's verbal engagements with his contentious mates, the humiliating gibes of his superior officers, and finally, the "red badge" he receives from one of his own maddened comrades, expedite his abandonment to the rage-driven, hysterical fever that, Crane ultimately argues, constitutes soldiering. In pathologizing soldiering, Crane mitigates Henry's responsibility for his murderous acts; perhaps this is why so many American reviewers found his version of the war comforting. Crane explained their barbarity in a way they could accept.

Initially it is the hysterical voice of wartime America, "the newspapers, the gossip of the village, [and] his own picturings" that "arouse" Henry Fleming to "an uncheckable degree" (*Red Badge* 414). He catches a fever from his community—a patriotism that Crane suggests is at heart irrational and even pathological—and is, then, made to feel important and self-indulgent because of his willingness to enter the ranks. The sounds of the village seduce him, for "one night as he lay in bed, the winds had carried to him the clangoring of the church bell as some enthusiast jerked the rope frantically to tell the twisted news of a great battle. This voice of the people rejoicing in the night had made him shiver in a prolonged ecstasy of excitement" (*Red Badge* 414). Henry's arousal is framed in illicit and corporeal terms. His body has an involuntary, sexualized response to the sensual goading of the community. The community itself is aroused to bloodthirsty joy by "twisted" news of the war, connoting the tangled, perhaps depraved nature of Civil War stories. Thwarting General Smith's efforts to distinguish good and bad excitations, Crane links sexual desire and warmongering in the way that they both, like disease, can overpower body and good sense. Ultimately, Henry's desire for individual attention is matched by the community's desire for his body, which is needed for the war machine. Such seduction encourages Henry to abandon himself, a pleasant experience initially. The regiment is "fed and caressed" in the stations on the way to the front, basking in the smiles of young girls and complimented by old men (*Red Badge* 417). Henry feels exceptional.

But army life eventually bears out Henry's mother's disappointing parting words: "Yer jest one little feller amongst a hull lot of others." Though his mother is right in articulating Henry's subsequent insignificance, she is wrong when she continues, "Yeh've got to keep quiet" (*Red Badge* 415). Joking, taunting, and above all, participating in gossip, is the linguistic glue that binds the regiment into one body and keeps them fighting—whether against each other or against the enemy. The rumors that fly continuously throughout the novel foster a mob mentality; they grow and transform, inciting the men to action. Appropriately, Henry's war story begins with such an incident. The tall soldier, waving his shirt, "banner-like," "swelled with a tale he had heard from a reliable friend, who had heard it from a truthful cavalryman, who had heard it from his trustworthy brother, one of the orderlies at division headquarters" (*Red Badge* 411). The truth of war experience is thus embedded in layers of narrative that dissipate its force—indeed, there is no confirmation that any truth lies at the heart of this convoluted tale. Less important than the actual news is the fact that it spreads discord among the regiment. One man claims, "It's a lie! that's all it is—a thunderin' lie!" The soldier who began the rumor feels called upon to defend its truth, and the two nearly come to blows. "Many of the men engaged in a spirited debate," Crane tells us. "They clamored at each other, numbers making futile bids for the popular attention" (*Red Badge* 412). The group splinters into smaller clumps of men who continue to bicker.[28] Such scenes are repeated in the novel, demonstrating how unreliable narrative leads to physical and psychological discord. Scientific historians sought precisely to eradicate such temperamental narratives by standardizing the form and method of their writing. In this way they could presumably avoid the dissension that resulted when truth became relative.

However, Crane shows that these often self-destructive utterances are crucial in moving people. The contentious mood keeps the soldiers from considering their powerless positions, their unending vulnerability. Nothing is more galling than a verbal assault or the thought that they may be killed in insignificant ways, for "without adequate ideological underpinnings," as Donald Pease argues, "battle scenes flare up as severe emotional and psychic blows without the consolation recognition brings."[29] For example, Henry's final rage is inspired by his superiors' observation that he and his comrades fight like "mule-drivers" and that their afternoon of battle has accomplished nothing in the grand scheme of things. The incessant trivialization of their efforts evokes a "nervous fear" and "anxiety that made [Henry and his comrades] frantic." The Civil War histories and memoirs flooding the market at the same time *The Red Badge of Courage* appeared reflected the regiments' uneasiness, anxiously insisting on the heroic significance of even the smallest actions of Civil War combatants. In his essay "The Red Badge of Hysteria," McClurg attacked the novel's "vicious satire" of the admirable American soldier, which was being spread through America—just as discord was spread among the troops—for the novel had "been so much talked about."[30] Thus McClurg is achingly aware of the power of words.

Henry's initial illness is caused by his unwillingness to participate in just such interactions. When the regiment is marching and they begin to argue and bellow, "the youth took no part in them. As he walked along in careless line he was engaged with his own eternal debate" (*Red Badge* 425). Henry's ability to extricate himself from the battle-sickness that afflicts his comrades allows him to note the "radical differences between himself and those men who were dodging imp-like around the fires" (*Red Badge* 426). Both Robert Rechnitz and Pease have argued that in extracting his "interpretive faculties" from the group, Henry is able to resist absorption in their narratives.[31] Here, Crane's imagery suggests that Henry has escaped incorporation into the circles of hell, where he would, like his comrades, succumb to primitive deviltry around the campfires. Instead, he studies the faces of his companions, searching for finer, "kindred emotions" in their faces. Disappointed, he concludes that some "ardor of the air . . . had infected" all in the new regiment but him, and he listens as they buzz with contentious tales of the certain victory to come (*Red Badge* 425).

Thus Henry's unwillingness to use language as a weapon and join in the mob mentality forces him to engage in an internal debate that itself eventually becomes pathological. Like Mitchell's injured patients who carry their hypersensitive, injured limbs carefully, Henry attends to his bothersome psyche. Provoked by the taunting of the veterans who prey upon the new recruits, despite his best efforts to tune them out, Henry tries to prove to himself that he will face battle bravely, "until a little panic-fear grew in his mind. As his imagination went forward to a fight, he saw hideous possibilities" (*Red Badge* 418). His rigorous self-examination leads to repeated anxiety attacks. In the darkness Henry "saw visions of a thousand-tongued fear that would babble at his back and cause him to flee, while others were going coolly about their country's business. He admitted that he would not be able to cope with the monster. He felt that every nerve in his body would be an ear to hear the voices, while other men would remain stolid and deaf" (*Red Badge* 428). Notice that babbling fear—words—are the weapons trained upon him, a multiple-mouthed monster that incorporates the taunts of many men. Even his comrades notice his illness; the tall soldier says, "You're looking thundering peeked. What the dickens is wrong with you?" (*Red Badge* 427). Henry's self-doubt becomes visible on his body long before he receives his "red badge." He joins a stream of wounded soldiers and wonders if they are "contemplating the letters of guilt he felt burned into his brow" (*Red Badge* 461). The tattered soldier finally recognizes the internal sickness that plagues Henry: "I bet yeh've got a worser one than yeh think," he advises Henry, "Ye'd better take keer of yer hurt. It don't do t' let sech things go. It might be inside mostly, an' them plays a thunder. Where is it located?" (*Red Badge* 468). As Mitchell's work showed, the wounds of war were always unlocatable; the tattered soldier adds that those who are visibly free from hurt are, perhaps, the deepest sufferers.

Eventually, Henry is wounded literally by the insufficiency of words—

both his inability to express the disquieting questions that plague him and his failure to be placated by unreliable gossip. During the regiment's frantic retreat, Crane writes, a thousand wild questions came to Henry, "but no one made answer." He grabs another fleeing soldier and tries to initiate a conversation:

> "Why—why—" stammered the youth, struggling with his balking tongue.
> The man screamed "Let go me! Let go me!" His face was livid and his eyes were rolling uncontrolled. He was heaving and panting. He still grasped his rifle, perhaps having forgotten to release his hold upon it. He tugged frantically, and the youth being compelled to lean forward was dragged several paces.
> "Let go me! Let go me!"
> "Why—why—" stuttered the youth.
> "Well, then!" bawled the man in a lurid rage. He adroitly and fiercely swung his rifle. It crushed upon the youth's head. (*Red Badge* 477)

Henry's vague questioning hinders the soldier's—and hence the army's—progress. The retreating soldier will not be engaged in disturbing internal debates. He wants only to "let go" of himself and succumb to the battle-sickness; his murderous reaction to struggling Henry's innocuous questioning is evidence of his illness.

One might argue, as Alfred Habegger has, that in sustaining his red badge, Henry sustains an irreparable moral injury.[32] At the very least, the flow of Henry's blood stanches his questions; he soon engages in the embattled conversation, eventually abandoning himself to the mob. Crane argues that warfare begins before the killing. Soldiers are steeped in violent, combative exchanges in camp that set the tone for later activities. Incessant peer pressure urges American white men to yield to incipient hysteria. Thus the symptoms of battle-sickness manifest themselves the minute the formerly withdrawn youth begins to expound publicly upon the idiocy of the officers. Henry is "secretly dumbfounded at this sentiment when it came from his lips. For a moment his face lost its valor and he looked guiltily about him. But no one questioned his right to deal in such words" (*Red Badge* 497). The way that Crane phrases this scene suggests that "such words" are powerful weapons—as destructive as the gun Henry later fires. The lack of consequences emboldens him.

By the end of the novel Henry is prattling unconsciously in "grotesque exclamations" (*Red Badge* 520). He allows himself to be driven into a "wild hate for the relentless foe. . . . He was not going to be badgered all of his life, like a kitten chased by boys, he said," and he develops "teeth and claws" in order to combat the increasingly provoking taunting (*Red Badge* 501). He finally relinquishes his individuality, becoming "not a man but a member. He felt that something of which he was a part—a regiment, an army, a cause, a country—was in crisis. He was welded into a common personality which was dominated by a single desire" (*Red Badge* 440). Battle-sickness diminishes Henry, making him into a fragment of a larger corporeal being—a "member" who sacrifices his idiosyncrasies to the common cant. He has a visceral reaction to the "war atmosphere" he breathes: "a blistering sweat, a sensation that his eyeballs were about to crack like hot stones. A burning roar filled his ears" (*Red Badge* 443). Henry allows himself to feel the "quiver of war desire," to be consumed by its fever, to become a creature of sensation: "In his ears, he heard the ring of victory. He knew the frenzy of a rapid successful charge. The music of the trampling feet, the sharp voices, the clanking arms of the column near him made him soar on the red wings of war. For a few moments he was sublime" (*Red Badge* 471). Henry lets his neurasthenic paralysis become inflamed into mindless, bodiless hysteria. He becomes incorporeal; like Bierce's Peyton, sensation divorced from form. Thus battle-sickness still takes men outside of themselves, estranging them from all they had known. Whereas for Mitchell this surrender to sensation signaled complete hysterical deterioration, Crane succeeds, as Andrew Delbanco contends, in "replicating the experience of war for the sensate individual."[33] I add that it is the nature of battlefield actions—of murder—that is reconstituted as sickness in these historical novels. Finally, Henry's "red badge" signals that he has become a good killer.

Whereas his comrades had earlier asked if the pale, forlorn youth felt okay, they now ask the savage soldier, with "his soiled and disordered dress, his red and inflamed features surmounted by the dingy rag with the spot of red blood," "Are yeh all right, Fleming? Do yeh feel all right? Ther ain't nothing' th' matter with yeh, Henry, is there?" (*Red Badge* 503). The narrator suggests that Henry "looked like an insane soldier," but Crane's imagery insists that to be a soldier is to suffer from a sort of nervous exhaustion, at the very least. Although the novel's ending allows the illusion that the corps is going to be able to "cast off its battlefield ways" and that its members will be able to "closely comprehend themselves and their circumstances," the verse the soldiers sing as they leave the fields suggests otherwise (*Red Badge* 534). "'A dog, a woman, an' a walnut tree, / Th' more yeh beat em, th' better they be!' That's like us," they chant (*Red Badge* 504). The hysterical sickness of battle will not be cured when the soldiers return home. Such barbarity simply cannot be cast off. Crane still marvels at the "battle reflection" shining in the faces of the regiment. "There was an appalling imprint upon those faces," he insists. "The struggle in the smoke had pictured an exaggeration of itself on the bleached cheeks and in the eyes wild with one desire" (*Red Badge* 440). Notice that it is not the actual battlefield experience itself but an "appalling imprint" an "exaggeration" that will stay with them—a distorted and perhaps even more virulent effect of war-era disease. It will emerge now and then as the "irritability" of which Mitchell's patients complain, provoking them to commit violent acts on the home front. After battle, Henry seems to regain his senses, feeling as if he will suffocate in the "foul atmosphere" of war. Yet when he looks around him Henry finds the men "leering at each other with dirty smiles" (*Red Badge* 445). The battlefield behavior to which the soldiers abandon themselves becomes a secret, perverse crime.

Though at the end of the novel Henry calmly reflects on how he has overcome the "red sickness of battle," I contend that he leaves the war terminally infected by the battle-sickness, for his body harbors sensate memories of his own murderous acts. Scholars have long debated the true meaning of Henry's final claim that he has acquired "manhood" on the battlefield. Henry does, indeed, become a man through his war service. The white manhood of which he speaks is associated with "touching the great death"—however, this seemingly sublime feat translates into fending off the violence of other white men, or killing them. In the hottest moments of battle Crane's soldiers move forward "insanely, burst[ing] into cheerings, mob-like and barbaric" and succumbing to the "delirium that encounters despair and death, and is heedless and blind to the odds" (*Red Badge* 510). The whole regiment is alternately unhealthily self-obsessed or dangerously abandoned.

Although the ending of the novel seems to suggest that the army as a whole, and Henry in particular, is triumphant, the dying body of the regiment negates such simple conclusions and signals how far battle-disease has penetrated social bodies. True, the regiment initially acts as an efficient, cooperative unit. And yet it is consistently personified as a malevolent entity. It "awakens" en masse and "tremble[s] with eagerness at the noise of rumors" like a dog picking up a scent (*Red Badge* 411). The regiment acts as one in all matters, for "whole brigades grinned in unison, and regiments laugh" and "whoop" together at jokes (*Red Badge* 425). Crane eventually reveals that "union"—perhaps like the political Union for which these murderous acts had been committed—is beastly, for when the regiment moves, he tells us, "it was like one of those moving monsters wending with many feet" (*Red Badge* 424). As more men are absorbed into the malicious creature, it becomes even more grotesque, with its scores of feet, multitude of grinning mouths, and its continuous buzz of voices. When the regiment engages in rough fighting, the injured men are described as a "flow of blood from the torn body of the brigade"; as it continues to bleed extravagantly, it also becomes "emaciated" by its loss of mass and men. In its final charge, the regiment appears to be in a "paroxysm, a display of the strength that comes before a final feebleness" (*Red Badge* 526, 528–29). The fact that the body of the regiment is monstrous when at full strength and that its once-vital body is dying by the end of the novel undercuts any positive associations with unionism and nuances the paroxysm of violence that overtakes Henry.

Crane tries to pass off his white men's barbarity onto the racial Other, conventionally pathologizing blackness and associating the barbaric behaviors of the Civil War with so-called African depravity. Henry and his comrades literally become blacker as they become more abandoned to their brutish work: "Moving to and fro with strained exertion, jabbering the while, they were, with their swaying bodies, black faces, and glowing eyes, like strange and ugly fiends jiggling heavily in the smoke" (*Red Badge* 526). Contemporary readers would have been fully aware of the racial stereotypes encoded in this and similar descriptions. Like supposedly savage Africans, their bodies enact their darkest fantasies, the internal rhythms of eroticized, murderous desires. Though such scenes were instrumental in solidifying postbellum racism, they did not suffice as explanation for the deviltry of white men. The Civil War was still a crucial event in the understanding of gender and race at the turn of the century, for the barbarity required of men on the battlefield exposed the essential inconsistency of a white racial identity premised both on civilized superiority *and* indomitable, violent shows of strength. Turn-of-the-century Americans apparently cherished the political, social, and racial Union that had been forged between white men through the gauntlet of the Civil War. However, Crane's novel teaches us that the male neurasthenia they shared was not ineffective; as Dunbar highlights, it mutated into a potent, destructive, and highly contagious force in American culture.

The Fanatics

I argue that Dunbar's work also seeks to expose the myths of the Civil War and the "heroics" of white soldiers in *The Fanatics*.[34] Critics have lamented that in this novel Dunbar chose not to showcase the experiences of heroic African American soldiers—among whose ranks could be counted his father, who had served in the Fifty-Fifth Massachusetts and had spent his final years in a home for veterans. Rather, they say, he chose to pander to his white audience with white characters, adhering to the "Plantation School" of turn-of-the-century fiction that reconstituted the mythical antebellum world the war had destroyed.[35] White critics writing in the spring and summer following the April 1901 publication of *The Fanatics* praised Dunbar's supposedly realistic portrayal of African American characters as they confronted freedom in the war era. The *New York Times* reports that, "in his treatment of the men of his own race

Mr. Dunbar shows excellent judgment. He tells us how pitiful were the conditions of those colored people who sought their freedom in the Northern states."[36] In Birmingham, Alabama, the reviewer insists that Dunbar even "magnif[ies] whatever good quality the negro displays" (*Bookworm*, June 1901, Roll 5, Box 18, Frame 475). More recent critical assessments of the novel have dismissed Dunbar's portrayal of war-era African Americans as conciliatory and racist. Ralph Story contends that Dunbar resurrects "someone else's nostalgia" in his characterization of the one substantive African American character, the offensively titled and buffoonish Nigger Ed. Though contemporaneous reviewers raved that " 'Nigger Ed' is a perfect representative of his race," most modern scholars agree that Ed is the biggest failure in the book (*New York Times*, April 6, 1901, Roll 5, Box 18, Frame 350).[37]

The question *The Fanatics* begs is what precisely Dunbar is doing with his passionate white characters and with the conspicuous Nigger Ed. I find that Dunbar's racial consciousness is focused on exploring the psychology of prejudice—in particular, how white culture cultivated the strand of racist violence that emerged during the Civil War at the moment of emancipation and grew as the nineteenth century wore on. Mia Bay has recently argued that Dunbar was not alone in his efforts to satirically reveal the "white problem."[38] Just as plantation fiction worked to naturalize black inferiority, Dunbar subtly exposes the violence that revealed itself in the diseased bodies and inflamed psyches of white Rebels and Unionists—his fanatics. In the novel, Unionist Bradford Waters and Confederate sympathizer Steven Van Doren have long-standing political disagreements, yet they and their children have lived peaceably in Dunbar's fictional Dorbury, Ohio; in fact, young Mary Waters and Robert Van Doren are engaged. However, once news of Fort Sumter reaches the town the two patriarchs—indeed, their whole community—come to blows and the lovers are torn apart. The regional conflict dramatized between the two clans later becomes intrafamilial in the subplot between rebel Colonel Stewart and his Union sympathizer son, Walter. Yet prejudice is not solely the purview of the white community in *The Fanatics*. True, when African American emigrants from the South enter Dorbury, racial bigotry supersedes regional bias and becomes a galvanizing force for the splintered white community. However, we find that the Southern refugees must be protected not only from white citizens but also from free African Americans who insist upon the difference "between people who had been free three or four years before and those just made free" (*Fanatics* 104).[39] Dunbar focuses on the *structures* of racism and prejudice, rather than on a particular ideological or political position, achieving a subtlety that has been lost on some readers.

The strategies Dunbar deployed in *The Fanatics* were well publicized from the novel's inception. In newspaper reports from the fall of 1899, when he began the novel, Dunbar told interviewers that he was working on a novel treating the plight of "copperheads" during the Civil War.[40] He emphasized to the *Chicago News* that his sympathies were "very strongly" with the Copperheads, explaining:

By that I do not mean that I believe as they did, or that I think they were in any way in the right. But they were acting conscientiously on what they believed to be the right. They were opposed to the war and they were not afraid to say so. They stood up for their belief and they suffered ostracism in many places and often bodily injury for it. (*Chicago News*, September 14, 1899, Roll 4, Box 17, Frame 977)

Dunbar's delicate criticism of prejudicial violence is so inoffensive that it is nearly invisible. A writer for the Topeka, Kansas *Capital* chides Dunbar for his seemingly Uncle Tom-ish sentiments:

When Lincoln issued his immortal proclamation of emancipation by which Mr. Dunbar's parents and all his race in bondage were made free, the copperhead press of the north exceeded all previous efforts in abusing "the nigger loving" government of Lincoln. All this Mr. Paul Lawrence [*sic*] Dunbar ought to know, and he ought never to forget that if it had not been for the men whom the copperheads most abused, his race would yet be in slavery. (September 21, 1899, Roll 4, Box 17, Frame 1002)

Surely Dunbar understood that the copperheads would have kept him enslaved. He insists in his public statement that he does not agree with Southern sympathizers or believe they were in the right. But he does support their right to peacefully express their opinions unmolested by those who disagree. It is not difficult to see that Dunbar's references to the "ostracism" and "bodily injury" suffered by those who express unpopular beliefs were nuanced by the racial climate in which he wrote. Copperheads were a thing of the past in 1899—agitators for racial equality, a present reality. Dunbar makes strange bedfellows of white racists and African American activists.[41] Like a member of the contemporary American Civil Liberties Union, Dunbar presents himself as an ethical and impartial champion of freedom of expression and equal protection under the law, no matter how loathsome the opinions expressed.

Dunbar's use of the Civil War was particularly apt. He knew of its fictional power, for his story "The Strength of Gideon" appeared in the October 1899 *New Lipincott* right next to the well-reviewed and popular *Love across the Lines* by Harry Sitwell Edwards. All of the reviews of Dunbar's story gathered in his scrapbook include extensive considerations of Edwards's Civil War novel. Dunbar knew the Civil War was being rewritten as the historical and psychological site of regional rapprochement and national identity—one that was forged on shared racist sentiments. Thus *The Fanatics* could be interpreted as reconfirming all of our nation's most cherished myths about the Civil War as the proving ground of white heroism and black incompetence. But Dunbar employs a clever narrative inversion where the behaviors traditionally attributed to African Americans—childishness, inconsistency, and violence—are pervasive and perhaps even inborn to white Americans. Contemporaneous representations of African American men made necessary Dunbar's narrative circumspection. At one point, Dunbar begins to tell of Ed's heroism during the war, but stops short, remarking, "But no more of that. The telling of it must be left to a time when he who says aught of a negro's virtues will not be cried down as an advocate drunk with prejudice" (*Fanatics* 34). Reviewers rewarded Dunbar for his "restraint." One criticizes Dunbar's lack of warmth in characterization but attributes this to "the studious impartiality with which he treats all parties and questions." His work "would do credit to an apostle of the modern historical method," the writer adds (*Town and Country*, New York, June 29, 1901, Roll 5, Box 18, Frame 480). If one extrapolates the reviewer's assumptions, it seems clear that depictions of disadvantaged African Americans and white gentlemen soldiers ensured proclamations of one's historical veracity.

But I see that Dunbar invokes the Civil War as the occasion for unleashed white violence that verges on race suicide. He shifts the seemingly unbreachable racial dichotomy from white-black relations to white-white relations—a feat that can be achieved *only* by the obfuscation of the conventional racial Other. The reviewer for the *Southern Workman* presciently notices, "It is perhaps a part of Mr. Dunbar's art and of his sense of proportion that the Negro plays so small a part in his book" (June 1901, Roll 5, Box 18, Frame 410). Clearly, Dunbar read his audience well. His move has profound implications for a whiteness conventionally understood to be a dominant, universal, and monolithic category in America. Dunbar's intricate orchestration of various racial/regional identities in *The Fanatics* prefigures Hazel Carby's dictum that we "make visible what is rendered invisible when viewed as the normative state of existence: the (white) point in space from which we tend to identify difference."[42] The Civil War is not the founding moment of national conciliation for Dunbar, but the occasion for whiteness to reveal its fault lines, exposing the constructed nature and hidden vulnerability of racial hegemony.

Dunbar depicts Nigger Ed as seen through a "white"—or at least a racist—consciousness, one that only dimly understands the subversive work in which he is engaged. For example, our first substantial description of Ed comes from the young female heroine, Mary Waters, who reflects, "For her part, she only knew one black man and he was bad enough. Of course, Nigger Ed was funny. They all liked him and laughed at him, but he was not exemplary. He filled, with equal adaptability, the position of town crier and town drunkard. Really, if all his brethren were like him, they would be none the worse for having masters" (*Fanatics* 10). For those readers steeped in the cult of true womanhood and inured to such racist sentiments, Mary can remain an admirable character, loyal and domestic. Her paternalism was standard in white-authored fiction of the day. But when one focuses on the politics of an African American writer creating such a passage, the seemingly conventional words become much more risky. Dunbar's public speeches, private papers, and editorial work reveal that even though he was conscious of class and regional differences within the African American community, he was a militant proponent of racial uplift. Putting what were surely to him odious words in the mouth of a true, white woman adds a critical edge to Mary's portrayal. She becomes bigoted and selfish.

Crispin Sartwell explains why Dunbar's dangerous depictions of white racism go unremarked: "One of the major strategies for preserving white invisibility to ourselves is the silencing, segregation, or delegitimation of voices that speak about whiteness from a nonwhite location; above all, we can't stand to be looked at, described, or made specific."[43] Whereas Dunbar's unflattering portrayal of African American characters garners almost all critical attention, his scathing critique of the cannibalistic nature of white characters goes unnoticed. As one of his characters explains, Dunbar's desire to put himself in another's place is "less the outcome of generosity than the result of a subtle selfishness. It was . . . the sacrifice which we make to the gods of our own desires" (*Fanatics* 36). Protected by the ingrained reading practices of the audience, as well as by Dunbar's delicate manipulation of racial stereotypes, Ed gains free reign to incite white violence throughout the novel. Particularly radical is Dunbar's insistence that racism is as virulent in the North and in the Midwest as it is in the South. Dunbar writes a Civil War novel that does not take us to the Southern battlefields, but focuses on the violent behaviors ravaging the home front "in a loyal and non-slave-holding state" (*Fanatics* 118). At the turn of the century, African American homes were firmly established as the new frontlines of civil unrest.

As far as we know, Dunbar began writing *The Fanatics* far from home while on a trip to Colorado during the summer of 1899, which he embarked upon to relieve his chronic tuberculosis. Addison Gayle reads the novel's feverish energy metaphorically as representing Dunbar's own deteriorating body.[44] I argue that racism and disease became inextricably linked to the Civil War in his work of this period. The novel meant a great deal to Dunbar, and he was anxious about its reception. On April 18, 1901, the *Chicago Advance* reviewer proclaimed of the new novel, "We have had war stories from the Northern and from the Southern standpoint: now we have one from the negro's point of view." Dunbar was surely disappointed by the way the reviewer simplistically supplanted his regional and national affiliation with his racial identity. Dunbar wanted the novel to stand as his magnum opus, a national—not Negro—piece about that most significant of national events. Thus when reviews of the novel began to appear while Dunbar was on a speaking tour/vacation in the South, he wrote to his wife Alice often requesting information about the critical response. On April 8, 1901, Dunbar asks, "Has the press begun to say anything about the Fanatics? I am very much afraid for it." Alice sent reassuring news, pointing out positive reviews and tempering critical ones.[45] The majority of readers were soothed by Dunbar's apparently sympathetic portrayal of Southern sympathizers, and his abandonment of the vexing "negro question," which, the *Louisville Post* claims "may be looked upon as an encouragement for the future" (April 30, 1901, Roll 3, Box 18, Frame 381). John de Morgan in the New York *Book World* asserts that Dunbar has "given us a book which will hurt no one's feelings, but will be read by Northern and Southern citizens alike, and each feeling better for its perusal" (June 1901, Roll 3, Box 16, Frame 424). Dunbar's apparently dispassionate tone successfully served to dissipate racist reactions to his fictional ventures. White reviewers throughout the country pronounced *The Fanatics* a safe book, an educational tool for the "new generation," which "deserves long remembrance and deep pondering" (*Boston Transcript*, May 22, 1901, Roll 3, Box 17, Frame 418). Dunbar surely noticed the deep irony of white reviewers recommending to young white America a book scourging the destructive powers of white fanatics.

Dunbar had already begun working out his reaction to the Civil War and the vocabulary of fanaticism before he started the novel. In *Lyrics of Love and Laughter* (1900) Dunbar's poetry explicitly links the Civil War and the racial inequalities that held sway over the country thirty-five years later. As he switched from the dialect work of "When Dey 'Listed Colored Soldiers" to the formal sentiment of "Robert Gould Shaw," Dunbar not only tested his novel's subject matter, but he also finessed the rhetorical strategies best suited to garnering white support for racial equality while at the same time neutralizing racial violence. In one of his most admired verses, an ode to the young white commander of the Fifty-Fourth Massachusetts, Dunbar lauds Robert Gould Shaw for his tempered heroism. "Far better," Dunbar insists, "the slow blaze of Learning's light, / The cool and quiet of her dearer fame, / Than this hot terror of a hopeless fight," for they redeem Shaw.[46] Dunbar's characterization of Shaw as a moderate, thoughtful man serves as a foil to the white-hot fanaticism of most white men exposed in *The Fanatics*.[47]

Two more poems in the collection celebrate the forgotten heroism of African American men during the war, rekindling, as James A. Emanuel puts it, "sublimated racial fire."[48] "Unsung Heroes" offers a conventional song of military courage and sacrifice. Whereas Nigger Ed is apparently emasculated by the white community's reaction to his Civil War service, Dunbar's unsung heroes are reborn: "God looked down on their sinews brown, and said, 'I have made them men'" (*Collected Poetry* 8). Here the Civil War makes African American men Adamic, as firmly engendered beings. "Unsung Heroes" brings the soldiers back to life, and "Dirge for a Soldier" provides an appropriate and long-overdue eulogy; according to the poem, catharsis ultimately enables one to continue the battle: "Now no time for grief's pursuing, / Other work is for the doing, / Here to-day" (*Collected Poetry* 44–46). Though the poem employs conventional Civil War imagery, it never mentions the war explicitly, making it as much about the perpetual battle for racial equality as this particular American war. Overall, Dunbar's Civil War poems of this period illustrate that he was fully aware of the important African American presence in the Union army and suggest that he was surely doing more than just pandering to white audiences in *The Fanatics*. Though writing of Spanish-American war veterans in his 1898 editorial "Recession Never," Dunbar articulates the persistence of racist attitudes toward African American troops when he mocks: "Negroes, you may fight for us, but you may not vote for us. You may prove a strong bulwark when the bullets are flying, but you must stand from the line when the ballots are in the air. You may be heroes in war, but you must be cravens in peace."[49] The sarcasm that I argue characterizes *The Fanatics* is undeniable here; even the editors of the muckracking *McClure's* magazine, which originally commissioned the editorial, found it too radical for their readers.

In *The Fanatics*, Dunbar outlines a complicated rhetorical juncture, insisting that fanaticism is a race marker that ensures the degeneracy of whiteness. Social violence is framed in the tropes of neurasthenic infirmity exposed through wartime pursuits—as "general madness in which no rule of sane action held" (*Fanatics* 27). In the novel, once news of Fort Sumter reaches Dunbar's Dorbury, the two patriarchs, Waters and Van Doren, come to blows and must be "forcibly taken to their homes" (*Fanatics* 6). As in *The Red Badge of Courage*, their violence becomes contagious; "rumors and stories of all kinds were passing from lip to lip" in a crowd gathered around the courthouse after the announcement, inflaming observers and spreading fear and anger through the community like a virus. The crowd's whispers swell to a roar as they begin "hooting and jeering." Predictably, the mob takes on a life of its own: "with one accord, they surged towards the newspaper office" of a Southern sympathizer "armed with horns, and whistled, hooted and jeered themselves hoarse" (*Fanatics* 11). Their aural weaponry soon is supplanted by rocks and fire bombs as the "madness seized them all and they battered and broke, smashed and tore, fired the place and fled singing with delirious joy" (*Fanatic* 12). Such a description echoes those employed by Crane to describe advancing Union forces.

The power of language is significant in these exchanges. Dunbar suggests that white culture needs only "words thrown at those swayed by emotions and [the] opinions of others" to incite violence. When a Confederate sympathizer is mocked, "a red mist came before his eyes and . . . he forgot everything but his fury." The crowd replies in kind, growling "like the noise of wild beasts" and "surging" upon the young man (*Fanatics* 29). Dunbar contends that the battle-sickness exceeds the boundaries of war in both space and time—it invades all aspects of American life, here reaching far beyond the frontlines to a seemingly insulated Midwestern town. Certainly it continued to manifest itself in the racially motivated mass hysteria that gripped the country as Dunbar was writing. In 1901, just as in 1861, "the enthusiasm of the time was infectious" (*Fanatics* 20). The Civil War remained a crucial point of reference. In an 1898 editorial piece, Dunbar comments, "You cannot turn back the years and put ten millions of people into the condition that four millions were in thirty years ago. You cannot ignore the effects that have ensued, the changes that have followed, and make the problem of to-day the problem of 1865." Dunbar marshals the expanded presence of the black body since the Civil War (4 to 10 million people) as solidifying the race's claim to national citizenship and equal protection. He makes the end of the war into an immovable benchmark against which subsequent progress will be measured. Yet his novel admits that the violent, uncivil behaviors that had been unleashed and encouraged during the Civil War continued to plague African American communities.

Although Dunbar writes of the Civil War, clearly his own contemporary moment was in his mind when he claims, "It was a moment when only a spark was needed to light the whole magazine of discontent and blow doubt and vacillation into a conflagration of disloyalty" (*Fanatics* 118). On August 12, 1900, an African American man ran into a New York cigar store, leaving his wife unattended on the street; when he emerged from the store he found a white man accosting his wife and stabbed her attacker in an ensuing scuffle. The stabbing victim turned out to be a popular member of the police force; when he finally died after three days of growing racial tensions, white mobs raged through New York unmolested by an indignant and racist police force. Dunbar, who was in the city at the time, was robbed of a diamond ring, a gold watch, and some book royalties as he fled the city.[50] Yet this event must have impacted Dunbar's view of white masculinity: a white policeman had attacked an unprotected African American woman, a whole police force was unwilling to protect their African American constituents from illogical mob violence, and a white mob ransacked and burned African American homes and tortured and murdered many individuals. The New York riot was not, of course, an isolated incident in 1900.

In an 1898 editorial that was widely syndicated, Dunbar highlights the way that white solidarity was being forged through racial violence:

It would seem that the man who sits at his desk in the North and writes about the troubles in the South is very apt to be like a doctor who prescribes for a case he has no chance to diagnose. It would be true in this instance, also, if it were not that what has happened in Georgia has happened in Ohio and Illinois. The race riots in North Carolina were of a piece with the same proceedings in the state of Lincoln. The men who shoot the Negro in Hogansville are blood brothers to those who hang him in Urbana, and the deed is neither better nor worse because it happens in one section of the country or other. The race spirit in the United States is not local but general.[51]

His rhetoric of health and healing mirrors Mitchell's: again, those doctors who claim the right to diagnose and prescribe cures for social ills supposedly contained in another "body"—here region—are imposters, for the disease they claim to treat also infects the doctors. Dunbar ingeniously inverts racialist discourse: the blood rules that were used to construct African American identity and the reconciliation of white Americans are invoked to express the genetic fanaticism coursing through white veins. Read within the context of his nonfiction, *The Fanatics* becomes a clear indictment of deep-seated American racism, which was so often rhetorically contained in foreign and more hot-blooded images of the South. As one Dunbar critic penetratingly remarks, "For those who viewed Ohio as the promised land, Dunbar certainly shattered the illusion."[52] Dunbar exploits the romantic sentiments that increasingly engulfed war-era memories, allowing them to camouflage his pointed criticism.

Dunbar uses his novel to remind white America that the Civil War was also a benchmark for them, a time when white society destroyed itself. In order to train our attentions on white-on-white violence, Dunbar casts his discussion of prejudice and disease through a nonthreatening white subplot. We never enter Ed's mind to understand the psychological wounds he suffers as a constant target of prejudice. Dunbar explains, "What [Ed] felt is hardly worth recording. He was so near the animal in the estimation of his fellows (perhaps too near in reality) that he could be presumed to have really few mental impressions" (*Fanatics* 115). Dunbar excises Ed's thoughts because in the "estimation" of his reading public, Ed would be "presumed" to have nothing of interest to say—at least nothing that they were willing or able to hear. Dunbar's strategies were much more subtle. The wounds of fanatical behavior are borne by a young white woman. Mary Waters's loyal love for Confederate Robert Van Doren causes her to be "forcibly, almost involuntarily" cast aside by her Northern community. She, not Ed, must "withstand contempt and reviling" (*Fanatics* 51). Mary's pain and alienation eventually make her sick, "alternately delirious and piteous"; her father's inflexibility causes a "raging fever" in Mary that "strains her weakened nerves" (*Fanatics* 59, 56). Mary Waters's vulnerable body is further enfeebled by the regional conflict enacted between her father and her fiancé; her father's steely patriotism impels Mary's brother to deadly service on the battlefield and almost kills Mary. Mary's illness is conventionally cured by her reconciliation with her family and her impending marriage to Robert.

Though I contend that Dunbar's main task is to probe the instability of whiteness, Ed's presence—as well as shadowy glimpses of anonymous Southern emigrés—are crucial, for, as Toni Morrison argues, the novel responds "to a dark, abiding, signing presence."[53] It is easy, then, for the white mob to proclaim that "the whole war is on their account" (*Fanatics* 105). The semiotics of race already at work in American culture provided convenient explanations for white postbellum citizens who used entrenched American racism to make sense of the ominous threats endangering their personal and cultural security—threats that were, as the novel shows, self-generated. In making the racial slur "Nigger" part of Ed's proper name, Dunbar calls attention to his perpetual marginality, as well as his singularity. As Morrison remarks of Mark Twain's Nigger Jim, "It is absolutely necessary that the term *nigger* be inextricable from Huck's deliberations about who and what he himself is—or, more precisely, is not."[54] Through the eyes of the racist white community, Ed *is* black America. "Upon one thing" all white characters, North and South, are united, and that is in their "hatred and disdain for the hapless race which had caused the war. Upon its shoulders fell all the resentment and each individual stood for his race. If their boys suffered hardships in the field, they felt that in some manner they avenged them by firing a negro's home or chasing him" (*Fanatics* 117). According to Dunbar, this perverted racist logic crystallized during the Civil War. It tied any violent breakdown of America to emancipated black bodies and consequently offered the destruction of those bodies as the cure to social ills.

However, Dunbar is not content to proclaim the unity of the "Africanist presence." He uses a constantly shifting array of racial, regional, political, and class alliances to highlight the invisible lines of identity politics that structured life in postbellum America. When the small town of Dorbury is deluged by a flow of emancipated slaves fleeing the South, "all party lines fell away, and all the [white] people were united in one cause—resistance to the invasion of the black horde" (*Fanatics* 102). In a hierarchy of prejudice, racial union supersedes regional bias. Even Mary Waters talks of "those people"—African Americans—"[who] are at the bottom of it all." "I wish they'd never been brought into this country," she continues, and a friend accuses her, "I believe you're getting a touch of hysteria." Mary replies, "It isn't hysteria, Nannie, unless the whole spirit of the times is hysterical" (*Fanatics* 17). Like Grant, Mary concedes that African Americans were brought to this country against their wills; however, she makes them into pathogens, permanently foreign bodies that are "at the bottom" of Civil War disease and its contagion. Crane's text imagines the end stage of this racialized disease in the blackened bodies and leering faces of his Civil War soldiers.

However, even the Northern "aristocrats," as Dunbar disparagingly calls Dorbury's free black citizens, try to distinguish themselves from the newly emancipated emigrants (*Fanatics* 104). But when the "embers of the [local white] people's passions had long smouldered and when a pseudo-politician in the glow of drink" goads them to mount an attack upon the African American community, "the whites made no distinction as to bond or free, manumitted or contraband" (*Fanatics* 104, 107). The threat of white violence then galvanizes the African American community; "artificial lines" Dunbar writes were erased between Northerners and Southerners. "Instead of a cowering crowd of helpless men," the "drawn, swollen, terrible" white mob that assaults the emigrant encampment is confronted by a "solid black wall of desperate men who stood their ground and fought like soldiers" (*Fanatics* 111). Here Dunbar seems to suggest that only African American solidarity can combat the battle-sickness still gripping white Americans. In his more overtly militant moments, Dunbar explains the crucial importance of such resistance. "Let those suffering people relinquish one single right that has been given them," he notes in "Recession Never," "and the rapacity of the other race, encouraged by yielding, will ravage from them every privilege that they possess. Passion and prejudice are not sated by concession, but grow by what they feed on."[55] Interestingly, Dunbar's reference to the rapaciousness of whites sexualizes violence, much as Crane's depiction of Henry Fleming had done. Given the frequency of the rape and castration of African Americans at the turn of the century, such rhetoric was apt.

Dunbar emphasizes that African Americans are indistinguishable to whites, foreign bodies that would take up valuable space and degrade the labor market. Dunbar's characters believe: "Pretty soon we won't have a place to lay our heads. They'll undercharge the laborer and drive him out of house and home. They will live on leavings, and the men who are eating white bread and butter will have to get down to the level of these black hounds" (*Fanatics* 105). Even to the present day, the threat of invasion by racial Others is framed in terms of economic security and national interest. Such descriptions lend credence to Lutz's observation that American nervousness is, at heart, an "economistic discourse."[56] Wealthy, neurasthenic Americans bemoaned their "nervous bankruptcy"; their attendant anxiety was projected onto an increasingly successful African American citizenry, which they perceived as in some sense leeching away the resources of a disturbingly enervated white culture.[57]

Despite critics' claims to the contrary, African Americans are not passive in this novel. Most striking, Dunbar asserts that they cunningly exacerbate the symptoms of white fanaticism, manipulating the incendiary speech that Crane, too, notes as the key component of the disease's potency. Dunbar is seemingly conciliatory when he writes that the "servant is always curious," and the "negro servant particularly so" (*Fanatics* 26). However, Dunbar celebrates the servants' ability to discern the shameful secrets of white culture and their willingness to use that knowledge to their advantage. The Confederate sympathizers in his novel lament that black servants are not what they used to be, for "they will talk and its few family secrets they don't know and tell." Wheras old servants had assumed the family pride of their "owners," the new "darkies have blown the father's business broadcast" (*Fanatics* 91). Dunbar insists that African Americans are not complicit in their own subjugation and in maintaining the myths of white culture. They stoke the embers of contention among whites, using carefully chosen words to encourage self-destructive behaviors.

Thus Nigger Ed is more than the buffoon the critics see. Rather than showing physical resistance, he uses his powerful position as town crier to incite discord among the white citizenry of Dorbury. Ed's versions of local gossip fan the flames of "popular anger" (*Fanatics* 27). After the assault upon Fort Sumter is announced, a mob gathers—"a combination of hot-blood and lawlessness"—to vent their rage against known Copperheads. Ed's cries of "Fiah, fiah" inflame an already angry mob so that "madness seized them all," and they destroy their own town (*Fanatics* 11–12). Like yelling fire in a crowded theater, Ed's actions may be construed as irresponsible. Yet Ed speaks the truth when he spreads the news that a known Copperhead is being hung—a clear case of murder in the minds of the white folks assembled in the town. When the angry crowd realizes that "they're only hanging him in effigy," Ed replies, "'Hit don't mek no diffunce how a man's hung, jes so he's hung" (*Fanatics* 17). This is a barely veiled reference to contemporary lynching. Dunbar reveals, as Bederman and Robyn Wiegman note, that the "lynch mob did not embody white manliness restraining black lust." The "black lust" here, as in contemporaneous lynching, is manufactured and fraudulent; instead, the event embodies "white men's lust running amok."[58]

Ed enters the army as a servant, but Dunbar allows him to be somewhat ennobled by the experience. The "new cap and a soldier's belt had had their effect on him, and he marched among his deriders, very stern, dignified and erect," Dunbar asserts. Ed tells local onlookers, "You got to git somebody else to ring yo' ol' bell now," for he has escaped their oppression (*Fanatics* 34). However, he is disappointingly neutralized on the battlefield; like Harriet Beecher Stowe's feminized Uncle Tom, Ed is limited to wartime activities in "hospital[s] and by deathbeds," where "his touch was as the touch of a mother" (*Fanatics* 34). One must read this characterization in the context of the unmitigated racial violence during which Dunbar was writing. Ed's is a soothing presence, both to the wounded soldiers and those readers who might become fanatical at the thought of armed black men, even the memories of those who had fought for the Union. By the end of the novel the once despised Nigger Ed has found a cherished place in the community as a walking signifier: in the remnants of his uniform he reminds soldiers of their battlefield experiences and local mothers and widows of lost loved ones he had nursed. Dunbar concludes the novel, "They gave him a place for life and everything he wanted, and from being despised he was much petted and spoiled, for they were all fanatics" (*Fanatics* 196). This ironic ending finally indicates that fanatical behavior is endemic to white culture, whether it is murderously violent in temper or smothering and benevolent. As Elizabeth Young also notes, whether Ed is bullied or "petted," he is still enslaved by his dependent community.[59]

The Relation of War to the Breed

I contend that lingering fears about the inherent fanaticism of the white race are the unspeakable core of turn-of-the-century Civil War narratives. It is the motivation behind criminal anthropologist and degeneracy theorist G. Frank Lydston's cryptic comment in *The Diseases of Society and Degeneracy, The Vice and Crime Problem* (1904) that "the War of the Rebellion" is "the most terrible crime in history"[60] In the end, it was clear that fanatical disease needed no one to cultivate it. Colonel Stewart's enthusiasm for the war "seemed to have turned its heat malignantly upon him to consume him." Such behavior is self-perpetuating, for "it was the spirit of [Stewart's] conscience to press the iron into his soul" (*Fanatics* 26). Dunbar suspects that this white-hot fever will eventually destroy those who harbor it. Translated as primitive masculinity, such behavior became increasingly attractive to an enervated culture when it was focused on barbaric, dark-skinned races or belligerent, immigrant hordes. Neurasthenia became a central tenet of such formulations according to Lutz, for it had "class and racial implications and was closely allied to the discourses justifying dominant American culture."[61] However, such primitive outbursts were unacceptable when white men killed each other. Thus Lydston and his fellow eugenicists, like their historical colleagues, make only veiled references to the shocking barbarity of the Civil War.[62]

Indeed, many postbellum medical theorists worked diligently to recast the invisible ills of the Civil War as a sign of American supremacy. George Beard, the "father of American Nervousness," argued that hysterical behavior was the result of "modern civilization" distinguished by "steam-power, the periodical press, the telegraph, the sciences, and the mental activity of women."[63] Because America was a leader in all of these fields, neurasthenia became a sign of the united nation's overachievement. Yet the disease was doubly marked by its invocation in narratives of the Civil War. Neurasthenia was not the unfortunate by-product of "progress" or evidence of the white race's accelerated evolution in Civil War historical fictions; rather, Civil War disease was evidence of a self-destructive degeneracy long engendered in white bodies. While eschewing direct discussion of the Civil War, Lydston and fellow eugenicists nuanced Beard's notion of American disease in this more negative vein. For example, Lydston argues that part of the American psyche's instability derives from its pathological hatred for authority—in some "civilized countries," Lydston remarks, "Americanism and lawlessness are synonymous" (*Disease* 234). Eugene S. Talbot in his work *Degeneracy: Its Cause, Signs, and Results* (1898) also notes that mental degeneracy is marked by the "removal of checks (which the race has acquired during evolution) and the explosive expressions of egotism and mentality" (*Degeneracy* 316). Talbot goes on to explain that degeneracy may remain latent "until the period of stress" provokes such "bio-chemic alterations as lead to diminished inhibitory powers" (*Degeneracy* 33). Thus battle-sickness was not necessarily caused by the Civil War but rather the war provided the trigger that merely activated the dormant traits of insubordination and violence.

Indeed, the exigencies of war sanctioned the lawlessness and passion that was latent in American men. In civilized society, "the individual is prohibited by law from stealing and murder," and yet "nations may do both under cover of a declaration of war" (*Disease* 257). The martial structures of war-time bred cultural disease to which most Americans were susceptible. War was particularly pernicious for it enabled the "natural-born coward" to become "permeated with the 'courage' of the living mass about him. By and by the savage, which usually lies dormant in man, comes to the surface, and his native cowardice is swallowed up in his lust for blood and glory. Of such stuff are some heroes made" (*Disease* 248). The war and its heroes were being reified in contemporaneous histories of the time, but Lydston, like Crane and Dunbar, suggests that the sacred causes of Yanks and Rebs were no more than the mindless cruelty of an unrestrained mob. Lydston particularly excoriates the rise of the "professional soldier," for in making "scientific" the act of murder, martial culture made the sickness of battle institutional and even profitable (*Disease* 264). As America rallied behind its troops—both its Civil War veterans and their modern-day capitalist and imperialist counterparts—it revealed that "an hysterical psychosis may affect an entire nation" (*Disease* 261).

Thus just as individual bodies succumbed to the sickness of war, so too are compromised social bodies forged out of the consuming fever. Eugenicists reasoned that the prodding of an extraordinarily degenerate leader and the mounting energy of even a mildly corrupted group of people could consolidate otherwise harmless individuals into a murderous creature.[64] "What a selfish, mean, cruel, unreasonable thing a mob is, to be sure," Lydston testifies (*Disease* 232). Lydston's work fortifies Dunbar's, for in the cases of lynching in particular he reveals that the "psychopathy of a mob surpasses the bounds of social hysteria . . . indeed, it transcends all bounds short of homicidal mania" (*Disease* 246). Like Dunbar, Lydston inverts common racist assumptions, arguing that it is the civilized white lynch-mob participant who runs amok "like any other savage" (*Disease* 246). However, even as he excoriates racially motivated lynchings, Lydston also exposes the racist core of eugencial theories, for "savages"—mostly members of dark-skinned races—were inherently degenerate. At the same time Lydston subtly critiques imperialist force in his explanation of the ways that degeneracy has managed to mask itself in discrete bodies throughout history: "It is not the ass in the lion's skin; it is the human hyena who has put on the garb of a nobler, if erratic, beast and gone forth 'to destroy, not to teach or reform." "This human hyena has been heard from before," Lydston continues, listing judges, saints, patriots, and martyrs among those who have "tortured, killed, and robbed" in the name of their sacred causes. Finally, Lydston insists that the degenerate "has ever been and is hydra-headed, and whatever name he has been known by,—and this has varied with his environment,—his true patronymic is Fanatic" (*Disease* 230). Lydston makes scienctific what had remained metaphoric in contemporaneous fiction: his hydraheaded monster is Henry Fleming's Civil War regiment; Dunbar's fanatics are men of all rank who hide a barbaric nature.

One of Bierce's most shocking tales of the Civil War, "Chickamauga," powerfully dramatizes these eugenical theories, as he presents moral degeneracy and its consequent physical carnage as the biological inheritance of white, Civil War manhood.[65] Bierce charts the misadventures of a six-year-old boy as he stumbles through a Civil War battle. He begins by seemingly celebrating the nameless boy's valiant pedigree, writing mock-heroically of his small excursions away from home into the forest. "This child's spirit, in bodies of its ancestry, had for thousands of years been trained to memorable feats of discovery and conquest," Bierce burlesques ("Chickamauga" 53). However, we discover that this "son of an heroic race" is not strong and indomitable, but dismorphic—a deaf-mute. Bierce reveals that centuries of "war and dominion"—the "heritage" which sprang from the "cradle of [his] race"—had not produced a highly developed individual, but a progeny who sustained not only the degeneration of his physical senses, but also of his empathetic response to others ("Chickamauga" 53). His hearing and speech impairments desensitize the boy so that he is oblivious to the suffering men who swarm around him. Thus he sees the prostrate, bleeding figures only as a "merry spectacle" reminiscent of the clowns who had amused him during a visit to the circus ("Chickamauga" 56). The men are solely instruments of his own pleasure, and so he mounts the back of one of the "crawling figures" just as he had "ridden" his "father's negroes." Even though he is only six years old, this boy is not an innocent, as so many nineteenth-century fictional children; Bierce depicts him as puckish, malevolent, almost inhuman as he "dance[s] with glee" among the wavering flames which have left "desolation everywhere" ("Chickamauga" 58). As Bierce concludes, "once kindled," the "warrior-fire is never extinguished," residing within even the youngest members of dysgenic races ("Chickamauga" 53). Thus, like his turn-of-the-century colleagues, Bierce too insists that the Civil War was not a genetic aberration.

The clear association of the Civil War and neurasthenia in Crane and Dunbar's historical fictions does not let postbellum America ignore the unpleasant ramifications of its ugly, costly regional conflict, either. According to Talbot's 1898 degeneracy textbook, hysteria is one of a variety of diseases—ranging from headaches to insanity—inherited through the "nervous system."[66] Scientists such as Mitchell had not been able to eradicate the disease, because it was firmly coded in white Americans' genetic material. Talbot writes, "A predisposition to certain diseases, seated in parts contiguous to the seat of insanity, often descends from parents to their children." The neurasthenic is degenerative, for "through the influence of various exhausting agencies the spinal cord and the brain lose the gains of evolution and the neurasthenic is no longer adjusted to the environment" (*Degeneracy* 39). Like Mitchell, Talbot vainly attempts to delineate the physical "stigmata"—visible signs of inferiority ranging from physical deformities to phrenological characteristics—which "may indicate how deep such degeneracy has penetrated" (*Degeneracy* 33).

With the advent of yet another bloody conflict, World War I, war and degeneracy finally and completely converged in the scientific literature. Two of the most prominent eugenicists of the early twentieth century, David Starr Jordan and Havelock Ellis, addressed the potentially degenerate effects of the new, modern war.[67] Both recur to identical romantic imagery when lamenting how the "flower of a nation's manhood" is being cut down by the "disastrous scythe of war" (*War* 9). And both trace this phrase back to an American forefather, Benjamin Franklin, who eugenicists invoke as the first to notice the "relation of war to the breed" (*War* 37). Jordan's text is punctuated by full-page photographs and short biographies of young, blonde, dead soldiers, most of whom, he writes, "died without issue." Clearly, the loss of the best and brightest of Europe's young manhood was cause for concern.

Yet neither explains why the most fit stock—Anglo-Saxons—are compelled to kill each other in such an atrocious manner. Like the Civil War, World War I is framed as an internecine war in these texts, for it pits one courageous white nation against another. Jordan explains that the soldiers on both sides of this conflict constitute a "brotherhood of men" united in "unquestioning devotion for homes and fatherland, for language, institutions, traditions, for all that they hold most sacred and most dear" (*War* 57). Ellis, too, contends that two "tribes" can come into a competition "which is acute to the point of warfare because of being the same" and, hence, "the conditions of life which they both demand are identical" (*Essays* 19). As such, both theorists seem reluctant to label the outcome of the war racial degeneracy. Rather, Jordan argues that World War I enacts the "reversal of selection," that is, "the process by which those organisms best fitted to survive under normal conditions are destroyed, while less well endowed types are thus left to reproduce the species." War is one of the "artificial" states under which such unnatural selection occurs (*War* 19). The weakening of the gene pool, which they both acknowledge must be the outcome of this war, is not due to any fault on the part of the warring nations. It is not the senseless "loss of the best strains of blood" that causes the "decrepitude in a nation," but their "replacement by recruiting from immigrants of the weaker races" (*War* 100). The internecine wars of white men were resolutely rehabilitated into the twentieth century.

The turn-of-the-century work of these disparate authors confirms, as Dunbar 'writes, that "the war was ended, but there were gaping wounds to bind up and deep sores that needed careful nursing" (*Fanatics* 194). Many African Americans faced pressing, life-and-death crises to ensure individual and community survival. Meanwhile, comfortable, Gilded Sge white Americans searched in vain for the cure to their internal conflicts. After being ordered to Europe for his health, Mitchell's Major Morton asks his wife," And I am to be carried about the world in search of health, Helen! . . . And where the mischief am I to go?"[68] (*In War Time* 180). Mitchell concedes that postbellum Americans were still chasing a figment, an intangible thing called health that would never be attained.

Chapter 6

Nursing Bodies: Civil War Women and Postbellum Regeneration

O women of America! into your hands God has pressed one of the sublimest opportunities that ever came into the hands of the women of any race or people. It is yours to create a healthy public sentiment; to demand justice, simple justice, as the right of every race.

—Frances Ellen Watkins Harper, "Women's Political Future"

And what, then, of the women? Were they infected with the sickness of battle? On the contrary, many turn-of-the-century women writers reclaimed Civil War nursing as a position of power and authority, one that superseded that of the patients they had tended. Although veterans' memories of war service were clouded by illness, by the turn of the century women nurses' vision of the Civil War was clear. Indeed, they laid a strong claim to historical authenticity via the unique healing abilities that were associated with their war service. In Frances Ellen Watkins Harper's address during the 1893 World's Fair, cited at the beginning of the chapter, she claims that women are the divine instruments of God's desire to create a "healthy public sentiment." God has literally "pressed" that responsibility onto women's bodies, specifically their capable hands. They are nearly divine means of rehabilitation. Harper and her contemporaries needed to exploit the trope of nursing in order to respond to contemporaneous theories of women's biological and racial disease solidifying after the war. The multifarious character of nursing activities during the Civil War—the counseling, secretarial work, cleaning, cooking, laundering, and, most important, the mothering performed—was detached from the war by medical theorists and eugenical scientists and recast as a sign of female irresolution and illness. White women were accused of maternal culpability—that is, their scattered attentions and compromised reproductive organs were responsible for the waning of the race. African American women were even more unfit, their bodies supposedly insensible and oversexed; miscegenation would tragically pollute the white race.

White nurses and memoirists Mary Livermore and Mary Gardner Holland, African American author Harper, and African American nurse and memoirist Susie King Taylor rehabilitate the maternal body through the trope of nursing, making women's corporeality a force of regeneration apart from their vexed reproductive capabilities. Countering the logic of hysteria, which focused attention on women's wombs, the word *nursing* implicitly moved the public gaze to women's productive breasts and capable hands. Of course none of the Civil War nurses depicted here are described literally as breast-feeding. However, the trope of Civil War nursing demonstrates that women's bodies produced metaphoric nutrients that infused the sick bodies of men and the body of the nation *without* diminishing their own corporeality. This interpretation of nursing resisted postbellum theories of bodily energy, which posited that bodies had limited resources: if a woman expended energy in one part of the corporeal economy (say, engaging in intellectual work) other body parts (e.g., the reproductive organs) would suffer. The Civil War did not induce corporeal lessening for nursing bodies; on the contrary, it fostered expansion. Only such multiple, aberrant, even mythical bodies were able to effect corporeal and cultural rehabilitation. Thus these women writers created restorative narratives, crafting a "healthy public sentiment" through the merging of images of prolific women with those of vanishing men. In their fluidity, nursing bodies both epitomized and transcended new corporeal and temporal norms, providing historical links between the antebellum era, the Civil War era, and the turn of the century.[1] Although turn-of-the-century Civil War texts teach that nursing bodies may not always be able to heal others' afflictions, they do enumerate women's generative properties.

War-Era Nursing

War-era writers initially detected the latent powers of women's bodies and the way that new Civil War work could unleash them. On September 6, 1862, *Harper's Weekly* printed a two-page illustration entitled "The Influence of Women," claiming to depict the roles publicly assigned Northern women during the Civil War period (Fig. 5).[2] The accompanying text describes "The Sister of Charity" tending to the spiritual needs of a dying soldier and the "lady-nurse" transcribing "home tidings" for a wounded man. Above these plain, middle-aged women float a group of young ladies darning socks. Their faces remain demurely downcast as their "fairy fingers fly along the work." They are all white women, perhaps members of the middle class who volunteered for the clean, labor-

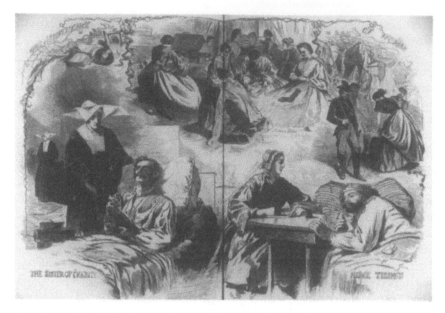

Figure 5. "The Influence of Women." *Harper's Weekly*, September 6, 1862.
Courtesy of the Rare Book and Special Collections Library, University of Illinois
at Urbana-Champaign.

free war work depicted in the illustration. And the tasks that they perform neatly fit within the cult of domesticity that women's historians
have used to characterize the mid-nineteenth century. As they sweat-
lessly labor for the Union cause, they are associated with home, piety,
and nurturance.

Whereas these first three images persisted into turn-of-the-century
Civil War iconography, a fourth image, tucked into the dark, upper-
right-hand corner of "The Influence of Women," suggests concurrent
dimensions of women's war work that remained largely obscured. Issues
of marital status, race, and class complicate the way women's actual war
labor related to this domestic ideology, the army patriarchy represented
by the threatening soldiers in this picture, and the corporeal complexities of the war era.[3] Here we have "honest Biddy" scrubbing clothes for
soldiers who stand near her while overseeing her work, their phallic
swords casually yet ominously drawn. The laboring Biddy's back is
toward the reader; consequently her race and age are obscured. However, the disembodied, dark face of a woman wearing a kerchief (apparently, an African American woman) peers behind Biddy's bent back
through the whitened laundry. The literal darkness and spatial marginality of this drawing represents its virtual invisibility in subsequent tell-

ings of the Civil War. These carefully framed and artfully composed drawings isolated and circumscribed the multiplicity of women's Civil War work and scripted their bodies in singular and limited roles. Indeed, the demanding physical and psychic work of Civil War nursing, the diversity of the women who performed that work, and the threat their prolific bodies were perceived as posing to the martial project are only hinted at in this illustration.

Despite this and similar efforts to differentiate white from African American women, the middle classes from the laboring classes, and middle-aged spinsters from young virgins, contemporaneous writers also anxiously reported the confusion of seemingly neat and delimited women's work. Though political dogma and battle updates took up most of the space in the publications of the day, many editorialized on the disturbing challenges faced by women—which, even more disturbingly, they seemed to be rising to admirably. A short article that appeared in *Frank Leslie's Illustrated Paper*, for example, undid the visual rhetoric of *Harper's Weekly*.[4] This short piece, simply entitled "Woman," laments the necessity of women's participation in the war and decries the disappearance of unambiguous boundaries of behavior. Clearly confused, the anonymous author (who I will take the liberty of assuming is a man) comments on the "women's rights" movement in the midst of war, complaining, "what they are to be 'emancipated from' does not clearly appear from anything that has yet been written, nor do we perceive precisely what rights they are denied, except those of driving omnibusses, attending primary elections and fighting battles. The truth is, woman has her own sphere." But the current state of affairs seems to unsettle the author most:

The misfortune of women is that of late they are expected to be both men and women at once. In the most earnest and distracting terms they are exhorted to make themselves cooks, artists, architects, doctors of every degree, carpenters, painters, glaziers, apothecaries, chemists, printers—every conceivable variety of human specialty; they are enjoined to be fascinating, to be graceful, to be feminine, to be self-asserting, self-denying, obedient, independent, emancipated— correct in all their accounts, moral and arithmetical—everything at once.

The boundless variety of skills, professions, and qualities flows out of the author's pen in an increasingly frenzied catalogue, ending despairingly in the summary that women are doing "everything at once." The writer evokes the image of many women all with multiple hands and many mouths multitasking before his very eyes. Woman's intellectual and physical productivity leaves the author dumbfounded. Rather than acknowledge that he is befuddled by their new multiformity, the author claims that omnipresent women create a "clamor" of "dull nonsense," which requires some "interpret[ation]." In doing "everything at once,"

Civil War women were not adhering to familiar chronology. The Civil War enacts a temporal compression here, as activities that should be accomplished one by one are performed simultaneously.

Women writing during the Civil War sought to exploit what Elizabeth Young would call this "topsy-turviness." Young is just one of the many critics, including Mary Capello and Jane E. Schultz, who have tackled the wartime multiplicity of Louisa May Alcott's *Hospital Sketches* (1863), a thinly veiled autobiographical account of her three-month nursing stint in a Washington hospital during the Civil War.[5] I argue, like the *Frank Leslie*'s correspondent, that the war did more than invert and mutate traditional gender roles—it momentarily multiplied women's vocational possibilities and revealed the capabilities of their fluid bodies. Alcott's war-era text demonstrates the rehabilitative power of Civil War nurses; however, she also dramatizes how their competencies strained the capabilities of narrative and ultimately waned in the immediate postwar period as women were removed from Civil War hospitals.

Female Civil War nurses were the first women to invade the previously male-dominated field of public health care. As Nina Bennett Smith suggests, through Civil War nursing "nineteenth-century women who would have been uncomfortable with radical feminism found their own justification for female participation in a male world."[6] The permeable parameters of that work have resulted in what Schultz calls the "institutional invisibility" of the estimated twenty thousand women who served in Civil War hospitals.[7] The role of the female Civil War nurse cannot be imagined in modern terms. Nurses had no clearly defined duties, little training, and no professional status. Not only were they required to clean wounds, administer medications, and assist in surgeries, they often cooked and served meals, laundered linens, and cleaned the hospital quarters. They also worked tirelessly as secretaries, transcribing letters for the soldiers; more generally, they soothed the wounded and dying. For all practical purposes Civil War nurses had no military rank; consequently, their place in the hospital chain of command remained ambiguous. African American women who nursed were not even granted the dubious title of "nurse," listed instead as "laundresses" in regimental records. The hospital zone became the site of constant negotiations between the women whose healing powers, many declared, could not be denied and the army patriarchy who wished to maintain that power as their own. Thus the amorphous professional status of nurses during the era both accommodated and hindered the newly realized multiplicity of women's bodies.

In *Hospital Sketches*, Alcott characterizes Civil War nursing by the power of the maternal role and the debilitation of her boys. Such transformations were possible only within the confines of the Civil War hospital.

For example, on the train ride to Washington, D.C., Alcott's alter-ego, Tribulation Periwinkle, notes how the neat, idyllic-looking homes she rides past "look like tidy jails" (Alcott 16). [8] And she observes that the ladies' shoes peeping beneath their sleeping compartments on the train "assert themselves as if their owners had committed suicide in body" (Alcott 14). Victorian women's imprisonment within the domestic realm and the social institutionalization of femininity the home literalizes constitutes gender suicide for her: traditional domestic roles dismembered women. However, nursing work allowed women to test their powers as they symbolically healed themselves through recuperating the fragmentary natures of their patients. Alcott claims that the nurses' healing work begins "when the poor soul comes to himself, sick, faint, wandering; full of strange pains and confused visions, of disagreeable sensations and sights." They must work not only to relieve physical pains, but also to restore "courage and self-control," to put the body and the soul of the broken soldier back together again (Alcott 69). [9]

Civil War nursing reinforced women's bodies by exploiting the popular belief in the magnetic power of mothers and extending that rejuvenation to women who chose to forego biological motherhood, such as Alcott and her fictional Trib. A woman's mere presence in the hospital was able to transform the uncomfortable, impersonal structure: "The matron's motherly face brought more comfort to many a poor soul than the cordial draughts . . . making of the hospital a home," Alcott testifies (Alcott 22). Thus nursing bodies are supplementary, emanating an indefinable essence that travels beyond the corporeal and imbues the environment with new meaning. Alcott briefly and vaguely alludes to the material inadequacy of Hurly Burly, writing of the "disorder, discomfort and bad management" of the hospital (Alcott 51). In reality, Union Hospital in Georgetown (Hurly Burly) was a dilapidated, converted train station cut into many small rooms with a few tiny windows. It was unventilated and improperly heated, and had no bathing facilities. Thus the hospital world created in texts such as Alcott's is a crucial aesthetic recuperation of the unsettling reality of war, a healing made possible through the presence of women's bodies.

Though Trib is often self-deprecating, she too has this power. Her favorite patient, John, longs for her attention, for she notes that he follows her about with his eyes and "now and then, as I stood tidying the table by his bed, I felt him softly touch my gown, as if to assure himself that I was there" (Alcott 41). John desires healing contact with a body that has magnetic qualities; yet his fear that Trib will disappear before his very eyes acknowledges that nursing bodies are only partly in one place, for they are everywhere at once. As she writes of her life in the hospital, "It was a strange life—asleep half the day, exploring Washington the other half, and all night hovering . . . I like it" (Alcott 34). In "hovering," Trib can be seen both as lingering near her soldier's sides and as, herself, wavering in an uncertain state. Alcott repeatedly catalogues the nurses' duties in an effort to conjure the fullness of their work. In describing how she tends three patients at once, Trib says that "she vibrated between the three beds like an agitated pendulum" (Alcott 38). It's almost as if her body moves so quickly that it becomes unlocatable. And her sense that she moves like an agitated pendulum suggests how her body relates to time differently during the Civil War. Notice also that Trib refers to herself in the third person, suggesting her essential multiplicity: she is both in and out of the scene, at once enacting and transcribing the events. When she claims that she is "looking about me with all my eyes," Trib alludes to the expanded vision the war affords her (Alcott 58).

Many critics have noted the way that women such as Alcott, who lived in a society predicated upon strict, stratified gender roles—where men inhabited hospitals and "true women" simply didn't—became somehow perverse and unnatural "masculine" women in pursuing their public work.[10] Fictional Trib attributes forbidden desires to some "inborn perversity," claiming that she is "naturally irascible," "born under an evil star" (Alcott 13, 8, 50). I argue that the mules she watches from her window while convalescing from typhoid symbolize more than a vexed gender duality but, rather, nursing bodies' disturbing multiformity. Trib later comments that nurses and mules vie for the title of hardest war worker, thus emphasizing their likeness (Alcott 72). She delineates four types of mules: moral, historical, pathetic, and jovial. One labors mightily under the delusion "that the food of the entire army depended upon his private exertions," whereas a more rebellious mule is "prone to startling humanity by erratic leaps, and wild plunges [and] much shaking of his stubborn head" (Alcott 56). Another is the weakest and most oppressed, "struggling feebly along, head down . . . eye spiritless and sad," and a fourth is the "peacemaker, confidant and friend of all the others" (Alcott 57). Nurses are clearly the mules of the army hospital, stubborn and rebellious in their resolve to participate in the war; they are also the hardest working and most frequently exploited hospital inhabitants. And they provide the emotional cement that holds the institution together. The mule also represents the nurse's prodigious gender; it is an "odd little beast," a "coquettish" "he." As the offspring of a mare and a jackass, an ultimately sterile creature, the mule is a fitting emblem of the woman who rejects literal marriage and motherhood and attempts to fit into masculine realms. And yet, as we've seen, Trib also lays claim to the hyper-feminized maternal role when tending to her boys. Thus she is at once fiery soldier and soothing mother, indignant protofeminist and reliable pal. In invoking not human bodies but mule bodies to represent Trib as a wartime nurse, and, then, not just one mule but many mules, Alcott suggests her truly preternatural, yet fully carnal, nature. Indeed, as Capello argues, Trib is also "proximate" to the pigs she sees on the street. In her characterization of Trib, Alcott cobbles together a protean identity that extracts its power from a variety of quarters.

Ironically, it was just such women, and only such women, whom the army allowed to nurse injured soldiers. Proscriptive dress codes, and the behavioral assumptions they entailed, attempted to divest the women who served as nurses of the more insurgent registers of their corporeal power. The Dorothea Dix guide for nurses required that "the applicant must be over thirty, plain looking, dressed in brown or black . . . and no bows, no curls, no jewelry and no hoop skirts."[11] The nurse's uniform functioned in much the same way as the soldier's uniform: it encouraged one to see the nurse, not as a multiform individual but as a unit, a symbol. In standardizing the nurses' habiliments, the army attempted to militate a similarly sedate, decidedly unsexual, almost mournful behavior. The fact that Tribulation has been "knocking about the world for thirty years," and that she wears her "cavernous black bonnet and fuzzy brown coat" signifies that she conformed her outward appearance to her nursing service (Alcott 2, 47).[12] Female sexuality and the potential for reproduction was perceived as threatening the ordered rehabilitation of soldier's bodies. Alcott admits in her journal that she was subject to flirtation, for one of the doctors "comes often to our room with books [and] asks me to his, (where I do not go)."[13] One might also argue that fictional Trib is attracted to John, who she describes as having "a most attractive face . . . framed in brown hair and beard, comely features and full of vigor" (Alcott 39). In her journal Alcott writes that she goes to nurse because she "*must* let out [her] pent-up energy in some new way" (Alcott 140).[14] Although she never specifies this energy as sexual, it is clear that Alcott's and Trib's bodies are nearly bursting with untapped resources.

I argue that the fluctuating narrative voice of Nurse Periwinkle, which Elaine Showalter views as the flawed result of Alcott's "perennial difficulty in constructing a serious female narrative voice," is, rather, an artful reconstruction of the way Alcott attempted to represent the potency and simultaneity of her nursing body.[15] Her generic heterogeneity indicates Trib's unwieldy nature. The chronological nature of narrative makes Trib discontinuous, rather than simultaneous and multiform. Alcott attempts to more accurately represent her nursing self, first by distancing herself from Nurse Periwinkle in fictionalizing her war experiences. After Nurse Periwinkle enters the hospital, she removes the romantic "rose-colored glasses" that had initially tinctured Trib's views (Alcott 4). Her sickness evokes a new, feverish view of the world. Then at the end of the story, Alcott writes a poem that claims Trib's nursing career is dead, "a 'nuss' had died too soon" (Alcott 61). After proclaiming her death Trib writes one more chapter of *Hospital Sketches*. And when this text ends Nurse Periwinkle—a character that Alcott chose never to use again—disappears.

Emphasizing Trib's fractured characterization helps to make sense of Alcott's decision to remove the sanction of autobiography from her story despite her pleas that we believe "such a being as Nurse Periwinkle does exist . . . that these Sketches are not romance" (Alcott 12). The war was at once real and surreal, romantic and alienating, funny and horrifying, and so too is *Hospital Sketches*. Trib writes, "Curious contrasts of the tragic and comic met one everywhere; and some touching as well as ludicrous episodes" (Alcott 27). And so she can starkly describe the horrifying chest wound of a man who is shaking in his bed "with the irrepressible tremors of [his] tortured body," and sixteen pages later claim he looks a "heroic figure" in death, "lying there stately and still as the statue of some young knight asleep upon his tomb" (Alcott 29, 45). The romance and realism are broken up by macabre, humorous observations, such as the one made by a young amputee musing upon the "scramble for . . . arms and legs" on Judgment Day (Alcott 25). All, Alcott suggests, are necessary to convey the fullness of Civil War experience.

Although the recuperative power of her narrative may be at issue, the fate of Trib's once-powerful body is not by the end of the story. Rather than infusing her patients with her bodily strength, Trib is eventually impressed by the men's diseased bodies: refusing to draw her hand away from John in his death throes, she discovers "four white marks remained across its back, even when warmth and color had returned elsewhere" (Alcott 45). She sickens immediately, infected with the sickness of battle in the form of typhoid. As Young contends, Trib's delirious sufferings became her own wartime wound replicating those suffered by the soldiers she tends.[16] Alcott herself contracted typhoid and was never well again, primarily because of the debilitating effects of mercury poisoning from the calomel treatment taken as a cure.

Productive Mothers

In gaining, as Young phrases it, a "wound of one's own"—that is, in claiming a soldier's battle injury rather than a woman's inherent disease—Alcott laid claim to a place in the postbellum nation. However, as we've seen, that privilege was dangerously conflated with battle-sickness when viewed through the gauntlet of the Civil War. Turn-of-the-century women writers configured the relationship between disease, gender, and the Civil War quite differently from their war-era precursors. In the ensuing years, theories of maternal culpability and racial degeneracy had coalesced, vitiating the power of nursing bodies, black and white. At the same time, as we've seen, consensual histories of the period rehabilitated the white soldiers' bodies. In response, women writers returned to the Civil War to reclaim the generative power of Civil War nursing. Writing in 1902, but reflecting on the patriotic fervor that swept the nation upon the commencement of hostilities, Livermore distinguished men's wartime sickness from women's stoutheartedness: "It is easy to understand how men catch the contagion of war, but for women to send forth their husbands, sons, brothers, and lovers to the fearful chances of the battle-field . . . involves another kind of heroism."[17] Whereas men were thoughtlessly infected by war fever, women's service was of "another kind"—a heroic choice that made them larger than life.

Holland's *Our Army Nurses: Interesting Sketches, Addresses, and Photographs of Nearly One Hundred of the Noble Women Who Served in Hospitals and on Battlefields during Our Civil War* (1895) and Livermore's *My Story of the War: A Woman's Narrative of Four Years Personal Experience as Nurse in the Union Army, and in Relief Work at Home, in Hospitals, Camps, and at the Front, during the War of the Rebellion* (1887) are two of the many memoirs of women's participation in the Civil War to appear as the nineteenth century drew to a close. Both texts proved quite popular; Livermore's sold between sixty and one hundred thousand copies according to her most recent editor, Nina Silber.[18] Livermore was one of the most well-known women of her time, speaking and canvassing tirelessly on behalf of the Union soldiers, and later in support of suffrage and temperance. Holland's call for reminiscences by Civil War nurses yielded far more responses than the ninety-two sketches she was able to include in her lengthy tribute to their service. Although both women were surely concerned, as Reverend A. Horton writes in the preface to Holland's text, with demonstrating that Civil War women were "ministers of light and love, passing and repassing over the dark scenes of these stormy years," their messages become much more complicated when read within the context of contemporaneous eugenical theories.[19]

Like the eugenicists and the consensual historians of their day, Holland and Livermore seem reluctant to include white war-era violence in their narratives. When references to battle do appear, Northern soldiers are figured as completely at the mercy of Southern aggressors. Holland tells us that Northern troops "bare their defenseless bodies to the shot and shell of our Southern brothers, whose big guns sweep furrows through our ranks" (*Army Nurses* 16). Because the Northern soldiers are not shown to be barbaric or aggressive, and because they are unable to

defend themselves, their subsequent wounds and illnesses are acceptable and even heroic. The Northern arsenal is erased and the Union
soldiers are vulnerable flesh at the mercy of "big guns." Livermore, too,
explains, "One can comprehend how, fired with enthusiasm, and
inspired by martial music, [Union soldiers] march to the cannon's
mouth, where the iron hail rains the heaviest, and the ranks are mowed
down like grain in harvest" (*My Story* 110). Livermore subtly acknowledges the aggression manifested by Northerners, though it is presented
as a coerced aggression. Finally, she naturalizes the soldiers as agricultural crops, the fruits of a fertile culture, powerless to the unnatural
"iron rain" that does not nourish but rather devastates the "grain."
Even actual Southern troops are removed from these scenes, replaced
by the weapons they presumably wield. War is made an admittedly
unsuccessful agricultural project, plowing furrows through and raining
hail upon a doomed harvest of men.

Although Holland's and Livermore's memoirs soft-pedal or skip over
battle scenes, they are dominated by the doings of Civil War hospitals—
even Livermore, who was not a full-time nurse but a United States Sanitary Commission (USSC) administrator, imbues her memoir with her
hospital doings and with male disease. Of course, Holland and Livermore's emphasis on diseased men might seem unavoidable, as tending
to the products of battles—providing supplies and aid to the suffering—
was the business of these women. Still, the vast majority of the men
depicted in these weighty tomes are weak-willed, delirious, puerile individuals in various states of ill health. The war produced an endless
stream of such men.

"Mother" Mary Ann Bickerdyke serves a pivotal role in these late-
century narratives of commanding women and infantile men. A noncommissioned nurse who aided several regiments during the war (she
was the only woman to accompany Sherman on his march to the sea)
Bickerdyke warrants substantial treatment in Holland's and Livermore's
texts: hers in the most extended sketch in Holland's compilation, and
she garners four long chapters in Livermore's autobiography. Several
shorter books are also devoted exclusively to her wartime heroics.[20] Bickerdyke emerges as a mythical figure in these works, possessing superhuman strength and endless ingenuity. Several stock tales constitute the
lore of Mother Bickerdyke. Many are conventional stories of the succor
she offered desperate soldiers and the innovations she developed to
obtain supplies for the troops. In one story she adds an emetic to her
stewed peaches in order to catch a pilferer; in another, she uses a frilly
nightgown to dress indigent soldiers. Perhaps mimicking the biblical
story of fishes and loaves, Holland's and Livermore's Bickerdyke is able
to multiply food, clothing, and other necessities.

However, the most apocryphal tale is of how Bickerdyke went out into the dark, stormy night following the battle for Fort Donelson to search for survivors who had been left for dead on the killing fields. As Holland tells it, her readers should admire "Mrs. Bickerdyke, who, with her lantern, was examining the bodies to make sure that no living man should be left alone amid such surroundings. She did not seem to realize that she was doing anything remarkable" and subsequently "walked over many blood-stained fields to save many a life fast ebbing away for want of immediate aid" (*Army Nurses* 521, 524). This image of her wending her way in the dark night through rows of the dead and mutilated is unique, primarily because it emphasizes Bickerdyke's ability to resist succumbing to nervousness. Holland explains that Bickerdyke would "tread the path of duty, outwardly unmoved by environments that must have unnerved less-determined persons" (*Army Nurses* 520). She is most remarkable for her calm, dispassionate manner, which serves as a stark contrast to the hysteria that had produced the slaughter she must tend.

Bickerdyke serves as an example to women such as Livermore, who initially shrink at the sight of hospital misery. Significantly, however, these women do not attribute their short-lived squeamishness to their own nature, but rather to the unnatural character of the carnage they are forced to witness. Livermore claims that it is "the manifold shocking sights that are the outcome of the wicked business men call war" to which she must become habituated and not the failings of her supposedly weak body. Livermore's and Holland's texts were particularly important given the way that S. Weir Mitchell had soon hidden his nerve injured soldiers behind the bodies of female hysterics. Although *In War Time* (1884) had exposed the sickness of battle, it was immediately superseded by his second novel of the Civil War, *Roland Blake* (1885), which features female neurasthenia.[21] Mitchell's eponymous, wooden war hero, Roland Blake, does not suffer from battle-sickness. Rather, Southern sympathizer Octopia Darnell is a textbook neurasthenic whose illness dangerously contaminates her innocent, young cousin Olivia Wynne. Octopia's name links her to the multilimbed octopus; however, rather than invoking the amazing amount of work so many arms and hands could accomplish, Mitchell associates Octopia's corporeal profligacy with her debilitating, tentacular grasp of all those who come in her path. Not only does Mitchell rewrite the nature of Civil War disease, but he also denies the regenerative power of female nurses. Caring for the "nervous, sickly," and cloying Octopia placed "too constant demands upon the brain, the body and the emotions" of Olivia, bringing about "gradual but certain degenerative changes" (*Roland* 57). Mitchell prescribes marriage as the happy fictional remedy that saves Olivia from the "malaria of the sick-bed" (*Roland* 57). It is not surprising that Mitchell argued here that female nurses were "an unfit and quite uneducated class" ill suited to medical work. In his 1894 speech to the American Medico-Psychological Association, he appealed to his male colleagues, "I wish to emphasize the fact that the nurse is by far the most important part of my organization. How can you hope for the best help from the class we usually see in your wards?"[22]

Mitchell's fictional shift reflected the emphatic re-engendering of nervous diseases that took place in the medical literature of the post-bellum period. His influential *Fat and Blood* (1877) similarly replaced enervated soldiers with "women of the class well-known to every physician—nervous women, who as a rule are thin, and lack blood."[23] Such women were incapacitated, "unable to attend to the duties of life and sources alike of discomfort to themselves and anxiety to others" (*Fat and Blood* 7). "Some local uterine trouble" always starts the "mischief," Mitchell tells us, insinuating that women's unstable bodies generated the disease. Since the disease emanated from women's wombs, they were all susceptible to sickness and vagary, and thus should be prohibited from participation in public life. Already in 1866 Susan B. Anthony was described in the *New York World* as "lean, cadaverous, and intellectual, with the proportion of a file and the voice of a hurdy gurdy."[24] Later readers would have recognized her as one of Mitchell's anemic, high-strung neurasthenics. Women such as Anthony—indeed, all women—needed to be "secluded" according to Mitchell, for any who sympathized with the self-deluded hysterics were merely "willing slaves to their caprices" (*Fat and Blood* 34). And because women's bodies were inherently unstable, they were eminently unsuited for nursing, which required dispassion, strength, and endurance. Sick women were human "vampires" who would suck dry the already susceptible bodies of female nurses. Female neurasthenia was highly contagious and nigh epidemic, Mitchell suggested.

During the latter half of the nineteenth century and into the twentieth century, Mitchell and his colleagues diligently prescribed the rest cure for their recalcitrant, hysterical female patients. At the heart of this therapy was enforced infantilazation, typified by bed rest and milk-rich diets. Turn-of-the-century women's narratives of the Civil War turn the tables, revealing white men as the rest cure's initial recipients, who required—even demanded—this therapy. When under duress, the patients become weepy and fickle; thus it is dealing with their patients' rages and puling demands that make women nervous—if they are affected at all. Though Livermore and Holland pay lip service to the heroic suffering of the men, their books are packed with detailed stories of childishness. For example, Livermore tells the story of one "forty-five-year-old 'boy' to whose uncertain appetite [she] was catering." He craves milk, and she procures permission from the doctor to give him some. As he tasted the milk, she tells us, "a sickly smile distorted his thin ghastly face, which was succeeded by a fit of weeping, his tears literally mingling with his drink. 'Is it good?' I asked. 'Oh,—*proper*—good!—jest—like—what—my—wife—makes!' with the drawl of long sickness and great weakness" (*My Story* 323). In this way she symbolically nurses the man, comforting him with milk and sympathy. When she asks another man what he would like to eat, he too bursts into tears. Though a "married man, as old as myself," Livermore says, "in his miserable weakness and discouragement, a mere puling, weeping baby" who finds it "an effort . . . to think or decide" what to have for breakfast (*My Story* 322). It is not only the combative fever of war that is infectious in Livermore's stories but also the indecision and tears that follow. Upon a kind word from her, a soldier breaks down; she tells us "weeping is contagious, and in a few moments one half of the men in the hospital were sobbing convulsively. I was afraid it would kill them." She finally calms them by giving them some milky tea and crackers (*My Story* 302). Yet another Major "burys [*sic*] his face in the pillow, and abandon[s] himself to hysterical weeping." "'I want milk too.' he sobbed bitterly," "after much soothing and coaxing" from Livermore (*My Story* 618–19).

Perhaps Livermore's most striking portrait is that of a mortally injured man who is terrified to die because, he says, "'I ain't fit to die. I have lived an awful life and I'm afraid to die. I shall go to hell'" (*My Story* 192). She is horrified by the man's passionate resistance. She tells us that he repeats, "'I can't! I can't! I *can't!*' And he almost shrieked in his mental distress, and trembled so violently as to shake his bed." This description contrasts sharply with Alcott's depiction of the saintly death of her beloved John. Livermore does not pause to consider the source of the man's distress; certainly, her narrative is committed to repressing the barbarity that, perhaps, motivates his contrition and fear. She concentrates instead on supplying the moral strength to help him die with dignity. Livermore drew close, placed her hands on his shoulders, and "spoke in commanding tones, as to an excited child: 'Stop screaming. Be quiet. This excitement is hastening your life. If you *must* die, die like a man, and not like a coward. Be still, and listen to me'" (*My Story* 192). Her laying on of hands and maternal commands have a calming effect on the man, helping him to accept his fate. Although Livermore eventually undercuts her story, explaining that most men faced death bravely, it is significant that she presents this story in such vivid detail. The man's battlefield experience clearly distorted his moral faculties.

The end result of these extended battles and inhumanity is a visible degeneration. Livermore reprints the remarkable letter of one nurse describing the men returning from Andersonville, a notorious Confederate prison:

> The appearance of these poor creatures is very peculiar. Their hair looks dead, sunburned, and faded. Their skins, from long exposure and contact with the pitch-pine smoke of their camp-fires, and a long dearth of soap and water, are like those of the American Indian. Their emaciated forms, with bones protruding through the skin in many instances, and the idiotic expression of their protruding eyes, tell of unparalleled cruelty and savage barbarity. (*My Story* 688)

The anonymous nurse draws on a multitude of well-known eugenical stereotypes to explain the complete deterioration of the soldiers. Their lifeless, faded hair resonates with characteristics attributed to the dysgenic families who were fast becoming the focus of anthropological study, according to Nicole Rafter.[25] The nurse's recourse to stereotypes of American Indians would have been unambiguous to her reading audience at this time: like the majority of Native American tribes who had by the 1890s been "relocated" to reservations, the once warriorlike soldiers have been reduced to an ignoble, primitive incivility. The horrors that they have seen have retarded their intellects. In referring to their "idiotic expression[s]," the nurse implies that the men have regressed to childhood, for the now obsolete term *idiot* was used to identify adults who had the mental capacities of toddlers. Finally, Livermore delineates the fates available to Civil War survivors after observing some "conquering heroes" returning from one particularly rough campaign: "The weary, famished, shivering, footsore conquerors painfully made their way back. Many sank on the march, and left their bones to bleach on the mountains. Others were so spent with fatigue that they reached Chattanooga only to die. Some live, testimonies to the hardships of that winter, utterly broken in constitution, and doomed to invalidism for the remainder of a reluctant life" (*My Story* 527). Death in the wilderness, death in the camps, or a living death at home are the results of war. Civil War history will be written in degenerate bodies, as the weakened forms of those who survive are the only "testimonies" to unspeakable acts. Thus history is imperiled without the women's rehabilitative powers, which both sustain the men's bodies and write their own stories. Though the women writers largely suppress the violence that had caused such suffering, white masculinity is still utterly compromised. Rather than the burning flame of battle-sickness, they depict the aftermath: either early death or lingering neurasthenia.

The consistent references to Bickerdyke and other famous Civil War nurses have troubling implications within the context of such dysgenic observations. Many scholars of Civil War women have already noted, as Schultz puts it, that "white women of all ages became 'Mother' to 'boys' of all ages" during the war. Ann Douglas Wood interprets this rhetorical move forcefully, arguing that "the myth of the bedside Madonna, still resplendent with her healing maternal power . . . pitted its potency against a masculine authority."[26] However, as stories about Mother Bickerdyke illustrate, turn-of-the-century writers did not believe that she demonstrated "true womanhood" during the war. Holland includes a scene that juxtaposes an ineffective, sentimental motherhood against Bickerdyke's muscular brand of parenting. In thanking Bickerdyke for saving her son's life, one mother praises:

"It is no wonder that you are called 'Mother' here, for you treat all these men with such kindness and patience. I owe to you the preservation of my darling's life. Oh, it would have broken my heart had I found him dead!" With that thought she burst into a passion of sobs, and buried her face in the pillow. [Her son] smoothed her silver hair with one hand (he had lost the other), and tried to comfort her. (*Army Nurses* 525)

Here even the soldier's biological mother acknowledges the superiority of Mother Bickerdyke's dispassionate mothering. Although Bickerdyke is able to attend to the soldier's needs, the "real" mother resorts to the tears that were traditionally employed to influence audiences in midcentury, sentimental narratives. However, her weeping makes her a hindrance rather than a help; the soldier's mother requires comfort from the one she is supposed to attend. Mother Bickerdyke ends up mothering her as well.

Bickerdyke's mothering is redeemed precisely because she is *not* the biological mother of these boys; her regenerative powers are cleanly separated from her reproductive capabilities through her nursing work. As Dale Bauer has observed in her study of Edith Wharton's engagement with eugenical theories, "maternal culpability" became the dominant cry of degeneracy debates as early as the 1880s. By this logic, "bad mothers," distinguished by both hereditary and behavioral degeneracy, were largely responsible for the "dysgenic decline" of modern America.[27] American women—in this case, particularly those who actively nurtured and encouraged the men during the war—were vitally aware of the imputations that could be leveled against them when Civil War barbarity and theories of heredity collided: if white men were degenerate, it was due in large part to the genetic inheritance passed through their mothers' wombs, according to the science of the times. Nurses had seen the war's savagery first-hand, tending to the mutilated bodies and enfeebled minds produced by the warfare; concurrently, they were fully aware of the wartime fervor that they themselves had cultivated. Documents such as Gail Hamilton's "Call to My Country-Women" had urged women to fill their men with "sacred fury" to stoke their male progeny's fiery passions.[28]

Because they are not the biological mothers of the boys they tend, Mother Bickerdyke and her counterparts cannot be held genetically responsible for the degeneracy of their boys. They are, then, exculpated of the soldiers' wartime crimes, and Civil War women are figured rather as instruments of recovery. As Livermore writes, "The transition of the country from peace to the tumult and waste of war, was appalling and swift—but the regeneration of its women kept pace with it. They lopped off superfluities, retrenched in expenditures, became deaf to the calls of pleasure, and heeded not the mandates of fashion" (*My Story* 110). Their frugal, tempered behavior is the opposite of the excessiveness of the men. In keeping with nineteenth-century theories of both monetary and physical economics, self-control was framed in terms of restrained consumerism. Thus women refilled the cultural coffers that had been depleted by wartime disease. Indeed, they are able to create new energy and life from a dearth of material (the "lopp[ing] off" of "superfluities" rather than limbs). Livermore phrases women's regenerative energies another way when she claims that they "strengthened the sinews of the nation with their unflagging enthusiasm, and bridged over the chasm between civil and military life" (*My Story* 9). Here they shore up the deteriorating national body with their tireless service. Livermore's reference to the "chasm" attending war echoes the volcanic imagery so many other war writers found compelling. In this way, nursing bodies helped cover over the cultural rifts and temporal discontinuities the war left in its wake.

Admittedly, this reading of women's Civil War nursing reinforces those eugenical theories that lay on women's doorsteps the responsibility for the quality of the race. However, it is important to note that their celebrated female productivity is unmoored from its hereditary and physiological consequences through the trope of the Civil War. Being a Civil War "Mother" does not emphasize white American women's angelic characters. Instead, they are forced to assume maternal roles when dealing with the childishness of their patients. As Livermore caustically comments, "I rarely rendered any service to these poor fellows that they did not assure me that I was like their mother, or wife, or sister" (*My Story* 355). One young man insists on making Livermore into his biological mother. "You have just her eyes, and her hair, and her way of talking and doing," he tells Livermore in his "lucid" moments (*My Story* 355). Consequently, these texts expose the gendered, cultural scripts that sought to keep women in service to their families and communities by assuring each individual mother of her unique significance.

Civil War women discovered that they were apparently interchangeable to men, merely instruments of the patients' recoveries.

Mother Bickerdyke is described again and again, not as being physically fecund, but as having a "fertility of resources": she is "unique in method, extraordinary in executive ability, enthusiastic in devotion, and indomitable in will" (*My Story* 479, 466). It is not her reproductive capabilities that empower her efforts but her prolific intellectual capacity that marks her mothering. These potent characterizations of Mother Bickerdyke might more properly be contextualized within the New Thought movements of the era that "sought to harness 'mother power' as a radical force."[29] Livermore tells us that Bickerdyke never backed down to medical superiors but scolded, threatened, and intimidated them. In one contest Bickerdyke tells a head surgeon, "'And, doctor, I guess you hadn't better get into a row with me, for whenever anybody does one of us two always goes to the wall, and *taint' never me!*" (*My Story* 509). Livermore likens Bickerdyke's character to that of the nurse's beloved General Sherman, for "both were restless, impetuous, fiery, hard working and indomitable" (*My Story* 516). Consequently, women war workers were less paragons of true womanhood and more accurately the true mothers of Progressive Era New Women.[30] It makes sense, then, that female veterans felt authorized to reclaim Bickerdyke in the 1890s, for the young women of that time were perhaps more likely to appreciate and emulate her multiform innovations. Civil War nursing offered turn-of-the-century Americans a model of nonreproductive, yet productive, womanhood.

Devotion in the Darkest Hour

Although many of the stereotypes regarding mothering pertained to African American nurses as well, they faced a different set of biological concerns than their white counterparts. Neurasthenia was coded as a white disease by medical scientists, the product of overcivilization. Significantly, when nervous disease collided with racial ideology it resulted in a pathological diagnosis that enlarged and distorted the neurasthenic symptoms evident in the white population. African Americans supposedly were not just unreliable, they were also mentally deficient and powerless to control their debased physical urges. Whereas doctors and biologists insisted that white Americans' nerves were exquisitely excitable, African Americans had a "nervous organization less sensitive to [their] environments."[31] Their blunted sensibilities—a congenital trait—presumably made African Americans more susceptible to madness and more fitted for physical labor than highly sensitized whites.[32] Sexuality provided particularly fertile ground for such oppressive discussions, for childlike African Americans had not only degenerate minds, but also ungovernable physical urges.

Harper's and Taylor's depictions of Civil War nursing counter the racial-sexual stereotypes that saturated turn-of-the-century America, for their female nurses gain power through their association with professional chastity and selfless devotion—characteristics that were presumably natural to middle-class white women.[33] What's more, Civil War nursing is reclaimed in these texts as the powerful domain of African American women.[34] Though African American women were often prohibited from entering the increasingly middle-class profession of nursing at the turn of the century, they have always been nurses. As slaves they were often required to breast-feed and nurture the children of their enslavers. Famous images of African American women's bodies, particularly Sojourner Truth's association with the bared, maternal breast, surely underlay subsequent references to the competencies and usages of African American women's bodies.[35] Civil War writers similarly exploit the persevering, generative power of African American nursing bodies. African American mother's milk had nourished the national body, black and white. As one of Harper's enslaved characters writes, he "loves freedom more than a child loves mother's milk," likening the nutrients from his mother's body and the cure to his social ills; ultimately he defers his freedom to stay on the plantation with his aged but powerful mother.[36] Thus African American nurses also served as unifying symbols at the turn of the century, connecting the slave past with the uplifting present through their palpable influence. Some turn-of-the-century African American activists, such as Fannie Barrier Williams, strained to erase the "stain and meanness of slavery" from stories of exemplary women, to blot out the "stress and pain of a hated past."[37] Still, the title of Williams's essay, "The Colored Woman and Her Part in Race Regeneration" acknowledges the etiological foundation of prejudice and the need for African American women's healing powers. Harper and Taylor return to the Civil War precisely because it was an optimistic, forward-looking moment—a moment when both freedom and stolen mother's milk could be reclaimed—in line with the aspirations of most turn-of-the-century activists.

Rather than eschewing African American women's bodies and their association with sexual abuse and forced pregnancy, Harper and Taylor's nursing bodies provide positive historical links between slave work, Civil War work, and contemporary racial activism. Nursing also took on a larger function in African American communities, according to nursing historians, where black women worked to cultivate the physical and mental health of their friends, families, and neighbors. From their earliest professionalization, African American nurses were asked by male community leaders to do more than tend physical wounds; they were also asked to teach personal hygiene, thrift, and morality.[38] Finally, to nurse can mean to harbor and sustain a feeling, most often a sentiment of malice or ill will. These stories of African American Civil War service continue to nurse racial outrage and solidarity, especially as violence against African Americans quickened and intensified at the turn of the century.

Many critics argue that African American women writers tended to foreground the heroism of black men in wartime, eventually embracing, as Claudia Tate notes, the rhetoric of manhood as an "emancipatory discourse to be mediated by both men and women."[39] Apparently, African American soldiers served as universal symbols of African Americans' fitness for citizenship. As early as 1866, in a speech delivered before the National Woman's Rights Convention, Harper offered "the bones of the black man bleaching outside of Richmond . . . the thinned ranks and the thickened graves of the Louisiana Second" as proof of the competence of all African Americans.[40] The fictional soldiers of her 1892 novel *Iola Leroy; or Shadows Uplifted* are equally significant. Here, Harper's Tom Anderson, a formerly enslaved and beloved member of the Negro regiment, heroically claims on his deathbed, "Some one must die to get us out of this" (Harper 53). Taylor, in her 1902 memoir *Reminiscences of My Life in Camp with the 33rd United States Colored Troops Late 1st South Carolina Volunteers,* repeatedly invokes the quiet heroism of her Company E. In one instance she praises her husband, Sergeant King; though "his hip was severely injured" in a dangerous fall, King refuses to let go his grip on a captured rebel.[41]

Yet African American women writers were not as self-effacing as some scholars have implied, asserting the persistence of their own bodies and their versatile war service as lasting evidence of African American fitness. Taylor is quite bold, explaining that she writes her memoirs in part because "there are many people who do not know what some of the colored women did during the war" (Taylor 141). Note that in the examples cited earlier, it is not the African American men themselves, but the barely legible traces of their efforts, that beg acknowledgment. The men are conspicuously absent from these wartime scenes; they are anonymous corpses, decimated ranks, injured bodies: only the graves of the Louisiana Second are "thickened." Instead, African American women are eminently present in the work of Harper and Taylor. For example, Taylor's memoir begins, not with stories of male heroism, but with a matrilineal legacy marked by the extraordinary longevity and influence of her foremothers: a great-great-grandmother who lives to 120; a great-grandmother, the mother of twenty-three daughters, who survives until the age of 100. Taylor's Civil War service and continuing efforts on behalf of war-era causes is part of this wonderful story of presence and perseverance. Men are absent here, too; Taylor's great-grandfather and his four brothers are consumed by the Revolutionary War, and her uncle James dies at the age of twelve, presumably succumbing to the rigors of slave life (Taylor 25). Finally, Taylor's first husband, Sergeant Edward King, mysteriously disappears from her narrative after the war. Only she remains to tell the war stories.

Harper's 1866 speech prefigured the corporeal claims of turn-of-the-century women war writers; after noting the erasure of African American male bodies during the war, Harper celebrates the accomplishments of Harriet Tubman. Instead of bleaching bones and thinned ranks, Harper draws our attention twice in one paragraph to Tubman's "swollen hands" made uncommonly large by Tubman's work as a trusted Civil War scout and underground railroad conductor. Harper's imagery suggests the great number and variety of tasks they had performed. She ends her speech by emphasizing Tubman's "courage and bravery," which "won recognition from our army" as fitting African American women, not men, for citizenship. In drawing upon the common synecdoche of "hands," Harper was surely drawing attention away from the sexualized parts of African American women's bodies, as well as celebrating Tubman's physical strength. The image of women's hands was also a symbol of potency for white nineteenth-century women activists, linking women's work across racial boundaries.[42] Harper's and Taylor's hands symbolize the multiple and simultaneous capabilities of African American women; the image reclaims their labor, and their nursing work in particular, as a powerful rather than shameful inheritance.

However, Civil War nurses most often were represented as middle-class, matronly white women in the popular press; Alcott's, Livermore's, and Holland's texts do not veer far from this script. African American women were invisible or relegated to the margins of the Civil War drama as laborers, as the *Harper's* illustration notes. Harper and Taylor attempt to reconfigure these representations; in some ways their African American nurses are no different than white women in their attention to the expectations of middle-class virtues. Iola and Taylor, as their hospital contemporaries remark, are also "born nurses." Even Booker T. Washington claimed that colored women had a "natural aptitude for that sort of work."[43] Thus in both Harper's novel and Taylor's memoir the army patriarchy is won over by the women's extraordinarily feminine appearance and deportment. Iola is initially recruited because the field hospital needed "gentle, womanly ministrations." The general "was much impressed by her modest demeanor, and surprised to see the refinement and beauty she possessed" (Harper 39). Taylor's male superiors are similarly "surprised by [her] accomplishments," and they tell her,

"You seem to be so different from the other colored people who came from the same place" (Taylor 33). Just as with their white counterparts, their mere presence as genteel women does more than qualify them for service in the field—it can heal. Iola's "presence was a balm to [Tom's] wounds," and later in the book maintains its "soothing effect" upon her Uncle Robert (Harper 53, 139). Iola's body is so potent that it produces a nimbus of healing energy, and her attentions can shore up flagging spirits.

Although Iola and Taylor's female bodies are integral to their ability to nurse, they also transcend the limits of the corporeal. Iola is described as "lookin' sweet an' putty ez an angel. . . . She sits by 'em so patient, an' writes 'em sech nice letters to der frens, an' yet she looks so heart-broke an' pitiful" (Harper 41). Above all, her "pitiful" sympathy affects her patients. Iola's heavenly influence supersedes the physical aid she offers, as well as the services she renders for her patients. As Deborah McDowell notes, "Every detail of Iola's life . . . is stripped of its intimate implications and invested with social and mythical implications."[44] Indeed, Iola is often described as ethereal, an angel whose tireless patience and sympathy mark her difference from those she tends. However, it is also her experience in slavery, not merely her conventional femininity, that gives Iola her power. As she testifies: "I have passed through a fiery ordeal [enslavement], but this ministry of suffering will not be in vain. I feel that my mind has matured beyond my years. I am a wonder to myself. It seems as if years had been compressed into a few short months" (Harper 114). Here Iola's slave work and Civil War work are amalgamated and compacted, making her a "wonder" who transcends time and age and circumstance. Taylor's personal nursing acts take on larger, mythical dimensions as well. Her devotion is such that she risks her own life to attend to a diseased soldier. Whereas no one else will go near the man's tent, Taylor visits him every day. She proclaims, "I was not in the least afraid of small-pox. I had been vaccinated, and I drank sassafras tea constantly" (Taylor 45). Taylor evinces an almost superhuman belief in her resistance to disease. Unfortunately, the small-pox sufferer dies, yet Taylor's body is impregnable.

Harper and Taylor employ the tropes of true womanhood encompassed within nineteenth-century nursing primarily to combat persistent racial stereotypes about African American women's sexuality. Harper represses the notion that the charismatic Iola would indulge in heterosexual desire, for such behavior precluded any women from nursing and, thus, could taint Iola's commitment to racial uplift.[45] Romance, like war, is often framed in the language of disease, as we saw in Chapter 3. Dr. Latimer, Iola's biracial and civic-minded husband, phrases his proposal of marriage as a "prescription" for Iola's "restlessness," suggesting that she "commit [her]self . . . to [his] care" (Harper 268). Latimer goes on to suggest a "change of air, change of scene, and change of name" to produce the "strong health and calm nerves" she will need to work as an activist (Harper 270). Although Harper seemingly reproduces cultural scripts of the female nurse as neurasthenic helpmate here, we might notice that it is Iola's "restlessness"—her boundless and multiple energy—that is pathologized by the medical patriarchy. Indeed, it is her desire to avoid marriage with white Dr. Gresham, not the weakness of her own constitution, that evokes an initial "general debility and nervous depression" in Iola (Harper 112).

Because Iola is so light-skinned, one might view her seeming susceptibility to nervousness as fulfilling stereotypes about African women's physical stamina versus Anglo-Saxon women's delicacy. Yet I would emphasize that the pressures of her life outside of the Civil War hospital bring on such apparent weakness, much as they had for Charlotte Forten. For the most part, Iola is characterized by her soothing, passionless behavior. Indeed, Harper invites comparisons between Iola and a nun, for a substantial number of white Civil War nurses were, indeed, sisters. The spiritual pledges of nuns to impartiality, obedience, and chastity are also invoked through Harper's descriptions of Iola's hospital ministrations.[46] Iola is worshipped "as a distant star" by the patients (Harper 40). Dr. Gresham falls in love not with Iola's personality or character but with a "deeply engraven" "image" of Iola in her severe "dove gray dress and white collar" (Harper 230). [47] There is no intimacy between Iola and her patients, no passion in her relationship with Dr. Gresham; rather, Iola is a religious icon to be worshipped from afar.

Taylor, too, represses heterosexual tension, reassuringly telling a new troop that "all the boys in other companies are the same to me as those in my Company E" (Taylor 67). Her benevolent statement and use of the diminutive "boys" denies attraction to the faceless individuals she tends. Such a strategy was surely deliberate, for Taylor's editors reveal that she was only fourteen in 1862 when she took up work with the South Carolina regiment. Despite the fact that she is still an adolescent, Taylor emphasizes that the soldiers address her as "Mrs. King," acknowledging her sexual unavailability as a married woman and associating Taylor with the respect accorded a professional. Her class position was quite different than fictional Iola's. One might even speculate that Taylor married Sergeant King at a young age to escape the suggestion of impropriety in the work she had taken on following the camp. Finally, one of the few remaining pictures of Taylor, reproduced with her reminiscences, depicts her in a costume that bears a strong resemblance to a nun's habit (Fig. 6). Not surprisingly, Catholicism has positive connotations in her narrative; her white childhood playmate, Katie O'Connor,

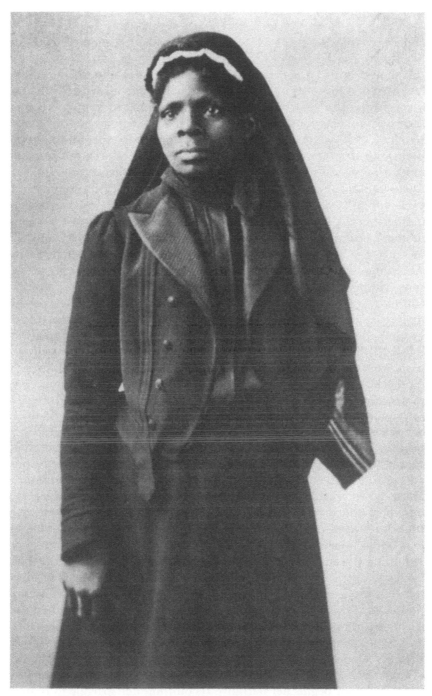

Figure 6. Portrait of Susie King Taylor, Civil War nurse. Courtesy of the
Photographs and Prints Division, Schomburg Center for Research in Black
Culture, The New York Public Library, Astor, Lenox and Tilden Foundations.

defies her father's wishes and passes her convent education on to Taylor (Taylor 30).

Although nursing bodies are denuded of passionate feeling, those feelings are transposed onto actual maternal bodies, which are the only forms allowed to elicit such dangerous emotions. As Young explains, "Harper embeds the Civil War in a trajectory of maternal quest and reunion." [48] Iola is devoted to her work and to her husband insofar as their joint devotion strengthens their individual efforts; but it is her mother for whom she works religiously to keep her heart pure. Indeed, Iola ostensibly rejects Dr. Gresham's proposal to search for her mother, exclaiming, "Oh, you do not know how hungry my heart is for my mother! . . . I have resolved never to marry until I have found my mother" (Harper 117). Iola's eventual husband, Dr. Latimer confesses too that it is his devotion to his "faithful and true" mother that convinced the light-skinned professional to cast his lot with African Americans (Harper 263). Certainly such sentiments were in keeping with the cult of true womanhood and traditional Victorian values. Iola's prominent speech "Education of Mothers," which refers to Harper's own essay "Enlightened Motherhood," invokes notions of Republican motherhood and the educative function of mothers. Tate adds that domestic plots, such as that found in *Iola Leroy*, "rely on a tradition of politicized motherhood that views mothers and the cultural rhetoric of maternity as instruments of social reform." Others suggest that the high regard for motherhood that permeates the African American literary tradition derives from persistent African traditions. Yet for both Iola and her brother Harry, the search for and reunion with the long-lost mother clearly supplants the heterosexual romance that organizes most women's writing of the nineteenth century. Harry's reunion with his mother, Marie, is remarkable for its intensity: "As she tenderly bent over Harry's bed their eyes met, and with a thrill of gladness they recognized each other. . . . Caressingly she bent over his couch, murmuring in her happiness the tenderest, sweetest words of motherly love" (Harper 191). Removing the adjective "motherly" from this passage exposes the most intimate, physical exchange in the novel. Mothers are allowed passion, for their capacious bodies are able to absorb and neutralize unchecked desire. For example, Harry is able to lavish emotion on his mother, and she ultimately heals his Civil War wounds; her "presence is a call to life" and her caresses and murmurs cause "new life and vigor" to "flow" through Henry's "veins," "calming the restlessness of his nerves" (Harper 191–92). In Taylor's text her grandmother constitutes the love interest; Taylor begins her narrative recounting her struggle to reunite with the ailing matriarch who had toiled and schemed to educate Taylor and her brother. It is her grandmother's steady "labor and self-denial" that evoke the strongest emotions from Taylor (Taylor 27). Though neither Iola nor Taylor garner their power from literal motherhood, the love of older African American mothers is ultimately rehabilitative, for their magnetic bodies fortify those they touch and galvanize families torn apart by slavery and war.

In fashioning powerful, influential mothers, Harper and Taylor combine the presumed healing power of African American mothers—and all African American women who have nursed—with that of white nurses. African American women then have a vast array of corporeal and cultural healing strategies at their disposal. Eugene Leroy, Iola and Harry's ineffective father, is initially described as "young, vivacious, impulsive, and undisciplined, without the restraining influence of a mother's love, or the guidance of a father's hand" (Harper 61). Though she is not his mother, Marie is able to quell Leroy's desire because she is his nurse. For his part, Leroy falls in love with Marie, not because he found her sexually attractive but because, as he testifies, she "followed me down to the borders of the grave, and won me back to life and health" (Harper 68). Marie's sanctified presence heals an uncontrolled soul. Leroy witnesses, "It was something such as I have seen in old cathedrals, lighting up the beauty of a saintly face. . . . In her presence every base and unholy passion died, subdued by the supremacy of her virtue" (Harper 69). Clearly, Harper works diligently to dispel the myth of the "Jezebel" or exotic mulatta seductress. Yet it is important that Leroy marries his "nurse," whose "devotion in the darkest hour had won his love and gratitude" (Harper 72, 76). Both of Iola's marriage proposals come from doctors who fall in love with her own devotion to her patients.

Of course there is one important difference between Iola's and Marie's nursing: Iola's is voluntary, whereas Marie's is coerced within the context of slavery. Reading Iola and Taylor's nursing history through slave work rather than domestic ideology recasts the significance of nursing in the lives of African American women. Nursing historian M. Elizabeth Carnegie argues that nursing was a role historically assigned to black women: "During the time of slavery, for example, black women were expected to take care of the sick in the families that owned them, breast-feed the white babies, and care for their own families and fellow slaves."[49] Many scholars have argued that the labor connected with slave culture—such as this important nursing work—was often marginalized. But Civil War service made explicit the fundamental link between antebellum and postbellum life. Nursing bodies become the solid, historical foundation of a cultural tradition not divided by emancipation; indeed, Civil War nursing became the nexus of this history, in which the various ways and means of African American women's work were fused into many multiform bodies. Taylor's great-grandmother was a "noted mid-wife" and entrepreneur; her own mother relinquished care of Susie and her brother so that they could gain education and freedom (Taylor 25–26). It is appropriate that Taylor's mother, a successful merchant, settles in "Doctortown." Thus Taylor insists on a long history of patriotism, sac-rifice, and healing, which culminates in her own Civil War service.

Harper explicitly notes the connection between slave nursing and postbellum nursing. Just as nurse Iola grasped the rough hand of the dying Tom Anderson and "*imprinted*" a "farewell kiss" upon his dusky brow, her mother notes how "the colored nurse could not nestle her master's child in her arms, hold up his baby footsteps on their floor, and walk with him through the impressionable and formative period of his young life without leaving upon him the *impress* of her hand" (Harper 55, 217, emphasis added). Rather than being a demeaning legacy, these quotes reveal nursing as a position of palpable influence in both the African American and white communities. Nurses literally mold bodies and characters. Civil War nursing validates the long and distinguished tradition of African American women as healers; yet in nursing African American men and children rather than white children during the Civil War, Harper evacuates that trope of its potentially demeaning associa-tion with Mammy stereotypes. Ultimately, nursing by African American women, in slavery and in Civil War hospitals, is reclaimed as a variegated legacy; whether exuding a delicate influence on their patients or a firm, corporeal impress, nurses' bodies have real effects on those around them.

Given the power of the nursing trope, nursing became a desirable profession for turn-of-the-century African American women. However, African American women's entrance into the profession was vexed according to most scholars. After the war, African American women were excluded from white nursing training programs, which sought to mark out nursing as a respectable, middle-class profession by excluding those whose bodies were associated with labor.[50] During the war, racial stereotypes about race, gender, and labor had prevailed. Taylor reminds us that though she served as both a teacher and a nurse in her "free time," volunteering for these extra duties in the understaffed hospital, regimental records list her only as a "company laundress" (Taylor 91). "I was glad, however," she assures her readers, "to be allowed to go with the regiment, to care for the sick and afflicted comrades" (Taylor 52). Schultz's efforts with the Carded Service Records of Hospital Attendants, Matrons, and Nurses from the war reveal that as many as eleven percent of Union hospital workers were African American women, though they remained identified as "laundresses" or "cooks" in the official records.[51]

Taylor even notes that her nursing work was supervised by Clara Barton, who was often on hand when she tended to her "sick and wounded" comrades in a Beaufort hospital (Taylor 67).[52] Like African American veterans, Taylor insists that she gave her services "willingly for four years and three months without receiving a dollar."

Yet the lack of remuneration could not vitiate the power of African American women's nursing work. In "Woman's Political Future" (1893), a "historic speech" delivered at the World's Congress of Representative Women during the World's Fair, Harper imagistically continued to expand nursing so that it encompassed more than the supposedly unskilled manual labor to which Taylor's work was reduced in the official records.[53] She repeats the imagery of women's "hands," noting that American women hold in their hands "influence and opportunity" ("Political Future" 223). Harper reiterates the palpable influence of women, remarking that it is the "women of a country who help *mold* its character, and to *influence* if not determine its destiny" ("Political Future" 223, emphasis added). Finally, she maintains that, like Eugene Leroy and Iola's Civil War patients, the public of 1893 had already felt the "*impress* of [the African American woman's] hand" through public proclamations, literary achievements, and legal maneuvering. This last statement entwines health, economics, and politics, investing African American women with broader nursing powers. Although African American women were shut out of the World's Fair and out of the mainstream nursing movement, Harper envisions African American women in homes, churches, legislative halls, literature, and society—they are everywhere at once ("Political Future" 223).

Although literal nursing would not be Iola or Taylor's fate, Harper and Taylor's imagery, read in conjunction with contemporaneous theories of African American women's nursing, encourages us to read their texts within a nursing paradigm of which various contours were set by Civil War service. Harper's Dr. Gresham describes the war as a "dreadful surgery by which the disease [i.e., slavery] was eradicated. The cancer has been removed, but for years to come I fear we will have to deal with the effects of the disease," he warns (Harper 216). Because contemporaneous African American culture was still apparently recuperating from that surgery, Harper suggests that nurses were still needed to tend to the patients. As Joanne Braxton has argued in her work on black women's autobiography, "In post-emancipation accounts of slaves, the central concerns for family and self-sufficiency do not cease but extend the ideal of service to one's community, state, and nation."[54] The Civil War hospital was represented as the original training ground, where skills and social lessons useful to contemporaneous society were learned. Iola tells us that it was in the hospital nursing the Negro troops that she learned "the latent and undeveloped ability in the race" (Harper 116). And Taylor's hospital experience teaches her how "our aversion to seeing suffering is overcome in war,—how we are able to see the most sickening sights, such as men with their limbs blown off and mangled by the deadly shells, without a shudder; and instead of turning away, how we hurry to assist in alleviating their pain, bind up their wounds, and press the cool water to their parched lips, with feelings only of sympathy and pity" (Taylor 88). Thus her narrative of 1902 could be directed toward those readers turning a blind eye to the unpleasant sights—the mangled bodies—of racial violence. Also, it could be a clarion call to African American readers not to become complacent to the suffering around them, to hurry still to "bind up the wounds" caused by economic oppression and racial violence. Like Livermore and Holland, African American nurses are unnerved by violence and not by their reproductive organs, and they thus have a responsibility to extend their energies to the suffering.

Taylor's Civil War nursing persisted until 1902, for she continued to care for Civil War soldiers. She writes that they have been her special charges ever since the war, for her "hands have never left undone anything they could do toward their aid and comfort in the twilight of their lives" (Taylor 133). Taylor insists that she receives letters still from her "comrades" with expressions of "gratitude for teaching them their first letters" (Taylor 141). Though too old to accompany the troops during the Spanish-American war, Taylor helps to "furnish and pack boxes to be sent to the soldiers and the hospitals" (Taylor 137). Later, Taylor explains that her participation in the women's relief corps has allowed her to use her nursing skills in a larger context, keeping track of the veterans' whereabouts and volunteering her efforts for money-raising benefits. Perhaps the most crucial part of her continuing nursing work is her effort to establish a stable and accurate history of the war.[55] She insists that not only should the exploits of men "be kept in history before the people," "but [also] those of noble women" who risked punishment and death "relieving those men" (Taylor 142). Like Livermore and Holland, she asserts that her healthy nursing body is best able to convey the war. "*I* have seen the terrors of that war," she testifies, sights that were so traumatic that they will never leave her until her "eyes close in death." "The scenes are just as fresh in my mind to-day as in '61," she insists, drawing attention to her remarkable memory and her text's historical accuracy.

Iola, too, continues to nurse after the Civil War, employing the ideology of influence developed in the hospital. Long after leaving her nursing duties, Iola's mere presence during a speech on moral goodness still evokes a visceral response in her audience. Harper writes, "Her soul seemed to be flashing through the rare loveliness of her face and etherealizing its beauty" (Harper 257). Such descriptions apparently reinscribe Iola's influence within the confines of moral suasion. However, like the new African American nurses of 1892, Iola will, "by her example of altruistic caring, self-discipline, and personal sacrifice, teach lessons of moral rectitude, cleanliness, order, proper diet, and deference to and respect for authority."[56] Thus when Aunt Linda calls for a teacher who will "larn dese people how to bring up dere chillen, to keep our gals straight, an' our boys from runnin' in de saloons an' gamblin' dens," she is calling for those versed in self-restraint, morality, and devotion, whose touch can exert a palpable influence on the African American community: Civil War nurses (Harper 160). Indeed, toward the end of the novel, one character, Reverend Carmichael, observes that he saw young ladies who had graduated as *doctors*—not nurses—on his tour of Southern universities (Harper 258). In her public speeches, Harper consistently catalogued the many women who had become doctors, advancing the healing tradition of African American women in new directions.[57]

Harper replicates the corporeal logic of nursing that undergirds the authority of Civil War texts authored by women throughout the nineteenth century. Soldiers' diseased and decomposed bodies were not sufficient to substantiate the war's reality. Women's bodies, too, were lost, not because they were diseased, but because their Civil War multiformity resisted contemporary biologism, social convention, and narrative form. Taylor's, Harper's, Livermore's, and Holland's texts suggest that Civil War stories are incomplete not only because of the missing dead but also because they turn a blind eye to the living bodies of women whose experiences remained unaccounted and unaccountable. A variety of physical labors and preternatural fantasies, the force of disease and the power of rehabilitation, simultaneously epitomize the war and reside in nursing women's tenacious bodies. As a trope that is embodied but not bounded, the Civil War persisted beyond its historical limits as well. As Jane Campbell puts it, in "reformulating history" into a "mythic future," African American women writers invoked the Civil War as a transformative and suprahistorical moment.[58] Magnetic, nursing bodies are the mediums of the war's multiple meanings.

Chapter 7

Historical Bodies: African American Scholars and the Discipline of History

> *A fervid imagination sometimes entirely upsets and supplants the plain and obvious teachings of common sense. In the glare of enthusiasm, fiction is often mistaken for fact, and what exists, somehow or other, is confounded with what ought to be. A state of mind analogous to this, leads some of our friends to assume that all distinctions founded upon race or color have been forever abolished in the United States.*
>
> —*Frederick Douglass, "Seeming and Real"*

Nowhere do the vexing instabilities of bodies, history, and the scientific, objectivist methods that were increasingly deployed to dictate both, come into clearer focus than in the Civil War histories written by African American historians at the end of the nineteenth century. These scholars returned to the Civil War precisely because of the diseases still sited there, and the attendant opportunities provided for dramatizing the rehabilitation of African American bodies before the eyes of the reading public. African American historians adhered to the same logic that impelled consensual white historians subconsciously aware of the fanatical impulses evident in white men during the Civil War: Civil War narratives stabilized by the discipline of history could produce stable, disciplined bodies resistant to the diseases the Civil War aggravated. Whereas white historians obdurately worked under the presumption that their racial identity ensured universal health—a presumption undermined by the Civil War, of course—African American Civil War historians had to contend with the belief that their bodies were already inherently diseased—a belief undermined by their exemplary service in the war. African American historians' insistent, meticulously supported stories of disciplined African American Civil War soldiers would dispel commonly held beliefs about their presumed racial degeneracy. Thus they attempted to rewrite battlefield ferocity as evidence of racial health and to redeem the many dead bodies of African American soldiers as the firm foundation of a vigorous people.

The new historical profession was crucial to such rehabilitation. In his *A New Negro for a New Century* (1900), the influential Booker T. Washington gathered "stories"—notably, those telling of the "black phalanx" during the Civil War and the Spanish-American war—"which once woven into the text-books of the Nation, will obtain for the brave contemporaries of our own time a place in history along with those of our heroic forefathers."[1] Washington concedes that African American experiences had been excluded from the historical record. But African American Civil War service, once appropriately "woven" into history, would merely confirm that African Americans were deeply interlaced into the fiber of American culture. As Washington's hopeful pronouncement demonstrates, African American historians were no different than any others in their subscription to the gap theory of historical praxis. That is, history was not necessarily a limited pursuit, but could—indeed, had a responsibility to—expand to accommodate newly "discovered" experiences or facts. The absence of African Americans from the historical record and, concomitantly, the race's perceived physical and mental deficiencies, were matters of oversight. Thus African American historians relied on the fact that history's stabilizing truth-claims could be extended to African American bodies.

But as Frederick Douglass notes in the quote opening this chapter, fact and fiction remained complicated categories for postbellum Civil War writers, the distinction between the two apparently muddied by the enthusiastic imaginings of the teller. Like the fleeing spectators and soldiers who left conflicting eyewitness accounts of the First Battle of Bull Run, those who attempted to transcribe the upsetting of racial categories during the Civil War could be seen as similarly undependable. The racist imaginings of white folks made them unable to perceive the "plain facts" of African American humanity, whereas African Americans and those sympathetic to the cause of racial equality were unable to see that exemplary African American Civil War service was still consigned to the imagination. In "Seeming and Real" (1870), Douglass presciently cautions that adherence to the claims of facticity can irresponsibly transform desire into historical "reality." His warning was even more relevant given the historical context in which he evoked it. True, fictions of race had shifted radically during the Civil War; bodies once understood as subhuman chattel were rhetorically transformed into persons. The radical nature of this bodily metamorphosis cannot be underscored enough. However, Douglass implies that the passage of laws did not ensure that such transformations had taken place in fact. The abolition of racial difference resides still in the realm of the fervid imaginary in Douglass's quote, whereas racial equality relies on a "common sense" that seems unmanageable to white bodies still infected by Civil War disease. The language of neurasthenia permeates this logic, allying the "seeming" with passion and the "real" with sensibility.

As African American historians have long noted, racial inferiority in America is not premised only on scientific discourses of health and disease. Indeed, throughout American history, many have argued that African Americans were not entitled to freedom nor equal rights because they had contributed nothing of note to the development of civilization and, thus, should share none of its privileges. As Benjamin Quarles points out in his assessment of black history's antebellum origins, African Americans have long been charged with having an "unworthy past."[2] This past is unworthy in at least two ways. First, racists claimed that Africans had achieved nothing noteworthy because they were genetically inferior; collaterally, they had no history, for they had made no progress. As such, those of African descent were an eternally undistinguished and indistinguishable race, their primitive bodies and minds ensuring that they were, as Quarles puts it, "destined indefinitely to lag below the historical horizon."[3] The implication of this statement is not necessarily that African Americans don't exist, but that they have no place in history. As Michel Foucault reminds us, humans have not always been subject to a distinct history[4]; Quarles adds that African Americans were denied historicity long after the white race had become its subject. Second, many white historians believed fervently that African Americans would never amount to anything, and, thus, their bodies and achievements could make no impression upon records of the past, leave no mark on the historical landscape. Indeed, the historicity of the white race was in part premised on the ahistoricity of presumably immobile black bodies. It was white Americans' distance from black that lifted them above the historical horizon. And in the histories I treat in this chapter, it is in part African Americans' proximity to whites, both physically and historically, that makes their Civil War work inherently historical. As such, these texts paint a surprisingly integrated picture of Civil War service, insisting that African Americans and whites inhabited the same historical plane.

In theory, because African American degeneracy and ahistoricity are intricately bound, a legitimate history could rehabilitate the race. Washington explicitly links medical and historical rehabilitation, contending, "As the surgeon must harden his heart while he probes the wound, that he may apply a healing lotion; so the historian must record the facts however heart-rending, that he may perchance suggest a remedy."[5] Incomplete or inaccurate history is likened to a wounded body, and the historians I treat here show how slavery-scarred, presumably degenerate

African American male bodies could be restored to health through recuperative Civil War histories. Washington also notes that such revisions might "rend" some "hearts" as they heal, suggesting that the destruction of a racist history could tear apart the corporeal fictions on which others' stable identities were founded and thus heal the social ills of a nation still suffering the wounds of the Civil War. Finally, Washington appeals to the promise of scientific method, insisting that it is possible for surgeons and historians alike to "harden" their hearts. In short, he asks these professionals to quell the individual sentiments that compromise their own bodies, and consequently, the bodies of the medical and historical texts they produce. The integrity of the race—indeed, the survival of contemporaneous African Americans—was contingent on the presumed objectivity and rehabilitative power of the historical project.

Civil War heroics, emancipation, and African American male enfranchisement seemed to promise health, history, and subsequent safety and prosperity for postbellum African Americans. That the war had not established such changes did not eradicate its power to signify them. Thus the Civil War served as a touchstone for those still battling unmitigated white ill will and racial violence a generation after emancipation. Although the initial wartime atmosphere of revolution had enabled Northern culture to accept emancipation and African American men's enfranchisement, the protracted length and disarray of Reconstruction, as well as the North's retreat from wartime racial liberality, led to dangerous and deadly lawlessness for many African Americans. At the turn of the century, the "nadir" of racial violence, typified by a full developed lynching culture, collided with the centennial aspirations of "the new negro in a new century." Susie King Taylor was one of the many writers who recognized that the Civil War was the pivotal moment in the modern constitution of African American bodies, though what it had inaugurated was still unclear. She insists on the possibilities of historical difference, even as she seems caught in the logic of the changing same: "The war of 1861 came and was ended, and we thought our race was forever free from bondage, and that the two races could live in unity with each other, but when we read almost every day of what is being done to my race by some whites in the South, I sometimes ask, 'Was the war in vain? Has it brought freedom, in the full sense of the word, or has it not made our condition more hopeless?'"[6] Taylor's forceful condemnation of contemporaneous racial violence is made more heinous by its contrast to the propitious birth of universal freedom during the Civil War. The differences between bondage and freedom, property and humanity, marked distinctly a past from a present and produced a discernible historical trajectory. Yet Taylor's desperate questions articulate the lurking fear that the historical trajectory from the Civil War to the new century might chart immobilization or descent rather than ascent, given the norms of historical progress. Despite the fact that African Americans were now free, the racial violence that gripped turn-of-the-century America served as stark contrast to the optimism that the end of the war brought. Taylor's attestation to the oppression still endured by many African Americans suggests that the physical and psychological "condition" of African Americans was still at issue during this volatile period. African American Civil War historians respond to a culture dangerously obsessed by the ever-changing round of answers offered to the vexing "Negro question."

Turn-of-the-century history provided paradoxical answers, given that black bodies, whether living or historical, were not granted the fictions of stability allowed white bodies and on which historical praxis was founded. Ironically, in efforts to efface this assumed corporeal difference, historians of the era spent their efforts distinguishing the Civil War service of African American soldiers from that of their white colleagues. Such projects of racial establishment are historically specific acts themselves. That the contested material and discursive site of the body was in great flux during the Civil War made the war the logical but dangerous location for efforts to both undo and rehabilitate African American bodies. Yet the very notion of *African American* history was premised on an irreducible corporeal difference. As Robert Reid-Pharr and others have argued, in order to produce such bodies of knowledge, one must "establish the stability of a Black American subjectivity by figuring the black body as the necessary antecedent to any intelligible Black American public presence."[7] That is, there must be an identifiable group of people whose dark bodies and/or genealogies (substitute any of the many elusory criteria used to establish the fixity of African American bodies in America) produce a discernible African American identity. Just as white American historians based their narratives on racial exclusions, so too did African American historians make crucial decisions about which bodies counted in their histories, implicitly attesting to the instability of race as a corporeal category in their efforts to decide who was in and who was out. For example, Quarles writes that in constructing African American histories that sought to reclaim a distinguished African heritage, "proof" of Negro ancestry proved difficult; some historians searched for evidence of "negroid" features in depictions of their historical subjects. In this way, the racial identity of ancient Egyptians was often in question.[8] Firmly barred from European narratives, African American historians had no choice but to craft alternative race-histories that emerged out of the founding historical logic of racial difference. Yet their efforts to show that the culminating Civil War heroics of individuals were enmeshed in a preexisting history became part of the larger ethnological project of the new science of race-history. Because of this distinctive historiography, even when African American Civil War soldiers performed the very same activities or suffered the same wounds as white soldiers, even when the very same language was used to describe their work, corporeal difference inflected their stories.

Equally important, the historians' racial identification nuanced their relationship to history and their ability to write it. In this way, Civil War histories written by African Americans demonstrate powerfully how bodies both grounded and troubled the modern historical project. These history books are particularly important, as they chart the collision between supposedly stable historical method and the supposedly unstable—and hence, unhistorical—bodies that employed that method. As writing bodies seemingly racially fixed in their unreliability, many African American historians eagerly embraced scientific method for the way it presumably erased the body of the historian. Yet in both dismantling and establishing racial difference through Civil War history, African American historians drew attention to their own bodies. Indeed, the questions raised about African American historians brought the reliability of all history-writing bodies into question. Civil War histories were particularly vulnerable under such scrutiny, given what the conflict had revealed about the ills plaguing white Americans.

The war remained a powerful trope for African American writers because of these varied instabilities. Many perceived that its stunning changes historicized black bodies, setting them into motion in ways that could not be denied. As an antebellum historian, H. Ford Douglass of Illinois, explained, "All other races are permitted to travel over the wide field of history and pluck the flowers that blossom there, to glean up heroes, philosophers, sages and poets, and put them into a galaxy of brilliant genius and claim all credit to themselves; but if a black man attempts to do so, he is met at the threshold" before he can embark on such temporal excursions.[9] Here history is spatialized, a vast, still uncharted land African Americans are prohibited from entering (forecasting the Jim Crow segregation policies of the South). The Civil War removed all barriers to this land, allowing African Americans significant mobility. The past accomplishments of African Americans are not contrived but natural, the fruit of a bountiful land. And they are preexisting, merely waiting for someone to recognize their beauty. Fittingly, many Civil War writers used the language of exhumation to express their historical work—that is, they wrote of digging up long-dead, unmarked bodies and bringing their stories to light. H. Ford Douglass, too, praised "the remains of ancient grandeur which have been exhumed from the accumulated dust of forty centuries."[10]

Ultimately, the racist premises of white historical praxis did not prove history's relativity for these writers but merely showed that prejudiced historians could misinterpret the facts, shine the light in the wrong directions. Civil War Negro historians pinned their hopes on the materialization of African American historical bodies and those visible bodies' ability to sustain a healthy racial identity. In searching for a historical past capable of rehabilitating the race, African American historians also ascribed to the notion of an original state of "health"—a mythical and more authentic racial past that history would restore to them. Indeed, Civil War rehabilitation was a particularly useful trope for African American historians, for the *re* in *rehabilitation* presumes a preceding state of health compromised, in this case, by historical circumstance. Given theories of historical progress and statistical biology, one grand, heroic act would not make African Americans historically visible. Extraordinary individuals could be dismissed as anomalies. Thus histories of the Civil War Negro regiments had to begin with an overview of African American participation during other wars in the nation's past. By situating the Civil War performance in a long and admirable historical context, these authors were able to reclaim "luminous flashes of martial glory," which cast light upon an "otherwise somber picture."[11] War service was particularly important to these projects of rehabilitation because of the way it focused attention on bodies. In particular, the press of the uncounted Civil War dead grounded the historical claims of African American and white historians alike. The dead bodies of African American soldiers are foundational in Civil War histories, their blood and bones mixing with the American terra firma as well as with the bodies of their white compatriots. Civil War heroism provided opportunities for African Americans to persist beyond the graves of the regional conflict in the American subconscious, and in this way they became historical.

In exploring the treacherous dynamic of African American history writing, I turn to the work of Negro historians (as they were called at the time) writing during the 1880s and 1890s. African Americans did write Civil War histories earlier in the century. In addition to numerous periodical accounts of Civil War service such as James Henry Gooding's letters, the public embraced history books such as William Wells Brown's popular *The Negro in the American Rebellion: His Heroism and Fidelity* (1867). However, in this chapter I am interested in how and why African Americans returned to the Civil War a generation after the hopes of the immediate postwar period were dashed. During the late 1880s and 1890s, two Negro Civil War history books dominated the popular literary market. The first is George Washington Williams's *The Negro Troops in the War of Rebellion, 1861–1865* (1888); a previous book, *History of the Negro Race,* had catapulted Williams into the national spotlight, and so his second effort was reviewed widely and mostly favorably. For example, in an early piece in the *New York Sun,* the reviewer comments that "Col. Williams has demonstrated at one stroke that the negro race possesses not only the gifts of a soldier, but those of a judicial expounder of events and of an accomplished man of letters."[12] Not only Civil War soldiers but also turn-of-the-century Civil War historians are validated in this comment. Subsequent African American historiographies have defined Williams as the first serious African American student of history; both Booker T. Washington and W. E. B. Du Bois emulated him in their early historical forays.[13] Joseph T. Wilson's effort, *The Black Phalanx* (1890), was released close on the heels of Williams's history; in fact, the two books were frequently advertised together and shared joint reviews. Wilson's history was also well received by both the critics and the public, going though three editions during the 1890s.[14]

Although these book-length efforts have garnered the majority of critical attention, a number of historical pamphlets also attempted to resuscitate the Negro Civil War soldier; though smaller in scope, I believe their intentions and methods are similar to those of the longer works. In addition to Christian Fleetwood's pamphlet, *The Negro As a Soldier* (1895), I will rely upon Norwood P. Hallowell's *The Negro As a Soldier in the War of the Rebellion,* which was read before the Military Historical Society of Massachusetts in 1892.[15] In yoking these writers together I do not mean to imply that there was one monolithic African American response to the war or that Negro historians shared a common historical (re)vision. As David Blight cogently argues, even prominent black intellectuals such as Frederick Douglass and Alexander Crummell struggled "over how and if to remember . . . the Civil War era."[16] Yet all four writers are linked by their common pledge to reclaim the tarnished Civil War veteran as part of the period's racial uplift sentiment.

Of particular interest are the authors' generic choices. It is not surprising that these aspiring African American professionals, like their white counterparts, worked to establish history as a more scientific, middle-class profession, trusting that the content of their histories would be validated along with the form. The texts I consider are meticulously footnoted and researched. The thickness of their authenticating machinery echoes the "attestations" familiar to students of nineteenth-century slave narratives. Thus by the turn of the century, African American writers argued that Civil War service showcased African American narrative skills that were already, and had always been, what was only in the 1880s and 1890s being termed professional employment. The professionalization of academic history writing implicitly sanctioned the innovations developed in those fields during the Civil War and the slave-era by African Americans, despite the fact that African Americans were denied membership in the American Historical Association at the time.

The historical context in which they were written, and their more substantial temporal distance from the war and from slavery, also lent a distinct set of meanings to these turn-of-the-century histories. Negro troops are praised again and again for their restraint and dignity, their ability to keep passions in check. At the same time, the historians' circumspect negotiation of racial stereotypes indicates that they wrote during a time that was equally as violent as the Civil War era for African Americans. Their politic characterizations of African American soldiers telegraph the continuing necessity of masking self-assertion and desire, especially in order to erase persistent stereotypes of African American men as murderers and brutal rapists. In white America's racist imaginings, African American men prowled the historical landscape, but they did not progress; instead they moved in frightening fits and starts as they tried to impress their bodies on white America through acts of physical violence spurred on by their unrestrained passions. Since war work is often violent and almost always impassioned, African American writers could not escape the racist imputations of the fervency of their national and racial commitments in Civil War narratives. The trope of exhumation allows Negro historians to symbolically "kill" the "Old Negro" and revivify the "New Negro." They do not erase the bodies of Civil War soldiers but, rather, attempt to use them as the site of corporeal and historical transmutation.

Luminous Flashes of Martial Glory

By the end of the war, nearly two hundred thousand African American soldiers and sailors had battled for their freedom. However, as Gooding's letters forewarned, military service was not always a liberating privilege. As the initial fervor that had fueled early volunteer rates cooled, and as African Americans won their hard-fought battle for admittance into the Union army, both former slaves and free blacks were impressed to fill draft quotas; whereas one in twelve whites in the Union army died of disease in the war, that statistic rose to one in five in the neglected Negro regiments. Williams reemphasizes the unequal pay accorded the Negro soldiers, telling of "Sergeant William Walker," who was shot for "leading his company to stack arms before their captain's tent, on the avowed ground that they were released from duty by the refusal of the Government to fulfill its share of the contract" (Williams 156). And perhaps most disturbing, the suicidal odds and huge casualties of many battles demonstrated, as Wilson gingerly put it, "the not unnatural willingness of the white soldiers to allow Negro troops to stop the bullets that they would otherwise have to receive."[17]

Even so, hopes were high immediately following the war that their sacrifices would be rewarded, for the African American soldiers' courage and fortitude clearly equaled, and in many cases surpassed, that of their white comrades. Further, the immediate political result of the war period—emancipation—was a revolutionary move, signaling the radical nature of the material and ideological changes taking place in American society.[18] In 1864, Union soldier James F. Jones captured the sense of potential and hope that accompanied military service and emancipation, proclaiming, "This will yet be a pleasant land for the colored man to dwell in. . . . One by one the scales that have so long blinded our race—ignorance and superstition—are falling off; prejudice, with all its concomitant evils, is fast giving way; men begin to reason and think of us in a rational and religious way. As a people, we begin to think of our race as something more than vassals, and goods, and chattels."[19] Jones is one of the thousands of Union veterans who believed that their exemplary performance as soldiers not only would disprove the racial assumptions of white Americans but would also bolster pride and confidence in the newly emancipated African American community. As important as the shifting climate of white opinion was the new vision African Americans presumably gained. The war effected bodily transformations as the once disabled ("blinded") became able-bodied. The preeminence of positive images of Negro troops in the popular white press seemed to ensure that their military exploits at least would be admired and rewarded by future generations. As Sidney Kaplan has persuasively illustrated with his vast display of war-era magazine articles, photos, and art works depicting the valor and manhood of the Negro troops, "the black presence in the Union army during the Civil War was common knowledge. The image of the Afro-American serviceman, fighting for his own and his nation's life, was then vividly and continuously in the public eye."[20]

Yet Kaplan argues that by the end of the century the visual image of African Americans during the Civil War had shifted from representations of upright, armed men in uniform to those of thankful slaves dressed in tatters kneeling to their white liberators.[21] Two famous monuments encased African American bodies, fixing them in subservient roles: the Freedman's Memorial in Washington, which depicts Abraham Lincoln standing with arm outstretched over a kneeling slave (1876), and the Robert Gould Shaw memorial in Boston (1897), where anonymous African American soldiers serve as backdrop to the white hero on horseback who towers over them. Williams recognized the importance of recasting African American bodies, offering a detailed design for a new monument to the African American soldiers on which would be inscribed the number of African Americans who had served in the army, the names of the engagements in which they had served, and the number of African American soldiers who had died in Civil War service (Williams 328–30). He understood the significance of the great Civil War accounting project in which turn-of-the-century historians were engaged; yet his plans came to naught. The Negro soldiers' achievements were ineffective in aiding the African Americans' transformation from property to citizen in the popular imagination for they were both visually and textually erased during the Reconstruction era. William Van De Berg observes that white histories at the turn of the century, from both North and South, either negated, derogated, or derided the idea of viable Negro heroism.[22]

Ironically, white Americans' concurrent denial of African American manhood and fear of its strength and ire prompted the Jim Crow laws, the economic terrorism, the lynchings, rapes, and castrations, that plagued the African American community, both North and South. Corporal "corrections" were particularly important, for they responded to persistent belief in the hereditary insufficiency and intemperance encoded in African American bodies. The African American bodily economy was at once too weak and too strong. Predictably, then, the response to Negro Civil War veterans was at best ambivalent, and at worst, disrespectful or violent. This attitude manifested itself most clearly in the government's reluctance to make good the pensions and back pay owed these soldiers or their widows and children. The distinction made between the value of white and African American war labor about which Gooding wrote was the model upon which all other economic relationships were forged; twenty-five years after the war, many African American veterans and their families still struggled to earn a living wage. The social transformation anticipated during the war period had failed to materialize, and concurrently, the exploits of African American soldiers faded from historical view. In 1895, Fleetwood laments that history has "absolutely efface[d] the remembrance of the gallant deeds done for the country by its brave black defenders," relegating them to "outer darkness."[23]

In response, Fleetwood joined the swelling ranks of a new army that was fighting to bring to light the tempered service of African American Civil War soldiers. Central to their historical texts are the vexed ideological implications of basing claims of a stable and healthy African American manhood upon military service. Pioneering twentieth-century historiographer Earl Thorpe argues that "the central theme of Black History is the quest for . . . manhood."[24] And African American manhood at the turn of the century was associated in the white imagination with laxity, laziness, excessiveness, and violence; the African American male was reduced to his unmanageable body. To this end, the histories respond to the anxiety inherent in allying African American manhood with military violence by creating the image of disciplined Negro citizen-soldiers. The image of the trained and controlled Civil War soldier, along with the insistence on the extraordinary facility of the Negro for such service, counteracted contemporaneous Darwinian assumptions and racial stereotypes. The historians argue that the current indictment of the race is unwarranted; rather, the circumstances of African Americans' underprivileged existences—especially their intensified economic plight—not a biological weakness, inspired accusations of excessive behaviors and appetites. Civil War service is offered as proof of this alternate theory of racial restraint.

These writers had to tread delicately as they asserted African American manhood and citizenship through the trope of the Civil War soldier. Particularly hazardous was the historians' attention to gender; in insisting upon the manhood of African American men, Negro historians defied the contemporary ideology of lynching, which sought to deny the gender of the victim through castration or other physical mutilations. For the purposes of this argument, Robyn Wiegman's work on turn-of-the-century lynchings will provide a model for theorizing the intricacies of manhood, racialized bodies, and discipline. As Wiegman explains it, "The decommodification of the African American body that accompanies the transformation from chattel to citizenry is mediated through a complicated process of sexualization and engendering."[25] The public spectacle of torture that comprised the lynching ceremony stripped the victim not only of his manhood; as Gail Bederman explains, African American men's "purported lack of manhood legitimized their social and political disenfranchisement." Ultimately, in denying their gender, particularly their reproductive powers, lynching culture denied African American men's ability to persist and their corporeal claims to history.

The real threat of violence that overshadowed the African American community at the turn of the century clearly informs the historians' textual strategies, as they seek both to expose the history of racial violence and to dissipate violent incidents in contemporary life. Consequently, even as Civil War historians uncover and excoriate the modern genesis of lynchings in the Confederate prison camps, their soldiers' masculinity is consistently tempered with attention to the gentler, stereotypical traits of docility, patience, and obedience. Yet in also emphasizing the ferocity and tenacity of the Negro soldiers and their wholehearted commitment to fighting for equality, the Negro historians suggest these might be qualities lying dormant in the contemporary African American community. They further exploit their tales of distant martial exploits by posing cleverly veiled threats of reprisal to unrelenting violence through them. Not surprisingly, they were sometimes caught in the delicate rhetorical webs they had woven. In concentrating on the established historical subtopic of military history, the Negro historians were able to suggest racial continuity and stability, as well as stake claim to the nationalist sentiments prevalent at the time. Still, there is no escaping the fact that war is violent work: to be a successful soldier is to be a good killer. Rhetorical posturing could not be disassociated from the realities of the racially segregated, potentially violent world that the historians' bodies inhabited.

The politics of negotiating textual responsibility lay at the heart of the African American historical project. In Henry Louis Gates Jr.'s terminology, the historians were required to become "masters of voice," incorporating the vocabulary of both racists and revolutionaries into their own. Such rhetorical adroitness was especially relevant to Negro historians working within the context of the emerging discipline of objectivist history in the 1880s and 1890s.[26] Histories that were meticulously researched and footnoted simply complied with professional standards in their pleas for credibility. Within this context, Negro historians cultivated the ability to throw the voices of other authorities and texts so as to create a smooth, strong historical fabric that would rehabilitate the race. However, it is also interesting to note that the authenticating techniques of citations and source-weaving were already familiar to African American writers in the nineteenth century. Thus the "attestation" of the slave narrative—that is, the insertion of corroborating statements by white observers—is here transformed into accepted academic practice. The historians ultimately succeeded in manipulating the codes of historical writing to benefit both the African American community in general and the discipline of Negro history writing in particular. It is the Negro soldiers' (and historians') forgotten, exemplary war service and their absent, long-dead bodies that entitle them to citizenship; additionally, Negro historians argue that it is the unique, difficult circumstances of African American life that make them the most effective American historians.

Put in the metaphorical terms of the historians themselves, the Negro historian's job was to transform what Hallowell terms "the full glare of the greatest search light"—the high beams trained unrelentingly on the Negro regiments during the war—into George Washington Williams's "luminous flashes of martial glory" dotting and enlightening the race's history (Fleetwood 14; Williams 332). According to Williams's biographer, John Hope Franklin, Williams had recognized the power of revisionist history long before the turmoil of the turn of the century. During the country's centennial celebration, Williams realized history could be used as a tool to make clear and comprehensible past glories; more important, it could be used to measure how the country had fared since the historical moment under consideration.[27] The Civil War became the primary yardstick. Though luminous light does not completely alter the object lighted, it can suggest shadings and dimensions—in historical terms, revisions—not seen in traditional light. Ultimately, the historians became luminaries themselves, taking up the militant role denied their soldiers and fighting their battles in text, relying upon ordered, disciplined historical sources as muscle. Wilson claims it is a "labor of love to fight many of the battles of the war of the rebellion over again" (Wilson, preface). And Thorpe concurs in retrospect, observing, "These historians have been influenced by the conception of Black history as a *weapon in the fight for racial equality*."[28] Because of the way it had initially unsettled bodies, the Civil War became the perpetual site of such contests.

Negro historians had quite a fight ahead of them. Peter Novick has argued that in presenting an "impartial" account of the Civil War, both Northern and Southern white historians based their accounts on the objective truth of scientific racism.[29] To reiterate, in this way historians were able to prove their objectivity to a society already convinced of the racist results they would demonstrate. In particular, according to Nina Silber, Northerners increasingly accepted the South's sentimental nostalgia for plantation days; largely in the interest of "financial bonding," white Americans "bowed to the racial pressures of reunion, to a process that depoliticized the legacy of sectionalism, overlooked the history of American slavery, and came to view southern blacks as a strange and foreign population."[30] African American Civil War service had not cemented an interracial, Northern community; rather, ahistorical black bodies became the historical means of ostensibly rehabilitating the fanatical white race.

Yet it is providential that antiromantic scientific history was emerging as a discipline at the height of African American intellectual reconstruction. In embarking upon objectivist historical projects at precisely the moment that their white counterparts were attempting to substantiate such practices within academic institutions, Negro historians ensured that even though they would be subject to stringent criticism, their work would rarely be nullified outright. In denying the work of Negro historians, white historians would have been, in essence, shooting themselves in the foot. Just as Civil War service had made strange bedfellows of white and African American soldiers, the vulnerability of the historical profession affiliated the plights of Negro and white middle-class historians. Before professionalization, full-time historians were most likely independently wealthy, upper-class gentleman amateurs. However, with history's installment in the universities and the profession's need for an army of journeyman researchers and instructors, historical research became a more widely accessible and acceptable bourgeois pursuit. Even more important, the standardization of historical-scientific method allowed marginal groups to claim autonomy, too; in theory, though their claims could be ignored or trivialized, they could not be invalidated if they followed the rules of historical method.

Although standards enabled Negro historians to engage legitimately in the practice of history, they did not ensure their entrance to the profession. Certainly most of the leading white historians of the time did not integrate the work of Negro historians into their own scholarship. And although this trend has not persisted, historiographers do suggest that American history and African American history have developed along parallel but ultimately distinct paths. Part of the problem stems from the institutional slant of most historiographies. In tracing the roots of their own institutional positions, academic historians have pursued the professionalization of history, along with its enthronement in the "best" academic institutions in the country. Negro historians such as Williams and Wilson who received no formal historical training are ancillary to such narratives of professional development. Though a number of African American universities were opened near the turn of the century, Negro historians were still prohibited from entering doctorate programs or participating in the famous seminars offered at schools like Johns Hopkins University. Presumably African Americans would not have been comfortable in William H. Dunning's famous Reconstruction seminar at Columbia in which students were encouraged to "detail the iniquities of the [Civil War] period" from a white Southerner's point of view. The end result was that African American history was initially premised on professional difference as well as an irreducible racial identity. Consequently, the key figure of Williams, pronounced the "greatest historian of the race" by Du Bois, is considered the progenitor of Black history—not American history.[31]

Embracing the objectivist tenets that perpetuated the Negro historians' professional invisibility and historical inferiority might seem counterproductive; nevertheless, there was more to be gained than lost by such a strategy. Primarily, Negro historians were able to back up their celebration of the soldiers with a strong network of corroborating voices—often white voices—removing the likelihood that their works would be dismissed as opinion. As African American men, their secondary sources not only served the purposes of historical scholarship, but they also functioned similarly to the authenticating mechanisms found in slave narratives. Robert Stepto observes about slave narratives that "in their most elementary form, [they] are full of other voices which are frequently just as responsible for articulating a narrative's tale and strategy."[32] African American writers were well aware of the historical significance of attestations and were willing to exploit and manipulate them for their own purposes. For example, Williams's last chapter, "The Cloud of Witnesses," simply lists the "testimony of friends and foe alike" as to the martial valor of the Negro soldier (Williams 320). Such appended materials were familiar to audiences of slave narratives. Williams suggests that the authenticity of his own historical voice, and hence the veracity of the story he tells, depends as much on the web of authoritative voices that frame the text as on the documents he has woven throughout. In choosing to buttress his own research with that of his white predecessors and contemporaries, Williams renders his version of history more persuasive to an otherwise hostile audience.

Once scholarly credentials were established, the Negro historians could attempt to educate an ignorant public on crucial issues in the lives of African Americans. Even as Negro Civil War historians consciously worked within historical paradigms, their integration of slave narrative techniques underscored the realities of Negro scholarship and life during the period. Fleetwood's tribute to citation method not only assuages readers' misgivings regarding his reliability but also calls attention to Negro veterans' efforts to collect pensions and back pay, in addition to the African American community's desire to establish economic viability. After marshalling a wide array of firsthand accounts and celebratory verse arguing for the valor of the Negro soldier in the Civil War, Fleetwood remarks how "the testimony . . . runs like a cord of gold through the web and woof of the history of the Negro as a soldier" (Fleetwood 11). Like Washington, Fleetwood likens history to a fabric that is still in the process of being woven. History literally becomes a habiliment in the making. Fleetwood's equation of citations with gold also suggests the precious value of historical practice, especially for African American writers. And his imagery signals the material circumstance at the base of rhetorical practice. Fleetwood's fellow pamphleteer, Hallowell, also expends some effort pleading for the monetary compensation still due the veterans and/or their survivors. It is no mistake that the testimony lacing Fleetwood's textual image of the Negro soldier is "golden," for such an image subtly pleads the economic value of those military efforts and also of subsequent African American labor.

These references reflect African Americans' serious efforts to assert themselves in a free market dictated by the gold standard. Michael O'Malley explains the connection between the resurgence of racism and the obsession with the "intrinsic value of gold" in the 1890s. O'Malley contends, "The essential value of specie [i.e., gold], like the essential character of certain races or occupations, helped resolve the ambiguity of identity in public by a resort to 'natural facts.'"[33] According to this logic, God gave gold intrinsic value; in weighting their stories with "gold," Negro historians clearly invoked a similar sense of natural merit for African American bodies. Their exemplary Civil War service was their gold standard, the essential signifier of value backing subsequent African American enterprise. However, this strategy could also backfire; instead of allying themselves with the inherent value of gold, African American historians also invoked the immutability of gold's economic status and, thus, of their own racial identification. As O'Malley continues, "Specie, like species, signified a belief in irreducible difference and final identity." Under slavery, African Americans literally were "specie."

Negro historians did not accept this traditional equation, instead revising the notion of historical specie and creating exciting innovations in the field of academic history. For example, Williams and Wilson conducted interviews as part of their research protocols. Williams traveled all over the United States interviewing African American enlisted men and noncommissioned officers, as well as white officers. Wilson, too, insists that in doing research "it was fitting to recall *their* [the veterans'] deeds of heroism" (Williams, preface). Franklin suggests that these interviews mark Williams and Wilson as pioneer investigators in the field of oral history, and are, perhaps, the first instances of academic oral history.[34] Yet they are also creative and utilitarian extensions of existing African American traditions. Oral testimony was often the only evidence available to the authors of slave narratives, for African Americans were traditionally absent and/or silent in the usual written records of antebellum America.

Despite their creative use of oral narratives, these Negro historians paid close attention to the tenets of historical authority, emphasizing written documents as reliable sources. The most widely used and influential manual of historical method from the period, Charles Victor Langlois's *Introduction to the Study of History*, explained how written documents created an illusion of historical truth merely by their physical existence—his motto was *"pas de documents, pas d'histoire."*[35] Without documentary proof—bodily traces—there is no history. Drawing from this manual, Negro historians insisted that the stories they told were already in existence, simply waiting to be discovered: "'found' and not 'made.'"[36] Wilson explains how earnestly he has embarked upon the work of "collecting the literature of the war, from which to cull and arrange much of the matter contained herein" (Wilson, preface).[37] Similarly, in relating an instance of racial heroism, Hallowell emphasizes that he is "literally" following the recital of the eminent white veteran, Colonel T. W. Higginson. Williams also exploits the authenticating power of the document. Franklin explains how he scoured libraries across the country, visited battle sites in Mexico, England, France and Germany, and perused the official records of the War Department in his search for proof; Wilson and Williams were also two of the very first historians to use newspapers as historical sources.[38]

Finally, the stance of objectivism fostered by citation-method enabled the Negro historians by metaphorically stripping their voices of bias; their particularity was obscured in the chorus of evidentiary material. More important in terms of the violently racist times, the historians were potentially de-raced. Their idiosyncratic bodies were not supposed to be the subject of debate, neither constant nor unreliable—ideally, they were invisible. Historical method erased the body and its presumed illogic. According to Peter Novick, the goal of the objective historian was to "rid oneself of preconceived ideas and so launder one's mind that it was capable of the immaculate perception."[39] This image of "laundering" one's mind gains new significance when read in the context of the Negro histories; it could imply the historians' personal "whitening" as the supposed stain of racial bias was bleached from their texts. For Negro historians fixed firmly within the racial uplift movements of their time, laundering could also imply the enlightenment that would come as the Negro soldiers' previously tarnished image was purified in the objective histories. Williams points out that during the great time of emancipation, "a thousand facts of history for five thousand years were flashing their certain light on the path of a bewildered nation" (Williams 146). Thus the Civil War was a historical lightening rod, educing and attracting the achievements of thousands of years to one temporal location. Williams suggests that the history coalescing in and during the Civil War was overwhelming—even blinding. Turn-of-the-century Negro Civil War historians hoped that their own work would organize and temper these flashes, lighting the way for an equally chaotic time.

While historians of the time were producing general histories of the Negro race, at least as many were dedicated solely to the martial exploits of Civil War soldiers. As Donald J. Mrozek points out, military life consciously tries to disengage itself from "the swift turns of civilian fashion and custom"; by extension, military historians have a much greater potential than other historians for creating the illusion of continuity and stability.[40] The military's distinction as a neutral, unchanging space, apart from the tumult of daily life and the threat of social change, became a distinction bestowed by association upon the Negro race in these histories. The Civil War in particular became a useful trope; in keeping with the historical trends of their time, Negro historians emphasized reconciliation in their reconstructions of the Negro Civil War soldiers' experience. However, they played up the commonalities among white and African American soldiers rather than their differences. African American historians could also reemphasize the other immensely important results of the regional conflict: emancipation and citizenship.

Thus the distinction conferred by Civil War military service was marked by both demonstrations of martial continuity and racial progress. The historians' emphasis on the significance of military life for the

Negro race—from Civil War service all the way back to the Egyptian army—allowed them to combat the image of the race as fragmented, chaotic, and hopelessly primitive. John Higham remarks that scientific historians' reliance upon evolutionary theory encouraged scholars to focus not on representative moments but on the "big picture," that is, moments as links in a great chain.[41] So although Negro historians were able to celebrate the significance of the Civil War as a "luminous flash," they were also encouraged by scientific method to place that moment within a context of equally luminous martial heroism, again creating continuity and stability for the Negro race. Negro historians consciously marked how African American participation in the Civil War encouraged a rediscovery of similar glorious martial exploits. In lamenting the lack of history about Negro soldiers in the Revolutionary War, Wilson rhetorically asks if the unwritten story "lies upon the soil watered with their blood; who shall gather it? [If] it rests with the bones in the charnel house; who shall exhume it?" (Wilson 21). His metaphors insist that the stories are already written, inscribed within the American/historical landscape waiting to be discovered and deciphered. Indeed, history is explicitly connected to the African American blood that had permeated the American firmament. It remains only for the scientific historians to employ their archival methods and "exhume" what may be interred right in front of their eyes. Williams emphasizes the need to hear the stories, rather than read them, remarking that "no doubt the Nile and the Delta resounded with the exploits of the Negro Army" in ancient Egypt (Williams 6). His own text is then figured as a historical reverberation of the same story. In short, the Civil War was the loudest sound and brightest spot on the historical landscape, the moment of heightened awareness through which other moments of racial stolidity became perceptible. However, Civil War service also allied African American men with modernity, signaling their distance from the past. Both strategies were needed to ensure African American historicity.

Although Negro historians used distant military exploits to create a proud heritage, their pre-Civil War stories can also be taken as warnings that Negro militancy had to be reckoned with. Williams's rendition of the doomed but heroic Haitian defense of Santo Domingo in 1802, for example, bears all the marks of the contemporary state of affairs in the United States. In doing so, the text literalizes the threat of rebellion encoded within military rhetoric. As the story begins, the newly emancipated Haitians have revolted against the plantation owners, who had denied "the enforcement of their newly acquired rights as citizens" (Williams 42). After overthrowing their oppressors in amazing feats of military courage, Williams claims that the "transition from bondage to freedom was effected without arrogance, pomp, or social convulsion"—

partly because it was engineered by the great black hero, Toussaint L'Overture (Williams 46–47). But proud Napoleon Bonaparte is jealous of the success and advancement of the Haitians and vows to "turn a revolution backward" (Williams 48). When their homes are threatened by French troops, Haitian men "who but a few hours before were as gentle as lambs in the imagined security of their homes, were now like wild beasts, stirred for the life of their young" (Williams 49). Williams's version of the Haitian defense—with its emphasis on the revolutionary nature of freeing the enslaved, the perils of transferring citizenship and power, the jealousy of demagogues and the destruction of families—certainly invokes the challenges facing turn-of-the-century African Americans.

This story is replayed in the next chapter, where the hearts of the mild, peace-loving Northern leaders are stirred to anger once provoked by the attack on Fort Sumter: "Men who had felt like exhausting every measure of pacification and concession were now eager for war" (Williams 64). Thus, even the most righteous people may be provoked to violence when their homes, families, and personal freedoms are threatened. Williams attempts to reestablish the Civil War ties of those of African descent and Northern whites here. It is not hard to imagine how these two stories might be read in the context of the Negro historians' time; the Haitian history suggests that African Americans were ready to mobilize if pushed too far. Men such as Toussaint L'Overture are not only physically strong but also brilliant strategists, capable of "broad plans and successful execution," knowing that "skilful planning is one-half of military success." The reader wonders, could Negro veterans be planning now? (Williams 44). Hallowell further suggests that a soldier's determination and willingness to take risks are heightened when he is fighting for a just cause. He remarks upon doomed Negro troops who rush into battle, "not with the intoxicated cheer of men who rush on to victory, but with the reckless shout that men give when they lead a forlorn hope" (Hallowell 13). Certainly, those surviving in the midst of unrelenting racial violence might have been just as reckless, believing they had nothing left to lose.

Various mechanisms of racial control emerged to monitor the perceived threat of African American freedom and advancement, for even these carefully constructed Civil War histories belie the resentment of the Negro community still under siege a generation after emancipation. Wiegman explains the symbolic/political meaning behind lynchings, the most horrifying and consequently effective means of racial terrorism: "Emancipation's theoretical effect—the black male's social sameness—is symbolically mediated by a disciplinary practice that literalizes his affinity to the feminine" through the act of castration. It is significant that the bodies and behavior of African American lynching victims are figured as "culturally abject, monstrosities of excess."[42] Albert Bushnell Hart, a prominent Harvard historian of the time, fervently believed that "the negroes as a people have less-self-control . . . are less affected by family ties and standards of personal morality, than the average even of those poor white people, immigrants or native."[43] The preceding stories argued precisely the opposite—that black violence emerged *only* when African American homes and families were threatened. Yet excess was most often figured within male sexuality; hence the castration that often accompanied lynchings "sever[ed] the black male from the masculine."[44]

The image of the Negro soldier directly combated the race's association with threatening passion figured in the Negro's body, because it emphasized how controlled both his body and behavior were under martial rule. In addition, the war situated the men in a homosocial context, which helped to dissipate fantasies of African American heterosexual violence. The soldier was the antithesis of the stereotype Jacquelyn Dowd Hall designates the "black-beast rapist," for, it was universally argued, he conformed easily—almost naturally—to military life and rule, and military codes were consistently associated with discipline and orderliness.[45] Evidence of Negro soldiers' remarkable adeptness for military life was offered by these historians as a demonstration of their disciplined natures and their citizenship. Gooding, too, had emphasized the calm doggedness of the African American troops; yet the context in which these Negro historians rewrite those familiar scripts inflects them differently. Regardless of its larger meaning, the "transformation" wrought by Civil War-era "military discipline" is, in the mind of sympathetic white observer Hallowell, "wonderful" (Hallowell 11). For example, "the aptitude of the colored volunteer to learn the manual of arms, to execute readily the orders for company and regimental movements, and his apparent inability to march out of time at once arrested the attention of every officer" (Hallowell 12). The Negro's body is so disciplined in his marching he can't help but match his motions to the required, controlled pace. Hallowell goes on to observe, "It is all very well of course to praise the bravery of these men as soldiers, but with what words may we express our admiration of the dignity, self-respect and self-control, they showed in their conduct as men as well as soldiers in the matter of pay" (Hallowell 16). Even when they are not counted as men, Hallowell testifies, Negro troops can be relied upon to behave like men in checking their anger and resentment.

By reasserting masculinity through the military association with restraint and bravery, the Negro historians also mitigated racial difference. For example, in writing of the Negro's Revolutionary War service, Williams asserts that "their splendid feats of valor covered their dark visage as with a halo of glory; and the only way to distinguish them from their white compatriots" is to go over their names in the roles (Williams 33). Hence, the military is a leveling mechanism, for the light of victory obscures racial difference, sanctifying African American bodies. Wilson is proud to recount that after one particularly fierce and victorious Civil War battle, "The whites were only too glad to take a drink from a negro soldier's canteen, for in that trying hour they found a brave and determined ally, ready to sacrifice all for liberty and country" (Wilson 219). The bravery and support manifested by the Negro troops on the battle-field is acknowledged by a pseudophysical contact between white and black troops—the sharing of the canteen. Apparently, fears that African American troops might turn against their white fellow combatants or that Negro excessiveness was contagious are allayed by exemplary battle-field service. This scene even suggests the white troops' reliance upon those whom contemporary society sought to protect them from, for the black soldiers offer sustenance to their white comrades after contributing their military muscle to the battle. Thus, these historians create a delicate balance whereby association with military success and discipline ensures the acceptance, and even invites the admiration of physical masculine behavior as it was defined by white martial culture.[46]

It is in this context that Hallowell proclaims the Negro's proclivity for imitation as a sign that he is "innately a gentleman," rather than as a mark of inferiority (Hallowell 11). Further, Wilson recommends the Negro to military life when he explains that "the taste with which negro soldiers arranged their quarters often prompted officers of white regiments to borrow a detail to clean and beautify" their own quarters (Wilson 128–29). The refinement and personal style of the Negro soldier were further proof of manliness, as defined by white, middle-class military norms. Yet these military associations, which had previously been the sole domain of white men, also invoked racial anxieties. The idea that Negroes have achieved "manhood" by the "fiery trials" of the Civil War is incessantly invoked (Williams xiv). The manhood these texts assert is very specifically associated with the military, yet the historians' rhetoric reveals that it is not the same "manhood" to which white men were entitled. Negro soldiers are not born men, nor even naturally inclined that way; the Civil War is presented as the fortuitous occasion during which "every element of manhood . . . could have full play" (Williams 327). Thus Negroes can only achieve manhood through military service. Admittedly, the military is often figured as a place where white boys become men, yet manhood is an explicitly de-naturalized category for Negro troops. Mirroring the strategies developed by war-era writers such as Gooding and Forten, Williams argues that the Negro had been "reduced to a machine" by years of slavery; military service "call[ed] . . .

into action" the soldier's mental capacities, transforming him into an "intelligent unit" (Williams 76, 130). The trajectory for African American manhood, then, is not chronological but evolutionary. The Negro soldier has been raised from mindless muscle to thinking creature through the gauntlet of the Civil War.

A significant implication of this model in terms of the postwar labor market is the historians' insistence on the Negro troops' trainability and educability. The Negro troops' ability to assimilate to military life, to hold his "bestial" passions in check and even sacrifice himself in the name of martial glory entitles him to humanity. Hallowell succinctly catalogues the primary characteristics of African American manhood honed during the war: "To stay, to endure, to resist, to follow, to work patiently, doggedly, to obey orders, never to skulk, or to desert their officers in trying moments,—what more do you expect, what more do you find in the mass of men" (Hallowell 22). The threat encoded in the story of Toussaint L'Overture, for example, is neutralized by such descriptions. African American manhood is associated here with loyalty, perseverance, and discipline; it is distinguished by absolute self-abnegation. In another example, Hallowell explains that the Negro soldier's "manliness" is demonstrated by the fact that he "fought without panic," "suffer[ing] severely before falling back" (Hallowell 25). All of the histories insist that Negro soldiers pushed themselves to the limit in "desperate deeds of valor" in order to qualify for that "new name"; yet taken to its logical extreme, this rhetoric suggests that the most manly Negro soldier is a dead Negro soldier. Thus African American rehabilitation was contingent on perpetual historical revisions of the meaning of the dead bodies of Negro soldiers. They had to fight, die, and be resurrected again and again in order to emphasize both African American men's remarkable adaptability and their stable characters.

Though Civil War service ironically facilitated acceptance of African American men's humanity at the expense of human life, it did not gain them entrance to the realms of white, middle-class, heterosexual masculinity; to fully negate the stereotypes underpinning lynching ideology, Negro manhood could not be sexual. In emphasizing the intellectual and self-effacing character of Negro manhood, the Negro historians disassociated the soldiers from their desiring bodies, along with the violent, sexual threat they were perceived as posing to the white community. Such had not always been the case. In the first enthusiasm of emancipation, one soldier was audacious enough to celebrate his body in an 1865 letter to the *Christian Recorder*. In describing a regimental bath, the author muses, "I was much amused to see the secesh women watching with the utmost intensity, thousands of our soldiers, in a state of nudity. . . . Our brave boys would disrobe themselves, hang their garments upon their bayonets and through the water they would come, walk up the street, and seem to say to the feminine gazers, 'Yes, though naked, we are your masters.'"[47] They garner their power not, as Michael Hatt has argued, despite their nakedness, but because of their nakedness. Their manhood is exposed with their genitals; their power accrues from their sense of sexual potency before the female audience in this scene.[48]

Such enthusiastic accounts had disappeared by the turn of the century. Lynching was predicated upon the belief in the hypermasculinization of the mythically endowed black rapist. And the naked soldier's imagery unfortunately links sexual and martial aggression through the image of the "erect" bayonet. Certainly Negro historians did not wish to fan the flames of lynch mobs. So it is not the presence of proudly displayed genitals that defines African American manhood at the turn of the century, but rather their physical lack, "their honorable scars," which plead their manhood before the white community (Hallowell 18). Hallowell echoes William Fox who also wrote of the signifying power of scars in *Regimental Losses in the Civil War*. Again, "scars" are intended to stand in for invisible hurts that cannot be denied yet at the same time cannot be fully substantiated—whether the sufferings of slavery, the wounds of the Civil War, or the painful persistence of racist belief and violence. The traces of pain are often erased; instances of flesh and bone bodies are replaced by de-humanized, dismembered parts in the Civil War histories. For example, in telling the story of the Negro's acceptance into the Union Army, Williams explains "the black arms of iron and fingers of steel that had lifted the burdens and held the hoe for the Confederacy were to be converted to the service of the United States Government" (Williams 109). Negro troops are mechanized resources that are passed from an agricultural to a military machine. Williams's emphasis upon the arms and fingers also recalls the common synecdoche of "hands," which referenced the enslaved. Whereas the hands of Civil War nurses had been full, capable, and nurturing, the hands of the soldiers are disembodied and allied with the castrations their scars signify.

Ironically, one of the few places where bodily suffering is specified occurs in the descriptions of the lynchings performed by Confederates upon captured Negro troops. Lynchings are not only historical subtext—they are integral parts of the stories these historians tell. Both Williams and Wilson devote lengthy chapters to detailing these atrocities in the prisoner-of-war camps. Though lynching remains a loosely defined phenomenon in current scholarship, I contend that the Civil War was the first time in American history when African American men were lynched in retaliation for their perceived claims to equality as citizens and engendered subjects. Lynching attempts to disembody, and, then, deconstruct the history that inheres in those bodies.

In 1905, Yale sociologist James Elbert Cutler situated lynching between "assassination and murder" on the one hand and "insurrection and open warfare, on the other hand."[49] Certainly, such efforts to distinguish among sanctioned and taboo types of murder seem pedantic at some level. Yet Civil War combat did follow a prescribed set of rules, rules that were deliberately ignored by Confederates when they faced Negro regiments. Negro military service particularly rankled Confederate troops, because it entitled Negro troops to manhood in the chivalric, militaristic codes of Southern society. Confederate troops sought to deny the manhood of the Negro troops by refusing to treat them according to the rules of warfare. Although prisoner exchanges were common, Negro troops were rarely relinquished for Confederates, for in doing so Confederates would admit that a Negro troop was equal to one of their own, white soldiers. Instead, Negro prisoners were simply murdered. Once a flag of surrender was unfurled during the Civil War, battle was to cease, yet rebel troops manufactured reasons to "indiscriminately slaughter" surrendering Union soldiers. Firsthand observers told of how men were called out like dogs to be shot down; of how the wounded prisoners were locked in houses which were then set on fire; of how live black sergeants were nailed to logs, which were then set ablaze. A mob mentality seemed to possess the Confederate prison keepers as they shot Union soldiers "just as fast as they could make their guns go off" (Wilson 332). The surrender at Fort Pillow produced the most infamous tales of extermination, where a "carnival of murder continued" for a whole day until 300 men, women, and children were butchered (Wilson 350). "Remember Fort Pillow!" was the call that rallied the Negro troops in subsequent battles, and it echoes through these texts as a reminder of the continued vulnerability of African American bodies to illegal but ubiquitous mob violence.

And the historians cannot ignore the physical, violent manner in which Negro manhood is forged. The image of the bestial black rapist/ murderer lurks beneath the Negro soldier's uniform, for in the racist ideology of the time, to acknowledge the strength of an African American man, for that man to exhibit passion, was for him to be a potential murderer or a rapist. And the carefully constructed self-discipline of soldiering must necessarily slip when one enters the battlefield. In Fleetwood's text, Negro soldiers are described as holding their positions "with set teeth, blood-shot eye and strained muscle" (Fleetwood 14). Fleetwood's description resonates with that of the mythical black rapist, whose barely leashed physical violence dominates him, implying that passion and brute force embody the Negro soldier. Moreover, because the only ritual access to the status of manhood is combat, Negro manhood is always associated with violence, "conflated with the power to kill and destroy."[50] Negro military achievement is at once the height of civilization and the most barbarous of human pursuits, reaffirming contemporary fears associated with African American physicality.

Because they are founded on the unstable logic of bodily rehabilitation, turn-of-the-century depictions of Negro Civil War service almost schizophrenically manifest both a subtext of rebellion and a rhetoric of restraint. Williams, for instance, seems exceedingly accommodationist and conciliatory in his description of "Negro Idiosyncrasies." Here he describes the Negro's powerful physique, his celerity and poetry of movement, his sentiment and love of music, his forming attachment to friends, his deep longing for freedom, his splendid courage and power of endurance, his patience in suffering and hope in despair, his trust in God and instinct for the right, his cunning aptitude and perfect obedience" (Williams 169). Perhaps the most telling feature of Williams's catalogue is his juxtaposition of characteristics—for example the Negro's longing for freedom, courage, and endurance placed next to his patience in suffering, or his cunning placed next to perfect obedience. Williams tiptoes around his subject, seemingly wanting to sing the praises of the Negro race, yet unable to relinquish the disabling racial stereotypes left over from slavery. But, again, we must consider the circumstances of many African American men's lives when these histories were written; the slightest sign of unmitigated resistance or militancy could spur random acts of violence. And the smallest indication of injudicious bias could taint Williams's whole historical project. So it is not surprising that Williams's critique of previous history is so tactful as to be almost invisible. He writes, "I have found it necessary, in the interest of history and science, to prick some bubbles of alleged history, and to correct the record" (Williams xiii). Williams's diplomatic approach was also more likely to win favor with his colleagues, for professional—still genteel—historical standards eschewed sharp controversy and criticism. African American historians clearly felt the imperative of rehabilitating specifically African American Civil War bodies for their readers. Yet white Civil War historians did not often delineate the racial disabilities of the white men in their texts—whiteness was the invisible norm. In making racial traits a topic of history, Williams and others made the disease of racial instability visible and their own bodies subject to scrutiny.

Despite all efforts to avoid conflict, to stay within the confines of historical writing and discipline the image of the Negro soldiers, these texts were still vulnerable to criticism, for excessiveness was figured as part of African American textuality as well as masculine sexuality. William J. Moses contends that we must recognize the complicated ways in which nineteenth-century black literature "had to fight against Victorian white liberals who sought to control the varieties of black literary expression."

Such forces have conspired to exemplify those writers who adhere to a "folksy," casual style, rather than writers who seemingly abandon the "vernacular of the street corner."[51] African American textual expression is then by definition informal, inconsistent, and spontaneous. Negro historians struggled against this paradigm. Though the more prominent Negro histories were reviewed favorably, those who did find fault with them imputed their shortcomings to lack of textual control figured in terms of inherent character. In the *Boston Post*, for example, Williams's ambitious work is described as "shiftless," a word more often ascribed to the behavior of lower class whites and racial minorities than to history books. Further, a reviewer in *The Nation* added that Williams and Wilson show an "inability to command their own materials."[52] Thus the characteristics often assigned to African American sexuality and character are transferred to their texts.

The publishers of slave narratives had averted such imputations earlier in the century by enlisting white editors as symbolic agents of control. Just as claiming manhood was a hazardous undertaking for the Negro historians, so too was claiming textual authority as their own perilous business; these authors document their constant awareness of the risks they run. In his preface, Williams acknowledges that it has taken "fortitude and skill to resist the insidious influence of interested friends and actors"; further, he expresses his resolve to "master the sources of historical information" (Williams ix). Although Williams received assistance from many historians, librarians, bibliophiles, and others, he remained fiercely independent. John Hope Franklin insists that the organization and interpretation of his materials were his own.[53] There is an important distinction made between the historian's explicit power to authorize his sources and arrange his texts and the restrictions traditionally placed upon nineteenth-century African American authors. Williams's work was presumably validated by the sources he integrated within his narrative; yet he also overwrote his own authority upon those texts, unequivocally commenting upon the utility and reliability of his sources. For example, he proclaims one of General Hunter's letters "admirable . . . the most concise statement on the question of making the Negro a soldier uttered during the war. It is splendid" (Williams 93). Though he might be accused of pandering here, the fact that he presumes to authorize General Hunter's source is notable.

Thus it was not the publisher or the editor who assembled and manipulated the authenticating machinery of the history; rather it was the Negro historian himself who provided an authenticating frame for his sources. In fact, Hallowell and Williams subtly emphasize the Negro historian's superior ability to speak and master many voices, as well as his ability to read and expose the codes of American society. Their profi-

ciency is not incidental: it is part of historical necessity. Hallowell contro-
verts the traditional conflation of African American bodies with lack of
control. The tattooed body of one exemplary soldier, which bears the
symbols of the Sudanese ruling class, is as "marked" as his linguistic ability; there is "no doubt he is the master" of nine languages, ranging from
English and German to Arabic and Turkish (Hallowell 3). The soldier's
linguistic control, as well as his social status as a ruler, is literally
inscribed on his body. Such imagery combats the bestialized markings
so often associated with African American men's bodies, for Hallowell
overwrites their traditional signifying power. The self-mastery of the
black body equals control of the historical text and vice versa. Further,
the tattooed soldier's command of both Western European languages
and Middle Eastern and African languages uniquely qualifies him to
translate and integrate any number of diverse voices. As Williams
phrases it, the Negro thinker's "power of assimilation made him
intensely American, and gave him, in his new home, his alphabet of
thought" (Williams 12). Dickson D. Bruce, too, has noted that Williams
shows "because of prejudice, blacks had become better Americans than
the whites themselves."[54] Most striking, however, Williams concludes
that Negro thinkers have always been superior readers, who "although
illiterate . . . read the signs of the time right" (327). Such claims sanction
the revisionist intentions of the objectivist histories and emphasize the
significance of Civil War service and turn-of-the-century Civil War historians. African Americans are the best historians, better able to "read the
signs of the times" than those who have all of the privileges of literacy
and money. The meanings and uses of the Civil War, in particular, were
discernible to African Americas, allowing them to demonstrate their corporeal and textual skills. Indeed, the Sudanese soldier's body extends
this historical facility: not only do black bodies underwrite American
texts, they are inherently diasporic, speaking for the vast experiences of
a people who span the globe.

It might seem counterproductive for Negro historians to embrace a
historical method predicated upon their degradation and inferiority.
Yet even as Williams's work carries not only the scars of Civil War service
but also those of centuries of racism and contemporary exigency, he
optimistically encourages his audience, "No people grow so rapidly in
the right direction as Americans" (Williams 89). Given the Civil War's
historicizing imperative, it seemed crucial that turn-of-the-century African Americans wrote Civil War history—again and again. They needed
to exhume African American bodies, to add them to the historical
record. In this way they could exploit the press of the dead, claiming the
stilling, rehabilitative power of the Civil War as their own. Yet the Civil
War's corporeal logic remained tenuous and so too did African American identity in the postbellum period.

Conjuring Civil War Bodies

Let me begin this epilogue by meditating briefly on two works—a particularly far-sighted text from the early twentieth century and one of its late twentieth-century successors—which direct us to the childhood fantasies and adult exercises that still seek to conjure the troubling bodies of the Civil War. Nearly a century and a half after the cessation of hostilities, the war, oddly yet fittingly, has become an attractive and appropriate topic of adolescent fiction and of adult diversion for some. Although Civil War history continues to compel any number of writers and thinkers in a variety of ways, it is through the serious playfulness of contemporarily imagined boy-soldiers and reenactors that the Civil War bodies of the nineteenth century are most powerfully rearticulated. In particular, contemporary writers attest to the persistence of the enervation, soul sickness, and battle ills the Civil War magnified, as well as to the war's potentially therapeutic, historicizing power.

By the turn of the century, the generation that had fought the Civil War was in its decline; yet memories of the war did not fade as Civil War survivors passed away but rather, were reconceived by a new generation. Well-known social reformer and Nobel Peace Prize winner Jane Addams devoted the second chapter of her autobiography *Twenty Years at Hull-House* (1910) to exploring the significance of the Civil War for Americans like her who had been children during the regional conflict. "The Influence of Lincoln" might seem an odd intrusion into a text that is otherwise dedicated to the development of Addams's social consciousness and the establishment of Hull House. However, it is not the fact of the war itself that interests Addams—not just its afflicted bodies and psyches—but also the symbolic value of those bodies and of the era's abiding icons. Addams's memories illustrate how central the Civil War remained to turn-of-the-century adults as they embarked, in James Marten's terms, upon a "quest for relevance—the need to make sense out of the war."[1] Subsequently, the Civil War was transformed into both a marvelous realm of romance and a benign instructional tool appropriate for children well into the twentieth century. Addams understands that resonant symbols of the war era epitomized the "search for the heroic and the perfect which so persistently haunts the young."[2] In Addams's case, an engraved roster of veterans' names that hung in the family living room; a local elderly couple who had sacrificed five sons to the war; and Old Abe (the Wisconsin state eagle brought into battle)— the object of a youthful pilgrimage to Madison—represent America's noblest aspirations. The hazy glow that surrounds these and other familiar symbols and that was cultivated by the tales of adults eager to shield their children from the ugliness of the war, obfuscated the war's horrifying legacy and made it an irresistible site of adventure and heroism for later generations.

Addams writes that "thousands of children in the sixties and seventies, in the simplicity which is given to the understanding of a child, caught a notion of imperishable heroism when they were told that brave men had lost their lives that the slaves might be free" (Addams 37). Southern children were taught of the equally intrepid conduct of Confederate war heroes. Although war might seem an inappropriate topic for children, Addams suggests that it is a trope particularly suited to the eager, impressionable natures of the young, for they are "as quick to catch the meaning of a symbol as they are unaccountably slow to understand the real world around them" (Addams 36). Thus children make few pretensions of grasping the "realities" of the time and place they inhabit and are more comfortable in the domain of the imaginary and suggestive intrinsic to the Civil War as its visceral reality faded. The war was doubly attractive because it represented a "connection with the great world so much more heroic than the village world which surrounded us through all the other days" (Addams 37–38). For millions of Americans quietly sequestered in rural areas such as Addams's hometown, Cedarville, Illinois, the Civil War represented travel to exotic places and courageous actions—in short, the romance of a world beyond, which could be found even in their own communities. Addams's Civil War links domestic concerns with those of the larger world—at once homey and wondrously strange. Even as an adult herself, Addams sees the Civil War through a child's eyes.

If Addams nurtured fond if inaccurate memories of the Civil War, those who grew up in the twentieth century were far removed from it, far enough to eschew Addams's sentimentality in favor of more unadulterated though equally benign versions of the great national conflict. A child during the 1960s rather than the 1860s, Pulitzer Prize-winning journalist Tony Horwitz similarly links his childhood to fond memories of the Civil War. In his best-selling travelogue *Confederates in the Attic* (1998) Horwitz attributes his early attachment to the regional conflict to the influence of his great-grandfather, an eastern European Jewish immigrant who arrived in America two decades after the war had ended. Together, they would pore over sepia-toned pictures of Civil War soldiers. "For me, the fantastical creatures of Maurice Sendak held little magic compared to the man-boys of Matthew Brady who stared back across the century separating their lives from mine," Horwitz reminisces.[3] Horwitz finds the very human participants of the Civil War more fantastic than the creatures of the most imaginative tales, their feats of heroism more unbelievable and enchanting. At the same time, those distant "man-boys" stare back at the young Horwitz, insisting that he see them as his peers—that he see himself in their faces. Like Addams, Horwitz realizes that the Civil War is inextricably bound to memories of family, even when no blood ties to Civil War participants exist. He recalls the comfort he felt when awakened by his father's war-era bugling as a child. Indeed, Horwitz concludes the book by telling us how he was been able to forge adult bonds with his father, a neurosurgeon, by attending a yearly conference on Civil War medicine with him (Horwitz 380). Thus his great-grandfather's fascination with a seemingly foreign history and his father's attraction to Civil War wounds bookend this reflection on the vitality of Civil War history in contemporary bodies and lives.

From the distant vantage point of the turn of the twenty-first century, the Civil War in many ways seems still a boyish enterprise. Like Addams almost a century before him, Horwitz also suggests that history is more available to the young; while on a memorable visit to Shiloh, he supposes, "When I was a boy, the field would have instantly filled with smoke and flame and shrieking rebels. But now, as a fantasy-impaired adult, I found myself glancing around self-consciously to make sure no one was watching" (Horwitz 170). Horwitz thus connects the conjuring of history to the artlessness and receptivity of unformed adolescent minds. I add that it is the changeable, unwieldy nature of adolescent bodies that also produces this affinity. Such a connection is not so surprising given that in the historical chronology of a personified nation, the Civil War is often explained as the country's troubled adolescence, characterized by its warring internal passions and uncontrollable bodies.[4] Although not properly ill, adolescent bodies are by definition transitional—capricious and insufficient, compromised beings on their way to becoming something steadier. In contemporary juvenile texts as varied as fact-based, imaginary diaries, history books, and time travel fantasies, which I survey in this epilogue, the mutability of the Civil War is conveyed through its attachment to these adolescent bodies. The protagonists' escapades rarely put them in real danger—their bodies prove impenetrable, while their adolescent foibles safely register the instability of a culture at war.

Rehabilitation is achieved, at least in theory, through the natural and inevitable maturation of those bodies. Boys and girls grow from temperamental and unpredictable beings into even-tempered, sure-footed adults. As such, the physical trauma and emotional unsteadiness the war epitomizes are neatly contained in adolescent bodies that presumably stabilize as the war passes into history. The white boys' bodies that dominate these stories, because of their whiteness and their maleness, also hold the place for persistent fictions of corporeal stability. The fact that, comparatively speaking, so few fictions imagine girls in a war context suggests that they have been discouraged from playing what is clearly a boy's game.[5] In boys' fiction, homebound white girls appear most commonly as plot devices, whereas still-enslaved African Americans are largely absent from the scene. Yet even young white men's bodies do not suffice to permanently steady Civil War corporeality and the stories that try to accommodate it. Ultimately, the promise of bodily rehabilitation through maturation is endlessly deferred, for if the Civil War remains the means of expressing amorphous, invisible ills as well as the site of bodily rehabilitation, then its expressive and healing powers must be forever lost at adulthood. The Civil War's corporeal and psychic (ir)resolutions are maintained as part of an unrecoverable past.

Horwitz concludes that his journey to Southern Civil War strongholds, which comprises the bulk of *Confederates in the Attic*, has been an "attempt to rediscover that boyhood rapture," that proclivity for imagination and transformation (Horwitz 386). "Rapture" seems an especially apt word to characterize twentieth-century revivifications of the Civil War: it implies pleasure, obsession, transcendence, and even bodily and spiritual transportation. Finally, I end this project by linking childhood renditions of the war and modern-day reenactments, but not to suggest that adult fascination with the war is inherently childish. Rather, I want to highlight the ways that the Civil War is still inextricably bound to the insubstantialities of bodies and histories—both to their insufficiencies and their potentialities. It is no coincidence that "encampments" sponsored by the Grand Army of the Republic (GAR)—the most powerful veterans' group of the late nineteenth-century—began appearing as a sporting and adventurous youth culture was emerging. Starting in the 1880s, GAR members would gather, wear old uniforms, sleep in tents, and stage sham battles.[6] These events were the precursors of modern reenactments described in texts such as Horwitz's that are, then, twice removed from the seriousness of the "real" war. Modern reenactors combat the mutability of history and the transience of historical bodies through their efforts to get all of the material details just right. Indeed, the most rabid reenactors approach the hobby as an extreme sport, losing weight and manufacturing physical discomforts in order to evoke a "period rush"—a moment of corporeal and historical transubstantiation. In this way, they attempt to get inside the heads of Civil War-era Americans, to get (un)comfortable in their skins. Ironically, the deprivations endured during Civil War reenactments are assigned rehabilitative power. Only the extraordinary bodily suffering of the Civil War—conjured now via the growing pains of adolescents or the self-imposed sufferings of reenactors—are seemingly able to express the inner ills of modern Americans.

I conclude that it is the bodies of the Civil War that attract us still, that are the core of its seemingly inexplicable, inexhaustible fascination. Many attempt to obscure the therapeutic potential of the Civil War for traditionally marginalized Americans emphasized in many nineteenth-century renderings of the event, instead reinscribing the apparently immutable differences between African Americans and whites, men and women. "Men were men and women were women. It was less complicated," one white female reenactor tells Horwitz while busily scrubbing clothes in a washtub (Horwitz 134). While some white women find performances of the "simpler" gender roles of the Civil War era comforting, few African Americans find respite in weekend excursions to the slave past. Though they still lay claim to the rehabilitative power of Civil War service through the production of history books, novels, and films, African Americans seldom participate in reenactments, eschewing the historical racism reanimated there. Ironically, Horwitz and others suggest that some neo-Confederates seem to have adapted to their own purposes the strategies of legitimization that I argue were developed by Negro Civil War historians in the nineteenth century. The persistent hurts of a defeated region (or of the instability of whiteness, economic disadvantage, personal crisis, and so on) are seemingly alleviated by the conjuring of Civil War bodies, while the revitalization of Reconstruction's consensual racism conventionally promises white vigor through the maintenance of the familiar racial Other. Yet the repeated resuscitation of these old prejudices suggests that they do not suffice; they do not effect the cure for regional or racial ills.

The contemporary texts I turn to here still attempt to manufacture palpable, material links to the past: accurate clothing, physical pains, blood ties, geographic sites. Many reenactors want to do more than remember the war and its heroes, and they wish they could do more than play at war—they want to be at war, to become Civil War-era citizens. Ironically, many reenactors seem to believe, at least implicitly, that inhabiting Civil War bodies can save them from the fragmentation, enervation, and moral ambiguity of modern life, of adult existence.[7] Again and again, both the authors of children's fiction and those who write of adult reenactments insist that the Civil War era was a "simpler" time or a "bigger" era: a time when life was less cluttered, affections and passions more sincere, and the delineation between right and wrong clearer (Horwitz 16, 30). Both adolescent fictions and depictions of Civil War reenactors value a culture of moral extremism, or at the very least yearn for a time without modern, adult responsibilities. However, Horwitz demonstrates that authentic, corporeally-based connection to the war is reached only fleetingly. Perhaps any sort of historical peregrination is only a self-induced hallucination after all, these texts suggest. The hallowed grounds the war was fought on, the clothing it was fought in, the language in which it was expressed, are seemingly never authentic enough. Civil War bodies are just always out of reach and so, then, is Civil War history and its rehabilitative power.

Living History

Recent historical juvenile fictions ably explore the connections between transient Civil War bodies and the historicizing imperative of the regional conflict. Powerful educational publisher Scholastic Books produces two related series: "Dear America," girls' fictional diaries situated at different points throughout American history, and "My Name Is America," boys' fictional diaries that are similarly constructed. Notice that girls address America as a national entity apart from them, whereas boys claim title to the nation—they are America. Predictably, then, whereas the "Dear America" books set in the Civil War circumscribe their heroines in domestic settings, "My Name Is America" books take us to the battle-front. In *The Journal of James Edmond Pease: A Civil War Union Soldier* (1998), Jim Murphy makes history writing necessary to his boy-soldier's war work and to his survival.[8] The textual substantiation of bodily experiences implicit in historical accountings thus remains at play in contemporary fiction. Our hero, sixteen-year-old James Pease, begins his diary, "I have been told to keep a record of what we do," and the rest of the text responds in part to the dictates of his commanding officer, Lieutenant Toms (Murphy 3).

Toms, who we later find out is a schoolteacher in civilian life (Murphy 28), instructs Pease throughout the war, occasionally reading over the journal and correcting his historical method. Pease's first entry reflects briefly on his own adolescent inadequacies and the monotony of the regiment's work. Toms pronounces it "all wrong" and tells Pease to "'Put in details'" and "keep 'an accurate and honest account'" (Murphy 3). In asking for "details" Toms reiterates modern historical method, wherein the gathering of a number of small observations will eventually be consolidated into a complete whole. Yet what Toms means by "details" continues to elude poor Pease. In efforts to help him out, Toms advises that he "'start with the date and the rest will follow naturally,'" setting a priority for Pease's efforts. Later, he asks Pease to list all of the men in the company, "being careful to give their proper ages and spell all names correctly" (Murphy 8). Finally, Pease is told to write "'brief histories of each of the men'" (Murphy 14). Thus Toms attempts to instill an ethos of statistical persons. Verifiable details—names, dates, parents, and professions—are the foundations of a proper history.

However, Pease's adolescent enthusiasms and emotional dramas inform his text, wreaking havoc with Toms's historical method. After reading Pease's account of his run-ins with the regimental bully, a spontaneous snowball fight, and a clumsy culinary accident, Pease tells us, "Lt. Toms read this journal and said, 'Good God, Corp., next you'll be putting in recipes for pie!' He then said I did not have to write so much and that when I did it should be something 'truly interesting or significant, and generally of a military nature'" (Murphy 49). Pease's attention to the soul sickness diagnosed by the USSC—to his own hopes and fears and to the dissension and attachments that distinguish his regiment— are feminized by Toms when he allies Pease's detailed sharing of emotion with the domestic act of exchanging pie recipes.

In "About the Author" Murphy confesses that he never found the Civil War history Toms seeks to elicit very interesting when he was in school. "The politicians and generals all seemed to write in the same stiff, florid style, and the war was always described in overly complex military terms" (Murphy 170). Thus Murphy concedes that traditional schoolbook versions of the war—the sort of history Toms demands of Pease—does not convey its fullness to modern readers. Murphy's aside is not insignificant, given that the Civil War stories that schoolbooks have offered during the last 100 years have great cultural potency.[9] For example, the powerful *Barnes's Histories*, which enjoyed perhaps the longest extended popularity of any school history during the late nineteenth and early twentieth centuries, typified the "catalog" style to which Murphy surely refers, featuring numbered paragraphs and bold print highlighting important events and individuals. The narrative of the Battle of Antietam is typical of the hundreds of textual items that comprised many catalog histories:

Battle of Antietam (September 17).—Lee fell back west of Antietam (an te'tam) Creek, and sent off couriers to hasten the return of his troops at Harpers Ferry. Fortunately for him, McClellan delayed his attack a day, and in the meantime Jackson arrived. The Union army was over 80,000 strong, and the Confederate but half that number. The Union right, under Hooker, advanced impetuously, but was repulsed. The struggle was long and obstinate. The Union left, under Burnside, advanced too late to relieve the pressure on the right. Night ended this bloody fight. The morning found neither commander ready to assail his opponent. That night Lee retired unmolested across the Potomac. Six weeks after, the union army also crossed in Virginia.[10]

This is monotonous fare by modern standards, at once overly specific and disappointingly vague, painting every little turn of the battle in broad strokes.[11] At the same time, Civil War generals' names are invoked again and again to stand in for all of the forces under their command, giving readers the impression that great warriors were pitted against each other in strategic battles. For example, another early schoolbook historian, D. H. Montgomery, writes, "From June 25 to July 1 (1862), Lee and McClellan were engaged in a number of desperate fights around Richmond, known as the 'Seven Days' Battle.' Lee captured many guns and prisoners."[12] This page is faced by a large portrait of General Lee. Thus the narrative encourages readers to follow the gaming exploits of extraordinary individuals. The many diseased, wounded, and dead bodies of the soldiers are obscured by the enlarged shadows of representative white men.

Murphy's text responds to the insistent efforts of early historians to stabilize Civil War history and reduce the corporeal complexities that inhered there; he links Pease's adolescent textual meanderings, and by extension the mode of historicizing most suited to tellings of Civil War bodies, to a modern ethos. For example, Pease notes that Lt. Toms is haunted by memories of a battlefield mistake. After another battle, Toms notices Pease transcribing the events of the day and asks to look them over. "He said I got it pretty much right except that he had not been nervous," Pease reports (Murphy 13). Thus Toms censors the history, attempting to excise debilitating nervousness—like other historians, he makes the story standard and his body stable. Pease's volatile body and heightened sensitivities prompt him to record the volcanic underpinnings of the inner life. In this way, he reconnects the Civil War, amorphous ills, and history in ways that hearken back to the nineteenth century.

At the same time, Pease's experiences also dramatize the potential rehabilitative power of Civil War history writing. Orphaned and then abandoned by his guardians, Pease fervently believes he is dogged by bad luck. Plagued now by obsessive thoughts of battlefield ferocity and of the omnipresent dead, he wonders, "Is this another part of my bad luck—to remember?" (Murphy 40). It is his ability to be haunted that distinguishes his mode of history writing. Yet Pease's penchant for remembering turns out to be good luck rather than a curse, for his journal literally saves his life. He is shot in battle, but finds when he removes his shirt that the journal had stopped the bullet: "The cover, which is of hard board, had a clean hole in it and the ball itself was lodged inside, having made a journey all the way to the entries about Gettysburg" (Murphy 36). The materiality of his memories saves him. History is symbolically solid, a defense against the specter of death. Pease later writes that he would like a new book—one without bullet holes—for "it has more history about it than I want to recall"(Murphy 59). Thus history and injury are linked; his Civil War journal literally bears the scars of battle. The extratextual meaning of the journal resides in its materiality as well. In this way Pease's sensibility echoes contemporary attention to the material traces of war and the power of objects to act as mediums of history, just as his remarkable ability to escape injury points to the relative safety reenactments provide modern warriors.

Like Crane's Henry Fleming, Pease's battlefield anxieties are cured by his passage from adolescence to manhood via his adventures in the Civil War. Initially, he is infantilized by his superiors, who tease, " 'When we come under fire, you hug the ground like a baby hugs its mother's teat' " (Murphy 4). However, as the days pass Pease is singled out for his thoughtless heroism, his quiet reliability, and, particularly, his valued "record-keeping" abilities. We learn that he has achieved the rank of second Lieutenant by the end of the war. Part of Pease's maturation derives from his ability to respond to the violence of another young soldier, Shelp, whose verbal threats and explicit challenges to Pease's authority make the pacifistic Pease "worry about the one who is marching along with me as well" as the enemy (Murphy 80). War service proves essential in teaching boys how to handle bullies. At the end of the journal Peace decides he can handle Shelp "just as I can handle Reb sharpshooters, my curse, and Army coffee" (Murphy 146). His survival through the gauntlet of the Civil War helps him conquer his adolescent insecurities and prepares him for the battlefields of the working world.

Indeed, Pease's burgeoning long-distance romance figures as prominently in his journal—and in his maturation—as his military endeavors. After receiving a letter from Sarah, his tent-mate's fourteen-year-old sister, Pease confesses the letter "was short and I am not sure Lt. Toms would think it 'truly interesting and significant,' but I certainly do" (Murphy 50). Johnny, the tent-mate, teases Pease that "he was going to write Sarah and say that I 'pined' for her so much that the earth shook and exploded under my feet" (Murphy 66). Adolescent lovesickness contracted through battlefield service is the volcano that shakes Pease's world. As his correspondence with the idealized Sarah proceeds, Pease dreams that he has asked her to marry him and awakes convinced that he has nothing to offer a wife or children. However, upon further thought he decides: "Well, James, you have survived a number of fights and even been made a sgt. over others, so maybe you are ready to be wed" (Murphy 125). His sheer persistence convinces him that he is an adult man, steady enough to take on the responsibilities of a family. At the end of the journal, as he heads toward Sarah and her family, Pease writes, "I am heading toward people who count on me and need me, even if just a little. I will probably never be a very brave soldier, but I think I can do my job and do it in an honorable way" (Murphy 146). He eschews his "bad luck" and becomes self-possessed and stable through the trials of the war.

Although Pease's new, white family will help make a man of him by relying on him, Pease's thoughtless reliance on an African American family teaches that African Americans are mere conveniences in the lives of white men. Separated from his regiment during a heated battle, Pease finds himself alone and injured, wandering through unfamiliar Southern territory. After almost being captured by rebels, he stumbles upon the cabin of a poor, enslaved woman, Sally, who, inexplicably, takes him into her home and shares her meager food supply with him. When he collapses on the cabin's one bed, Sally sings gently to him, making the orphaned boy feel safe and mothered. "No one who sings you to sleep would just forget about you," the boy reasons (Murphy 126). In this way, the text reinscribes traditional stereotypes about African Americans, and African American women in particular; Sally and her family exist in the text solely to serve Pease's needs. Indeed, Sally speaks French, a language that is foreign to Pease; her comments go untranslated in the text, and her thoughts remain incommunicable to us. Later, when Sally and her family decide to run from slavery, Pease becomes one of their party; indeed, Sally's nephew, Davie, rubs mud on Pease's hands and face so that he will not be recognized by the rebels. His blackface performance merely represents Pease's own vulnerability and does not apparently undermine racial difference. Although his experience with kind African Americans is supposed to teach Pease and his young white audience racial tolerance, it implies that African Americans were extraneous to the war effort, kind Uncle Toms and Aunt Chloes who nurture white boys and yet make no demands on them. At the end of the narrative the African American family that had ensured Pease's survival to manhood has been whisked away to St. Louis by the Union Commission, never to be heard from again (Murphy 151).

I believe that the messages conveyed through children's histories and fiction, particularly the war's alliance with unstable bodies and the foundations of history, were instrumental in nurturing the twentieth-century psychological function of the Civil War and in authorizing reenactments. Adolescents' bodies are as mutable as the Civil War history we seek to know; like the historical project, they evolve toward a seemingly definitive end. Yet adolescent adventures in the Civil War, like reenactments, pose no real threat to the safety of those who participate. Though their practiced exertions leave them tired and dirty, reenactors don't bleed and they don't suffer from war-inflected illnesses. As Elizabeth Young notes, authenticity is observed insofar as the "wounds are make-believe, battlefields have been sanitized as tourist sites, and actors play roles that are only as permanent as their costumes."[13]

Transforming dangerous, real-life situations into the imaginative playground of the young is clearly a convention of the adventure genre—the Civil War is not the only historical event that receives such loose treatment. However, Civil War narratives gain additional resonance when one notes the development, first of turn-of-the-century pageants sponsored by the GAR and, subsequently, of Civil War reenactments. Young Pease's adventures in some ways mirror the history of Civil War pageantry: just as his harmless escapades are crucial recitals of the "real" war, twentieth-century reenactors recreated the rituals of the GAR veterans who gathered at turn-of-the-century encampments and engaged in military theatrics.[14] Certainly reenactments are not merely the childish play of grown men and women: as many Civil War scholars have shown, reenactors consider themselves serious students of the Civil War and practitioners of "living history." Indeed, reeanacting is a logical realization of nineteenth-century Civil War bodies and histories. It is here that we can see how the barbarous carnage of the Civil War has become not only a popular hobby, but also the site of adolescent adventure, a visceral tragedy, a psuedoreligion, and a national obsession.

A brief look at some contemporary representations of reenactments may reveal what Civil War pageantry offers weekend warriors and explain why the Civil War is still allied at once with unnerving instabilities and the possibility for rehabilitation. In a fascinating statement defending reenactors, *Camp Chase Gazette* publisher Bill Hoschuh argues that reenactors pursue their hobby because they want to do more than read about history: "They want to *feel* what happened."[15] Once the imaginative site of ontological unease—of nineteenth-century Americans' *inability* to feel—the Civil War is now often associated with invigorating diversion. As the reigning popular expert on reenactments, R. Lee Hadden writes, "Doing without modern clothing and incidentals will teach you more about the time period than books. It is an excellent break from modern stress, too."[16] Through bodily discomfort, the amorphous ills of modern Americans will be eased. The material accoutrements of the Civil War have become so crucial to reenactors because they are used to elicit the appropriate sensations from their participants' bodies. Best-selling books such as Juanita Leisch's *Who Wore What? Women's Wear, 1861–1865* (1995) and *Illustrated Catalog of Civil War Military Goods: Union Weapons, Insignia, Uniform Accessories, and Other Equipment* (1985) make habiliment a primary source of historical truth. Hadden continues, "It is enjoyable to wear different clothing, and to learn and talk about what you feel and find out when you live another lifestyle" (Hadden 14).

Here the performance of living history functions like a talking cure, leading reenactors back to their bodies and to their feelings.

Neil Johnson's juvenile history book *The Battle of Gettysburg* (1989) affiliates history, performativity, adolescence, and adult reenactments. According to the introductory "Author's Note," this book was written in part to commemorate the 125th anniversary reenactment of the Battle of Gettysburg. Although the text of the book conventionally relates the military details of the three-day battle fought at Gettysburg, the accompanying pictures tell another story. The book is copiously illustrated with black and white photos of the 1988 reenactment. Johnson reasons in his "Author's Note," "I like to think that if the Civil War photographers had used today's cameras and film, their photographs of the battle might have looked like these."[17] Thus he implies that the bodies and actions of the Civil War are precisely commensurate with those of the 1988 reenactors. Horwitz believes photographs of Civil War soldiers are a crucial part of the event's signifying power, for they make the event seemingly accessible: "Without photographs, rebs and Yanks would seem as remote to modern Americans as Minutemen and Hessians" (Horwitz 386). Civil War photos serve as mirrors in contemporary tellings of the Civil War, allowing modern boys and girls to "see themselves" in those who lived so long ago. Thus photography makes the Civil War knowable to us in a modern idiom; the bodies of the Civil War, the personalities that are conveyed through eye and expression, are made imaginable and ultimately replicable. Indeed, Johnson suggests that cameras and film, not immutable people, make and frame historical difference. He asserts that contemporary photographs of the 1988 reenactment might be more accurate than those taken during the Civil War, for the primitive photographic equipment of Matthew Brady, Alexander Gardner, and Timothy O'Sullivan did not allow them to photograph actual battles—"they could not freeze movement" (Johnson "Author's Note"). Contemporary cameras are better able to capture bodies in motion, and, then, to historically rehabilitate them by fixing them accurately and clearly for future generations.

Given the clarity of the photos lacing the book, it seems evident that they depict contemporary people and events. However, the preeminence of the contemporary Civil War—of the war's incessant reiteration—encourages one to read the text of the book differently, more like a script describing how the battles were restaged than a history book detailing what happened more than a century ago. Contemporary bodies upstage historical veracity. For example, when Johnson writes, "After two years of fighting, many of the soldiers were poorly clothed. Some were even marching barefoot," he not only evokes the circumstances of the Civil War soldiers in 1863 but also directs reenactors as to how to

habil themselves in order to evoke those events most powerfully. Johnson goes on to tutor his young readers:

For the reenactors, it was truly a chance to live history. We can read about what
the soldiers ate in 1863, but actually eating roasted chicken around a campfire
is learning what history tasted like. We can read about what the soldiers wore
into battle, but actually marching in the hot sun wearing scratchy wool uniforms
is knowing what history felt like. We can read about the crackle of musket fire in
battle, but putting a musket to your shoulder and firing the black powder charge
inches from your ear is hearing what history sounded like. (Johnson "Author's
Note")

Thus Civil War reenactments ensure universal sensibility; our sentient
bodies are the means of historical knowledge. Johnson contends that we
can know what history "tasted like," "felt like," and "sounded like."
Evoking those sensations in our own bodies conjures history. Apparently, the Civil War tasted like chicken, felt like a woolen uniform, and
sounded like a charged musket, though the prominence of the simili-
tude "like" reminds readers that there is an authentic core that remains
out of reach. History here is not words on a page, nor a lecture from an
expert; rather, history becomes perceptible through the evocation of the
"feelings" of the bodies one seeks to know.

The conjuring of the Civil War is echoed less seriously in recent juvenile novels that take as their topics time travel to the Civil War. Time-
travel fiction points both to the reality of history, implying that modern
bodies can know the corporeal sensations endured by human beings in
another time; yet time travel is, of course, fantastic, and so too remains
the Civil War. In a recent juvenile-time travel novel, *Brothers at War*
(1997), by Margaret Whitman Blair, the main characters are two feuding
brothers, Rob and Jamie, who participate in Civil War reenactments
such as the one depicted at Gettysburg in Johnson's text, one as a Rebel
and one as a Yank.[18] A third character, a young girl named Sarah,
becomes the point of friction between the brothers in the opening of
the story. While on a break from their reenacting performances, the
three notice a photographer's tent labeled with the sign "QUICK-
SILVER IMAGES. Relive the Past through the Magic of Authentic Civil
War Photographs" (Blair 9). Like Johnson's history book, this sign
advertises photography as a means of assuring authenticity. However, in
this novel the photography is really magic. The mysterious, heavily
bearded photographer, "Alexander G" (later revealed as a feisty and
recognition-hungry Alexander Gardner) appears and explains that he
uses actual Civil War-era photographic equipment to create an "authentic" effect. The youngsters are puzzled but not overly worried when the
photographer begins to speak of Robert Lincoln and Matthew Brady as

if he knew them personally. After trespassing into Alexander's darkroom, the brothers wrangle over Sarah's attentions, tip over some chemicals, and break their photographic plate. As the "three ghostlike figures gradually emerge onto the plate," they all pass out and awake to find themselves transported to the Civil War. Here, the ghostly forms of Civil War soldiers are not transferred to the present; rather, contemporary adolescents "ghost" the past, suggesting their affinity for the Civil War's internecine violence. The angry brothers slip seamlessly into their roles as warring countrymen, while thoroughly modern Sarah bravely nurses the soldiers.

Awakening on a Civil War battlefield, the three notice initially that "everything seems so pristine, so . . . pure" (Blair 23). Such a claim supports the underlying assumption of Civil War reenactment that implies there is some great good to be derived from historical access, that the Civil War era was a less cluttered, more sincere and authentic time than our own. Reenacters often frame the necessity of their historical mission in terms of education—their wholesome examples of Civil War life will reveal this "pristine" and "pure" historical and psychic space to their audiences. In this juvenile novel, the children's thorough and accurate knowledge of Civil War history helps them to negotiate Civil War battlefields and find their way back home. Thus the historical knowledge that contemporary Civil War buffs cultivate today has real use in the Civil War; it becomes a means of survival. One brother is able to recall the location and time of one of Gardner's famous photographs, leading the finally reconciled trio back to his magic photographic tent. More important, Gardner reveals that they have time traveled because they "were wearin' something original, something real, from the Battle of Antietam period when [he] took [their] picture" (Blair 49). Thus the imperative to material authenticity has real effects here—it becomes the literal means of their corporeal and historical peregrinations.

Yet these children discover, "truth be told, living in the Civil War was no picnic. This [their time travel] would teach Rob to stop romanticizing about the Good ol' days!" (Blair 37). Weevil-infested hardtack, ubiquitous lice, body odor, exposed excrement, and the stench of dead corpses all offend the sensibilities of modern adolescents. Gardner reveals that he had time traveled to the future because he wanted to learn about modern photography: "Y'see, if I can make truly powerful pictures of the dead and wounded, and folks see the true horror of it all, maybe men will stop marching off to war" (Blair 71). Again, modern photography is posited as the means of conveying the suffering of war. Yet the children reveal that many costly wars followed on the heels of the Civil War—Gardner's photographs had no effect. On the contrary,

Horwitz emphasizes that he, like many other young boys and girls, thrilled to the pictures of the Civil War.

Though the Civil War does not offer the heroism and romance the three had expected, it does effect reconciliation between the brothers. After unlikely adventures where they meet some of the most famous figures of the Civil War (Generals Stonewall Jackson and McClellan, and Clara Barton), they become sick of the "bloody nightmare" they've stumbled into and they return to the future. "The past stinks," one of the brothers claims as he wrinkles his nose at the stench from the corpses at Bloody Lane. "Aye, but it will make a powerful picture, won't it now?" counters Gardner (Blair 140). In this way, the author suggests that it is the war's profound representability that makes it valuable and not its horrifying reality, per se. One of the brothers is injured in battle, and his infected wound is mystically healed as he time travels. Thus the war is the source of disease, but it is the *process* of history, the unpredictable interplay between past and present, that effects rehabilitation.

Reenactors know, of course, that their staged dramas do not resurrect the Civil War. However, some do seem to believe that their bodies can feel right, that proper habiliment will lead to rehabilitation. The promise of Civil War history resides in the possibility that bodily sensations are universally apprehensible and that they can be reliably and repeatedly elicited and, finally, re-membered. Yet the dramas continue—the Civil War persists in this way only through continued reenactment. We might borrow from Judith Butler to theorize the repetition necessary to create the illusion of corporeal truth. Butler argues of gender performance that it must be endlessly reiterated for "it is always and only an imitation of an imitation, a copy of a copy, for which there is no original."[19] Her work makes sense of the fact that the reestablishment of seemingly sure, previously existing gender roles is a crucial part of the reenactment. As Young suggests in her exploration of female reenactors who cross-dress as soldiers, the search for gendered and historical authenticity are affiliated through the culture of reenactment.[20] Yet the ethos of Civil War reenactment suggests that the bodies of Civil War history are similarly sustained; gender is just one component of the corporeal authenticity required of participants. A rigid adherence to minutae, a boundless knowledge industry, and incessant reenactment, among other things, obscures the lack of corporeal integrity with which Civil War texts grapple. In this context, I posit a corporeal subjectivity created by the exigencies of Civil War history.

The essential, illusory aspects of Civil War histories are evoked by reenacting expert Hadden as well, for he claims that reenactments might even be supernatural, literally raising the dead. He begins his introduction to the world of reenacting by noting that reenactments historically are tied to religious pageantry. "Because of this connection to religion, many reenactors have a mystical bent toward the hobby"; he continues:

Ghost stories and supernatural events are discussed around the campfire. Many reenactors openly discuss visions or weird experiences on battlefields and historical sites. Unknown reenactors visit campfires and then vanish with morning light. Extra soldiers are recorded on film marching in lines, who aren't recognized or remembered by the troops marching next to them. Living historians camping at historic sites mention hearing unexplained gunfire at night, smelling gunpowder fumes, and seeing apparitions. (Hadden 2)

I quote this passage at length because of the many registers of Civil War history it evokes. First, in connecting Civil War reenactments to religious rituals, Hadden makes explicit the perceived sacred nature of both events. His book functions as a bible of sorts, instructing neophytes on reenacting dress, accoutrements, behaviors, and etiquette. Though he claims that reenacting is fun, he also insists that it is a serious, pseudoreligious activity. Like spiritual pilgrims, Civil War reenactors yearn for the sublime—and for them, this is found in moments of complete authenticity. Hadden's passage implies that if properly performed, Civil War reenactments might conjure the (holy) ghosts of long-dead soldiers. Thus Civil War soldiers inhabit a half-way world, both discernible to human sense and ethereal. Phantom soldiers march side by side with the "living historians" as embodied markers of the reality of the past. Yet like ghosts and religious miracles, the reality of the Civil War can only remain a matter of faith.

Horwitz more explicitly claims the religious registers of Civil War reenactments to make sense of the compulsion of his Southern Civil War enthusiasts. Admittedly, many of the individuals he highlights in *Confederates in the Attic* are not typical of the estimated forty thousand Americans who participate regularly in reenactments. One "average reenactor" tells Horwitz, "This is a hobby, not a religion," in explaining why he refuses to eat rancid bacon. Yet it seems that the "hardcore" enthusiasts to whom Horwitz is drawn, particularly his "missionary or guru," Robert Lee Hodges, are the most keenly attuned to the enduring rehabilitative power of the Civil War (Horwitz 140). Horwitz writes of the "evangelical fervor" of Hodges, the "odd magnetism" that draws "acolytes"—including, for a time, Horwitz himself—"to the hardcore faith" (Horwitz 8, 140). Hodges's penchant for period clothing distinguishes his sacred commitment to historical authenticity. He admits, " 'I'm obsessed with my clothes. It's like I'm searching for the Holy Grail, except it's not a cup, it's a bit of gray cloth with just the right amount of dye and the exact number of threads' " (Horwtiz 388). What links the Holy Grail and a piece of cloth is faith: Hodges believes that the right piece of clothing, like the mythical Grail, will bring him closer to a divine state, for they have both touched the bodies of those whom the "disciple" seeks to conjure. It seems no coincidence that at the end of sham battles the order comes for the men to "Resurrect!" from their play-deaths on the battlefield (Horwitz 133). These performances enact historical events again and again, promising an embodied afterlife of sorts through the trope of the Civil War. Both the agonies of death and the joys of revivification are simulated in these scenes.

Throughout his travels Horwitz is also shown honored "relics" of the war—a piece of shinbone from a relative (Horwitz 32), a lock of Robert E. Lee's hair (Horwitz 56), the hide of Little Sorrel, General Jackson's horse (Horwitz 272). In these cases, actual bits of bodies are preserved and invested with historical powers. By this logic, even the sites of long-gone battles become sacred ground. One man clings to Fort Sumter, intoning, "These are the original stones and the original cannonballs." Horwitz continues, "He pressed his palms against the sun-warmed bricks and closed his eyes [singing] 'Break on through to the other side'" (Horwitz 49). Though not bodies themselves, these material markers of a significant battle touched and were touched by Civil War-era bodies, and thus contain holy residue capable, the tourist hopes, of helping him to another state of consciousness.

Given that the tourist to Sumter quotes a lyric from The Doors, a psychedelic band of the 1960s that openly experimented with drugs, it is not surprising that the "high" garnered from contact with the Civil War (via the objects that touched Civil War bodies) is often expressed as feeling the same as a drug trip. One hobbyist jokes, "I tell women I don't do drugs, I do the Civil War" (Horwitz 14). Here the reenactor testifies that he is mentally and physically altered by his reenacting exertions; though we don't know if the Civil War "drug" is meant to be recreational or medicinal, to numb or to heighten sensation, the Civil War is clearly a curative for many of Horwitz's enthusiasts. "The only Scarlett they knew back then was fever, not O'Hara. We're pussies compared to them," another buff complains (Horwtiz 138). Such a comment uses the specter of physical illness to express a larger fear about modern gender confusion and weakness. The rigors of reenactment are meant both to recall and to cure the illnesses of the war era, making men and women of those who participate.

Horwitz's hardcores profess that "absolute fidelity to the 1860s: its homespun clothing, antique speech patterns, sparse diet and simple utensils" are crucial to producing a Civil War high (Horwitz 7). Some believe that not only material accoutrements but also modern bodies themselves must conform to Civil War codes. Horwitz reports that some reenactors starve themselves in efforts to slip into the bodies of their malnourished objects. Hodges leaves his tent at a reenactment and chooses to sleep outdoors in torrential rain in order to know "what it's like to be soaked and cold on the night of battle" (Horwitz 140). Others look to place to provide fidelity. One of the men Horwitz meets at Shiloh hopes that his great-grandfather's Civil War rifle will work like a dowsing stick: "I'm half hoping this gun will start glowing and shaking and getting real heavy. You know, telling me exactly where my great-grandfather picked it up" (Horwitz 163). Horwitz's travels through Southern battlefields reveal how important precise geography is to the project of rehabilitating Civil War bodies, and yet how elusive such a project proves, as suburban sprawl has covered over the great landmarks, many of which, he discovers, were mismarked in the first place. One Park Ranger points out the "'ghost marks' on the landscape" that the war left behind, and seems to promise that these previously overlooked geographic markers of burial pits and trenches might be able to show where events "really" happened (Horwitz 176).

Still other Southern enthusiasts see themselves as connected to the event through blood. Horwitz notes, much as turn-of-the-century Negro historians had of African American troops, that Confederates have "a blood tie to a patch of American soil that I never would," for the blood and bones of their ancestors mingle literally with the soil (Horwitz 175). Indeed, Horwitz writes that half of modern white Southerners are descended from Confederates. One of these women claims she cannot help but care about the Civil War, for her family lives on through it: "But they [Northerners] don't have the family Bibles we do, filled with all these kinfolk who went off to war and died. We've lost so much" (Horwitz 26). Thus she implies that the wounds of war are still felt in modern bodies. Like the bone and bits of hair that make reliquaries of many Civil War museums in the South, the bloodlines of thousands of modern Southerners corporeally tie them to the past—indeed makes it alive in them. These folks see their connection to their ancestors as providing a solid foundation in a terrifying modern world. One man turns to Civil War genealogy at a low-point in his life: "I was trying to get my life back together," he claims. He is saved by "connection with [his] past that [he] can reach out and grab hold to" (Horwitz 29). Thus, the familial bodies of the Civil War are the means of re-membering contemporary lives, of putting things back together again and healing modern ills.

What seems to attract many of the people Horwitz interviews to the Civil War is the desire for a "period rush," as the hardcore reenactors describe it. A successful reenactment should produce a moment of corporeal and temporal transcendence that takes the reenactor (or even the common visitor to a battlefield) out of time and space and solves the problems of history. Several of the Civil War enthusiasts Horwitz interviews talk about how, ideally, history becomes more real to them than the present. "Sometimes after weekends like this, it takes me three or four days to come back to so-called reality," one reenactor brags about his success in transcending reality (Horwitz 11). Even those who immerse themselves in books instead of battlefields are susceptible, one writing, "When I'm reading, I feel like I'm there, not here. And when I finish I feel content, like I've been away for a while" (Horwitz 30). Why psychic travel to one of the bloodiest and deadliest eras in American history should provide "content[ment]" is ultimately explained by a theory of Civil War rehabilitation. As Dennis Hall contends, the "tactile, sensual, aesthetic, the material culture of reenacting" that persuade the reenactor that he or she can "participate in the Civil War world" is "not different in kind from that allowing the reenactor to participate in the 1990s world."[21] Yet the Civil War is invested with magical, religious, and, most important, healing powers that counteract the bodily instabilities that plague us now, as they plagued the Civil War writers I've examined.

At the center of *Confederates in the Attic* is Horwitz and Hodges's "Civil Wargasm" a "dreamy, religious . . . holy trek" through the Civil War battlefields of the mid-Atlantic states and upper South. In calling the trip a "Wargasm" and talking about the craving for historical "hits" (visits to identifiable historical sites) that propels the trip, Horwitz likens the sensations evoked by the trip to a sexual or chemical buzz. In doing so, Horwitz, via Hodges, translates the experience into corporeal language that makes it more apprehensible to readers and also duplicatable. The trip is completed quickly in order to get as many "hits" as possible in the shortest amount of time. Horwitz and Hodges travel in fetid period uniforms; they eat little food, take no showers, and sleep rarely and fitfully, camping out of doors in order to heighten the period rush. The physical discomfort is, in large part, the means of transcendence. Hodge claims that on the Gasm, "bug bites are spiritual. You're lying there listening to mosquitoes buzz in your ear, trying to sleep, and thinking, 'This is what They experienced. This is the real deal'" (Horwitz 212). Like monks, hardcores scourge their bodies in order to feel the suffering—and to beckon the divinity—of their heroes. The body does not lie, apparently; in this world, its pains, not its pleasures, seem the only ahistorical markers of a knowable past. After days of deprivation, Horwitz experiences his own period rush at Gettysburg: "My heart began thudding, more from excitement than exertion. I felt suddenly *lightheaded. This is it. Plunging over the world's roaring rim*" (Horwitz 278). He feels himself thrust out of this world and into . . . we know not where, for the sight of a plastic sword and the sound of camera shutters bring him back to the present. Yet Horwitz's rhetoric likens his experience to a death of sorts; the italics indicate that he is speaking in another voice, at the very least.

However, bodily deprivation is not the only means to the past. Horwitz also suggests that the Civil War is ever present in the correct environment and can be revealed to those sensitive to its presence. As Jane Addams had claimed in 1910, children are more attuned to the "meaning of a symbol" than to the "real world around them"; this is a psychic state cultivated by Civil War enthusiasts. For example, Horwitz details his predawn trip to Shiloh battlefield on the anniversary of the engagement fought there. Popular historian Shelby Foote had described his own extrasensory experiences there to Horwitz: "If the light and the leaves and the weather are right . . . I swear I can see and hear soldiers coming through the trees" (Horwitz 155). Notice that Foote's environment is largely responsible for allowing the vision, whereas his preternaturally keen senses are responsive to the bodies of history. Later, in the predawn light and the easy company of strangers also visiting Shiloh to commemorate the battle, Horwitz himself sees a shape in the dark and confesses, "There was a murmur of voices and I thought I could see the silhouette of a rifle. It was just as Foote had described; you could almost see soldiers coming through the trees" (Horwitz 161). One of Horwitz's companions summons such reincarnations, bringing to mind a scene from the movie, *Patton*, in which the general hears trumpets on an ancient battlefield "like he's been there before, way back when" (Horwitz 162). Ironically, such yearnings, expressed on the ground of a brutal slaughter, might be read as efforts to stave off death and to stabilize history: if there is some mystical or genetic connection to the past, some inner ear attuned to Civil War battle, then history is never remembered or reenacted—it does not suffer the instability of the *re*. Rather, those experiences are always alive in modern bodies and lives. Concurrently, the men who stand on the field of Shiloh today know that their "battles" will echo through the lives of those who follow. Perhaps the fear of being soft and unequal to the rigors of the battlefield signal the anxiety that their exploits will not be loud enough to reverberate through time.

Indeed, Hodges and his compatriots object to the term "reenactor," preferring "living historian" or "historical interpreter." Although the preference is never explained fully, one can connect the *re* in *reenactor* to the *re* in *rehabilitation*: both words signify a solid, healthy, originary body or action that one is trying to recapture. Even the term "hardcore" connotes something definite and concrete at the center of it all. Living Civil War historians still adhere to the logic of health and history that compelled nineteenth-century writers of the Civil War, for they look to bodies as marking the existence of the event. Like their nineteenth-century precursors, hardcores also want to eliminate the *re*, to sever it from *enact* and *habilitate.* Indeed, the *re* marks both the existence and the essential instability of history—its unbridgeable distance from us. Thus the goal of "doing it right" must become an end in and of itself; one reenactor claims "I'd take the chance of being killed just to see what it was really like to be under fire in the War" (Horwitz 16). Yet Horwitz reveals that by the end of his journeys Hodges and his compatriots rarely participate in reenactments anymore because "the most authentic moment of any battle couldn't be reproduced"—gunshot, wounding, and "real" death, the sheer number of which distinguish this war and constitute its fascination (Horwitz 126). Here, again, lies the essential and conjoined instability of bodies and histories.

Injury, dismemberment, and especially death, suffered within the context of battle are the bodily experiences that hold the war's deepest meaning. Death is the beginning and the end of history. But it ultimately is the place we cannot go and return to tell the tale. Even if injury is sustained at a reenactment (as it often is) it does not conjure the "real" and profound rehabilitations the war epitomizes. Thus the Civil War continues to fascinate and confound, providing resonant shorthand for the vital issues that coalesced during the regional conflict and remain unresolved to this day. From volatile, formative teens to unyielding, aged veterans, from statistical persons to fantastic travelers, and from unnerved to rehabilitated forms—the Civil War's corporeality continues to elude and yet to accommodate. We return to the Civil War in search of health through disorder, home through travel, maturity through youth, safety through danger. As a historicizing trope, the Civil War is the place we desperately want to get back to, and yet it is also the place we have never really been. In this way, it represents the (im)possibility of corporeal knowledge itself. As many Civil War enthusiasts proclaim, they continue to pursue knowledge of the conflict because they want to keep the "true story" "alive" (Horwitz 318). Such claims imply that the stories of the Civil War require a body of some sort, or at the very least a sentience, an unpredictable liveliness that makes the writing of Civil War history possible and yet endlessly changeable. Ultimately, it is the uneasy and uncounted dead of the Civil War that are the foundation of subsequent American cataclysms and histories, pressing the unnerved bodies of those who remain to an accurate accounting: to the promise of rehabilitation.

Notes

Introduction

1. "The Lounger," editorial, *Harper's Weekly* August 10, 1861: 499.
2. This excerpt from "Battle of Bull Run, July, 1861" is in Whitman's *Specimen Days*, a series of diary-like sketches published in 1882 but written over the course of the previous twenty years. In *The Portable Walt Whitman*, ed. Mark Van Doren (New York: Penguin, 1973) 407.
3. *Harper's Weekly* August 10, 1861: 491.
4. See "Year That Trembled and Reel'd Beneath Me" and "The Wound-Dresser" in *The Civil War Poems of Walt Whitman* (New York: Barnes & Noble Books, 1994) 55, 56–59.
5. John William De Forest, *Miss Ravenel's Conversion from Secession to Loyalty* (1867; New York: Holt, Rinehart & Winston, 1955) 11. Rebecca Harding Davis, *Bits of Gossip* (Boston: Houghton, Mifflin, & Co., 1904) 110.
6. Fittingly, renowned Hudson River school painter Frederick E. Church shifted his artistic focus from majestic visions of sublime American landscapes to oversized paintings of roiling, red Central American volcanoes during the war era. Nothing familiar or native could represent the panic gripping Americans. One art historian claims Church's 1862 masterpiece *Cotopaxi* was a "painted parable of the Civil War." See *Frederic Edwin Church: An Exhibition Organized by the National Collection of Fine Arts* (Washington, D.C.: Smithsonian Publications, 1966) 17. In *Creation and Renewal: Views of Cotopaxi by Frederic Edwin Church* (Washington, D.C.: National Museum of American Art and Smithsonian Institution Press, 1985), Katherine Manthorne agrees that Church "associated war and national strife with geological upheaval." In particular, Manthorne supposes that the "lifeless landscape" surrounding Church's Equadoran volcanoes might have reflected the devastation of the American South (48).

As Cecelia Tichi demonstrates, postbellum writers further developed a "volcanic geopolitics" to represent subsequent upheavals of social bodies. See her "Pittsburgh at Yellowstone: Old Faithful and the Pulse of Industrial America," *American Literary History* 9.3 (Fall 1997): 522.
7. "The Real War Will Never Get in the Books," *The Portable Walt Whitman*, 482–84; Daniel Aaron, *The Unwritten War: American Writers and the Civil War* (New York: Oxford University Press, 1973). In his excerpt from *Specimen Days*, Whitman proclaims that it is best that the "real war will never get in the books," for he does not wish the "seething hell and the black infernal background of countless minor scenes and interiors" to continue to wreak its havoc on American psyches (483). Aaron reinterprets this literary void as the outcome of "spiritual censorship," which encouraged the excision of the more unsavory aspects of war from popular narratives (xvii). Aaron applies traditionally historical criteria to Civil War literature, looking for texts that "say something revealing about the

meaning, if not the causes, of the war" (xviii). Whitman finds the war much more amorphous and ultimately unwritable than Aaron, suggesting that the war remains "untold and unwritten," for only a "few scraps and distortions" are possible (484).

8. In "National Uprising and Volunteering," in *Specimen Days, The Portable Walt Whitman* 406.

9. Michel Foucault is the most famous scholar to similarly delineate a "network of analogies that transcended the traditional proximities" of the human sciences (xi). Such pursuits, he reminds us, are never without their costs. It is a neat coincidence that in uncovering the discursive power of the human sciences Foucault claims, "I am restoring to our silent and apparently immobile soil its rifts, its instability, its flaws; and it is the same ground that is once more stirring under our feet" (xxiv). *The Order of Things: An Archaeology of the Human Sciences* (New York: Vintage Books, 1970).

10. Hayden White writes of the utility of historical narratives: they offer "that what cannot be explained is in principle capable of being understood." *The Content of the Form: Narrative Discourse and Historical Representation* (Baltimore: Johns Hopkins University Press, 1987) 54.

For more detailed explanations of the nineteenth-century evolution of the professions of medicine and history, see Peter Novick, *That Noble Dream: The "Objectivity Question" and the American Historical Profession* (New York: Cambridge University Press, 1988); Bonnie G. Smith, *The Gender of History: Men, Women, and Historical Practice* (Cambridge, Mass.: Harvard University Press, 1998); Paul Starr, *The Social Transformation of American Medicine* (New York: Basic Books, Inc., 1982); John Harley Warner, *The Therapeutic Perspective: Medical Practice, Knowledge, and Identity in America, 1820–1885* (Cambridge, Mass.: Harvard University Press, 1986).

11. Quoted in B. Smith 105, 139, and Novick 33.

12. Foucault offers a structural explanation for the intimacy between history and medicine, positing that "history constitutes for the human sciences a favorable environment which is both privileged and dangerous. To each of the sciences of man it offers a background, which establishes it and provides it with a fixed ground and, as it were, a homeland." See *The Order of Things* 371.

13. White contends that "the normal body can have no history" because it is mythically static and exhibits no changes; without movement, there is no story. "The normal or healthy body is a negation that exists solely to mark the visibility of the abnormal form," he continues. "So let us try to think of history as inhabited by vast congeries of types of monstrous bodies," White exhorts his readers (233). Hayden White, "Bodies and Their Plots," *Choreographing History*, ed. Susan Leigh Foster (Bloomington: Indiana University Press, 1995) 229–34.

14. For an extended explanation of this move, see Novick and David Blight, *Race and Reunion: The Civil War in American Memory* (Cambridge, Mass.: Harvard University Press, 2001). Blight's project explores the many ways in which American racism was used to make memories of the Civil War palatable to postbellum survivors. He writes, "A segregated society demanded a segregated historical memory. The many myths and legends fashioned out of the reconciliationist vision provided the superstructure of Civil War memory, but its base was white supremacy in both its moderate and virulent forms" (361).

15. Most historiographical overviews of the development of the historical profession agree, as Robert J. Evans writes, that "the emerging historical profession was dominated by the view that the historian's task lay principally in the study of

the origins and development of [nation-]states and in their relationship with one another." See *In Defense of History* (New York: W. W. Norton & Company, 1999) 22. Such pursuits took on a particularly racist form in the United States. B. Smith adds that when scientific method infiltrated historical practice, it yielded "highly gendered fantasies of historical work," premised on the pliancy and/or resistance of the feminized historical archive and the potency of the masculine historical adventurer (103).

16. Introduction, *Literature and the Body: Essays on Populations and Persons*, ed. Elaine Scarry (Baltimore: Johns Hopkins University Press, 1988) xxii. Scarry focuses precisely on this notion of matter as effect: "When 'matter' goes from being a noun to being an active verb—when we go from saying of something that 'it is matter' or 'it has matter' to saying 'it matters'—then substance has tilted forward into consequence" (xxii).

17. Judith Butler, *Bodies That Matter: On the Discursive Limits of "Sex"* (New York: Routledge, 1993) 30. Gender theorists have been most intensely engaged in recent efforts to reclaim bodily matters from the void to which they supposedly have been relegated by poststructuralists. Butler does not necessarily reaffirm the primacy of matter but rather argues that to deconstruct matter is not to negate it. Indeed, like Scarry, she employs the phrase "to matter" in order to connote both "to materialize" and "to mean" (32).

Butler and others attend to sex and gender because of the way the differences encoded therein trouble universalizing theories of corporeality. Gender and sex are effects that ensure the stability of mythical origins—in this case, of fixed bodies. Although I remain keenly attuned to gender difference in this book, I want to examine it as one of an array of supposedly embodied sureties that remain troubled in texts written during the Civil War and, later, about the Civil War.

18. Evans 90, 66.

19. I employ Susan Leigh Foster's notion of "choreographing history" here, though my notion of disease links physical and psychic moves more explicitly than Foster's dancing forms. See "Choreographing History," *Choreographing History* 16, 4.

20. *Regimental Losses in the American Civil War, 1861–65* (Albany, NY: Albany Publishing Co., 1889) 575.

21. Elaine Scarry, *The Body in Pain: The Making and Unmaking of the World* (New York: Oxford University Press, 1985) 13.

22. "Unnamed Remains the Bravest Soldier," a selection from *Specimen Days* in *The Portable Walt Whitman* 425.

23. In his fine work on Whitman's relationship to medicine, Robert Leigh Davis argues that Whitman "likens the ideal democratic polity to an infirm, rather than a healthy, body. He construes as a restorative political value the incompleteness and uncertainty of the suffering body, a body subject to the constant change and rendering provisional the conditions of its care" (8). This loss of sure knowledge and endless deferral—expressed in what he terms Whitman's "convalescent writing"—produces the possibility of a "therapeutic condition" (21, 12). I agree with Davis that the indeterminacy Whitman seeks allows for the rehabilitation of those who were labeled deviant by social norms. *Whitman and the Romance of Medicine* (Berkeley, Calif.: University of California Press, 1997).

24. I refer here to the subtitle of James M. McPherson and William J. Cooper, Jr., eds., *Writing the Civil War: The Quest to Understand* (Columbia: University of South Carolina Press, 1998).

25. Recent social historians reclaim, among other things, women's experi-

ences of the war, the impact of war on the Northern home front, the war's role in the Industrial Revolution, and Northerners' formation of postbellum conciliatory culture. See, e.g., Elizabeth Leonard, *Yankee Women: Gender Battles in the Civil War* (New York: W. W. Norton, 1994); Phillip Shaw Paludan, *"A People's Contest":The Union and the Civil War* (New York: Harper & Row Publishers, 1988); J. Matthew Gallman, *The North Fights the Civil War: The Home Front* (Chicago: Ivan R. Dee, 1994); Nina Silber, *The Romance of Reunion: Northerners and the South, 1865–1900* (Chapel Hill: University of North Carolina Press, 1993); and Blight, *Race and Reunion.* Such works diverge from previous historical endeavors in their effort, as Paludan explains, to explore "the impact of the war rather than to chart its course" (xi). This social approach finds its most varied articulation in Catherine Clinton and Nina Silber, eds., *Divided Houses: Gender and the Civil War* (New York: Oxford University Press, 1992).

26. *Writing the Civil War* 7.

27. For a brief treatment of hobbyists, see James McPherson, "The War That Never Goes Away," *Drawn with the Sword: Reflections on the American Civil War* (New York: Oxford University Press, 1996) 55–65. McPherson claimed in 1996 that more than 250,000 Americans described themselves as hobbyists (55). Jim Cullen, too, addresses the general popularity of the Civil War in *The Civil War in Popular Culture: A Reusable Past* (Washington, D.C.: Smithsonian Institution Press, 1995).

28. "Nineteenth-Century American History," *Imagined Histories: American Historians Interpret the Past* (Princeton, N.J.: Princeton University Press, 1998) 166.

29. C. Vann Woodward, *Battle Cry of Freedom: The Civil War Era* (New York: Oxford University Press, 1988) xvii.

30. Robert A. Lively, *Fiction Fights the Civil War: An Unfinished Chapter in the Literary History of the American People* (Chapel Hill: University of North Carolina Press, 1957); Edmund Wilson, *Patriotic Gore: Studies in the Literature of the American Civil War* (New York: Farrar, Straus and Giroux, 1962); Aaron, *Unwritten War.*

31. Elizabeth Young, *Disarming the Nation: Women's Writing and the American Civil War* (Chicago: University of Chicago Press, 1999) 19. Sweet is interested in the "transformation of wounds into ideology" during the war, a crucial rhetorical and visual recuperation that took place in poetry and photography. See *Traces of War: Poetry, Photography, and the Crisis of the Union* (Baltimore: Johns Hopkins University Press, 1990). Diffley employs a similar approach in her consideration of magazine fiction. Here it is domestic rhetoric that "register[s] the lacerated status of Revolutionary compromises and the persistent resuscitation of Revolutionary ideals" as it negotiates the disturbing racial makeup of the new American family. See *Where My Heart is Turning Ever: Civil War Stories and Constitutional Reform, 1861–1876* (Athens: University of Georgia Press, 1992) 12. Their projects prefigure my own, for disease and wounding are clearly a subtext, saturating the critics' language as well as that of their subjects. In his study of war-era literature, Gregory Eiselein also uses the term "patients" to describe those who receive war-era benevolence. See *Literature and Humanitarian Reform in the Civil War Era* (Bloomington: Indiana University Press, 1996).

Young asserts that a more accurate consideration of Civil War literature reveals that the Civil War represents the essential instability of gender. In this way my work echoes, for we are both interested in the slippage of bodily norms evident in war-era literature. Young fills the gap in which the great war novel is supposed to reside by rewriting the literary genealogy solidified in the scholarship by Wilson and Aaron to originate with women.

Alice Fahs, a historian rather than a literary critic, also revises Aaron's pronouncements, arguing that the war was not unwritten but, rather, that the profusion of "popular war literature was vitally important in shaping a cultural politics of war" (1). The implication is that in adding new literature to the canon we will more accurately understand the war. See *The Imagined Civil War: Popular Literature of the North & South, 1861–1865* (Chapel Hill: University of North Carolina Press, 2001).

32. Historian John E. Hallwas argues that "factual" accounts of the Civil War "are not valued as self-expressions, as reconstructions of personal experience, as literary artifacts, but as contributions to our understanding of the war." This generic inflexibility in Civil War studies has cut two ways. On the one hand, as Hallwas observes, "factual" texts describing the Civil War have "not been read so much as looked into—scanned for information." On the other hand, so-called fictional accounts of the war have been valued primarily to the extent that they can reveal practical information about the war. See "Civil War Accounts As Literature: Illinois Letters, Diaries, and Personal Narratives," *Western Illinois Regional Studies* 13.1 (1990): 48.

33. Stewart Brooks, *Civil War Medicine* (Springfield, Ill.: Charles C. Thomas, 1966) 57.

34. Louisa May Alcott, *Hospital Sketches, Alternative Alcott*, ed. Elaine Showalter (New Brunswick, N.J.: Rutgers University Press, 1988) 12.

35. Introduction, *Literature and the Body* xxi.

36. "Nineteenth-Century American History" 181.

37. Hayden White, "Historical Emplotment and the Problem of Truth," *Probing the Limits of Representation: Nazism and the "Final Solution,"* ed. Saul Friedlander (Cambridge, Mass.: Harvard University Press, 1992) 38, 52. I find compelling White's exploration of the narrative and ethical limits placed upon particular historical events. However, White ends his assessment by asserting that the Holocaust is not unrepresentable but, rather, that it "requires the kind of style, the modernist style, that was developed in order to represent the kind of experiences which social modernism made possible" (52). Thus, he is not willing to abandon narrative's ability to communicate. Rather, he privileges another form of narrative.

I do not mean to effect a similar bait and switch. Indeed, Civil War historicism has proven quite useful, and my own project is contained within its limits. I do not, however, argue that because historicality has been so prominent in tellings of the Civil War that it must somehow be better suited to conveying the war's reality. Rather, I seek to explore the embodied complexities of this one powerful event.

38. Cullen, *Civil War in Popular Culture* 3.

39. Transcribed in F. B. Carpenter's *Six Months at the White House with Abraham Lincoln* (New York, 1866) 76. I am indebted to Young's work for pointing me to this quote.

40. *The Inner Civil War: Northern Intellectuals and the Crisis of the Union* (New York: Harper & Row Publishers, 1965).

41. Joan Burbick, *Healing the Republic: The Language of Health and the Culture of Nationalism in Nineteenth-Century America* (New York: Cambridge University Press, 1994). Burbick lays claim to the period 1820–80, demonstrating how health professionals asserted themselves in a variety of forums during the period to monitor and instruct a burgeoning citizenry increasingly perceived as unable to take care of itself. Although Burbick charts a subtle shift from confidence in the

nation's citizens and their apparent good health to a clear cultural anxiety about the nation's bodies, the Civil War does not figure largely in her story.

Young begins her treatment of Civil War fiction with Harriet Beecher Stowe's *Uncle Tom's Cabin*, published a decade before the Civil War began. Because of the novel's ability to elicit abolitionists' sympathies and slaveholders' ire, Young argues that any analysis of Civil War writing has two starting points: the start of the war and the publication of Stowe's novel. *Disarming the Nation* 25.

42. Historians Mary Dearing and Gerald Linderman have labeled the postwar years stretching until 1880 the "quiescent years," a time during which the wounded country and its traumatized citizenry tried to forget the war. Gerald Linderman, *Embattled Courage: The Experience of Combat in the American Civil War* (New York: Free Press, 1987) 270–71; Mary K. Dearing, *Veterans in Politics: The Story of the G.A.R.* (Baton Rouge: Louisiana State University Press, 1952) 185. Fewer novels about the Civil War were published during the 1870s than during any other decade in American history. Still, Kathleen Diffley's important excavation of Reconstruction-era magazine fiction about the war demonstrates the war's enduring appeal throughout the nineteenth century.

43. S. Weir Mitchell, *In War Time* (1884; New York: Century Co., 1912) 226.

44. Joel Pfister, "On Conceptualizing the Cultural History of Emotional and Psychological Life in America," *Inventing the Psychological: Toward a Cultural History of Emotional Life in America*, ed. Joel Pfister and Nancy Schnog (New Haven, Conn.: Yale University Press, 1997) 27.

45. Robyn Wiegman, *American Anatomies: Theorizing Race and Gender* (Durham, N.C.: Duke University Press, 1995) 4.

46. Although Lears's claim may hold true for some varieties of "martial ideals"—e.g., the Gilded Age craze for medieval knighthood—Civil War experience repudiated the "authentic life" for which his modern knights searched. T. J. Jackson Lears, *No Place of Grace: Antimodernism and the Transformation of American Culture, 1880–1920* (Chicago: University of Chicago Press, 1981). See particularly his chapter entitled "The Destructive Element: Modern Commercial Society and the Martial Ideal."

47. The senator was Carl Schurz. Cited in Eric Foner, *Reconstruction: America's Unfinished Revolution, 1863–1877* (New York: Harper & Row Publishers, 1988) 499.

Chapter 1

1. S. Weir Mitchell, Letters to Elizabeth Kearsley Mitchell, August 1864, ms. 2/0241–03, Box 4, S. Weir Mitchell Papers, The Francis Clark Wood Institute for the History of Medicine, The Library of the College of Physicians, Philadelphia, Pennsylvania (I will refer to this collection as SWM Papers). This letter is dated August, 1864. All subsequent references to Mitchell's personal correspondence refer to this collection unless otherwise noted. Mitchell's sister was an extremely important figure in his life, serving as an intellectual mate and spiritual guide. In November 1873 Mitchell wrote to his son John, "there is some gain and some disadvantage in having an outside conscience. In my case it is called Aunt Lizzy." Mitchell, Letters to John K. Mitchell, Box 5, SWM Papers.

2. Quoted in Mitchell's medical biography by Richard D. Walter, M.D., *S. Weir Mitchell, M.D., Neurologist: A Medical Biography* (Springfield, Ill.: Charles C. Thomas, 1970) 200. For complete biographies of Mitchell, see Anna Robeson

Brown Burr, *Weir Mitchell: His Life and Letters* (New York: Duffield & Co., 1929), and Ernest Earnest, *S. Weir Mitchell, Novelist and Physician* (Philadelphia: University of Pennsylvania Press, 1950). Joseph P. Lovering supplies a short biography in his survey of Mitchell's literary oeuvre in *S. Weir Mitchell* (New York: Twayne Publishers, 1971).

3. See Walter vii. For a discussion of Mitchell and his female patients, see, for example, Suzanne Poirier's work in "The Weir Mitchell Rest Cure: Doctor and Patients," *Women's Studies* 10 (1983): 15–40, and "The Physician and Authority: Portraits by Four Physician-Writers," *Literature and Medicine* 2 (1983): 21–40. In her autobiography, *The Living of Charlotte Perkins Gilman* (Madison: University of Wisconsin Press, 1988), Gilman caustically explains that "The Yellow Wallpaper" is "a description of a case of nervous breakdown beginning something as mine did, and treated as Dr. S. Weir Mitchell treated me with what I considered the inevitable result, progressive insanity" (119).

4. S. Weir Mitchell, M.D., George R. Morehouse, M.D., and William W. Keen, M.D., *Gunshot Wounds and Other Injuries of Nerves* (Philadelphia: J. B. Lippincott & Co., 1864) 25. All subsequent references are from this text and are cited parenthetically as *Gunshot.* Though Mitchell is listed as only one of three coauthors, most scholars agree that as the senior doctor and mentor of his two colleagues, Mitchell was the primary author of the text.

5. David B. Morris, *The Culture of Pain* (Berkeley: University of California Press, 1991) 15. Morris's work has been instrumental in shaping my own thinking on the cultural and temporal meanings ascribed to illness and pain. For a discussion of the doctor's role in shaping cultural norms of pain, also see Leon Eisenberg, "The Physician as Interpreter," *Comprehensive Psychiatry* 22.3 (May/June 1981): 241, 245.

6. As the story goes, Mitchell's friend was no longer surgeon general when the war ended. Consequently, the government commandeered all of the research Mitchell and his colleagues had gathered during their years at Turner J. Lane. Mitchell and his assistants painstakingly handcopied more than 2,000 pages of case studies and other notes.

Mitchell sandwiched his hospital research among the myriad duties he took upon himself during the Civil War. On July 26, 1863, he complained to his sister of the many tasks he had taken on: inspecting the 9,000 imprisoned rebels held at Fort Delaware, "attending a mélange of other folks['] practice—I say Mitchell you are going to be in town a while," as well as attending to his hospital cases. Mitchell, Letters to Elizabeth Kearsley Mitchell, Box 4, SWM Papers.

7. Deborah Journet, "Phantom Limbs and 'Body-Ego': S. Weir Mitchell's 'George Dedlow'," *Mosaic* 23.1 (Winter 1990): 89. For more detailed discussions of the tremendous influence of Mitchell's text, see Earnest 50–51, 226, Burr 112–13, and Paludan, *"People's Contest"* 326.

8. William W. Keen, M.D., S. Weir Mitchell, M.D., and George R. Morehouse, M.D., "On Malingering, Especially in Regard to Simulation of Diseases of the Nervous System," *Philadelphia Medical Journal* (October 1864): 367–94. All subsequent references are from this text and are cited parenthetically as "Malingering." Keen was given top billing on this paper.

9. "The Case of George Dedlow," *Atlantic Monthly* 18 (July 1866): 1–11. All subsequent quotations from this story are referenced internally as "Dedlow."

10. Mitchell, *In War Time* 226. All subsequent references from this text are cited parenthetically as *War Time.*

11. Morris 73.

12. On the connections between hysteria in the two periods, see Leslie Katz, "Flesh of His Flesh: Amputation in *Moby Dick* and S. W. Mitchell's Medical Papers," *Genders* 4 (Spring 1989): 1–10, and Erin O'Connor, "'Fractions of Men': Engendering Amputation in Victorian Culture," *Comparative Studies in Society and History* 39.4 (October 1997): 742–78. Katz argues that Ahab's phantom limb and its "hysterical" behavior is transformed into the body of the female hysteric in Mitchell's medical writings (6). And in her fine treatment of midcentury amputation and prostheses, O'Connor argues that dismemberment "unmanned amputees, producing neurological disorders that gave the fragmented male body—or parts of it anyway—a distinctly feminine side. Thrashing, twitching, and suffering from phantom pains, stumps showed a deep-rooted propensity for theatrical malingering that rivaled that of the hysteric herself" (744).

13. Eisenberg 241, and Howard Brody, *Stories of Sickness* (New Haven, Conn.: Yale University Press, 1987) 87.

14. Morris 42. He goes on to support this claim by citing twentieth-century studies conducted with World War II veterans, which show that soldiers do not perceive pain to the same degree as civilians.

15. See William J. Winslade, "Taken to the Limits: Pain, Identity and Self-Transformation," in *Dax's Case: Essays in Medical Ethics and Human Meaning*, ed. Lonnie D. Kliever (Dallas, Tex.: Southern Methodist University Press, 1989) 118.

16. William F. May, "Dealing with Catastrophe," in *Dax's Case: Essays in Medical Ethics and Human Meaning*, ed. Lonnie D. Kliever (Dallas, Tex.: Southern Methodist University Press, 1989) 133.

17. Brody observes, "If sickness leads us to see our bodies as being something foreign, thwarting our wills by their intransigence and unmanageability, then sickness has fundamentally altered our experience of self and has introduced a sense of split and disruption where formerly unity reigned" (27).

18. See Burr 71, and Walter viii.

19. S. Weir Mitchell's unpublished autobiography, ms. 2/0241–93, Box 16, SWM Papers

20. Journet 87.

21. Quoted in Burr 104–5.

22. Earnest tells us that each case history took five to nine pages of foolscap and recorded "name, place of birth, general health before the wound, place (geographic) wounded, description of wound, length of time before treatment, nature of treatment, extent of recovery, sensation, motion (of limb), comparative sizes of limbs if wound was in limb. A single case might be followed for as long as two years" (49).

23. Mitchell's unpublished autobiography 34.

24. Submitted to the *Atlantic Monthly* by friends without Mitchell's knowledge, "The Case of George Dedlow" was chosen as the lead story in the very next reader. [The medical department in the Civil War]: address before Physicians' Club, Chicago, Ill., Feb. 25, 1913, Box 17:22, SWM Papers.

25. See Richard Malmsheimer, *"Doctors Only": The Evolving Image of the American Physician* (New York: Greenwood Press, 1988) and Starr, *Social Transformation.* Mitchell was passed over three times for various professorships at medical universities early in his career. One supporter framed Mitchell's rejection within the terms of this professional debate in a note to his young colleague: "You know as well as I do what deep struggle is going on in scientific circles among us, and how deeply the future prospect of science in the U.S. is involved in the context. Those who study books whose chief claim to success lies in their familiarity with what others have done v. those who progress knowledge [*sic*]" Earnest 78.

26. Morris 31.

27. Stephen L. Daniel, "The Patient As Text: A Model of Clinical Hermeneutics," *Theoretical Medicine* 7 (1986): 202. Daniel claims doctors confront the "double task of interpreting both the patient and the patient's story."

28. Karen Halttunen, *Confidence Men and Painted Women: A Study of Middle-Class Culture in America, 1830–1870* (New Haven, Conn.: Yale University Press, 1982).

29. See *Gunshot Wounds* 21, 37, 113 and 115 for examples of Mitchell's "treatment" of malingerers.

30. Also see Brody 36.

31. In 1864 Thomas Frank Cullen read a paper before the Medical Society of New Jersey in which he decried the "evil" that had been advanced during the war by the "influx of all kinds of pretenders into the medical corps of volunteer forces." Cullen describes the military doctors in specifically class terms, complaining that "men who, quitting the grocery-store, the blacksmith's shop, or the factory, after a few weeks or months of real or pretended study, had boldly assumed the responsibility of human life." He then warns his audience that instead of using the tools of the doctors—the "scalpel and bistoury"—the untested tradesman might use the tools more familiar in their trades—"the catilin & the saw"—in butchering "living heroes." It is ironic, given Mitchell's and his colleagues' penchant for administering painful, unnecessary tests to their patients, that the profession was concerned that tradesmen would inflict needless suffering on the soldiers. See "Observations on the Influence of the Present War upon American Medicine and Surgery," speech read before the Medical Society of New Jersey, 1864, Library of the College of Physicians of Philadelphia. The citations in this paragraph appear on page 22 of the pamphlet. In 1869 Mitchell published another short novella, *The Autobiography of a Quack*, in which he reveals the subterfuges and moral degeneration of a man who passes himself off as a doctor. This is certainly in line with the professional crisis with which Mitchell and his colleagues seemed to be wrestling.

32. As Brody explains, "A diagnosis is indeed a gnosis; a mode of self-knowledge that creates a cosmos in its image" (10).

33. S. Weir Mitchell, Letters to William W. Keen, February 8, 1865, Box 8, and Mitchell's unpublished autobiography.

34. Cited in Earnest 46. Also see [The medical department in the Civil War], SWM Papers.

35. David Rien concludes that the ending must have "appealed to Mitchell's sense of humor." *S. Weir Mitchell as a Psychiatric Novelist* (New York: International University Press, 1952) 32.

36. Mitchell, Letters to Elizabeth Kearsley Mitchell, August 8, 1861, SWM Papers. Mitchell later found it quite amusing that "spiritualist journals seized on" George Dedlow's ending as "new proof of the verity of their belief." "Imagine that!" he amusedly writes. [The medical department in the Civil War], SWM Papers.

37. Mitchell, Letters to Elizabeth Kearsley Mitchell, SWM Papers

38. S. Weir Mitchell, Letter to George M. Gould, December 9, 1899, ms. 2/0241–93, Box 8, SWM Papers.

39. S. Weir Mitchell, Letters to W. D. Howells, December 17, 1905, University of Pennsylvania Library. Quoted in Lovering 51.

40. Mitchell's unpublished autobiography.

41. Letter from W. D. Howells to S. W. Mitchell, October 20, 1885, University of Pennsylvania Library. Quoted in Lovering 60.

42. Eugenia Kaledin, "Dr. Manners: S. Weir Mitchell's Novelistic Prescription for an Upset Society," *Prospects* 11 (1986): 202; journal excerpt quoted in Kaledin 205.

43. Tom Lutz, *American Nervousness, 1903: An Anecdotal History* (Ithaca, N.Y.: Cornell University Press, 1991) 32. For example, William Muldoon's exclusive spa offered "militaristic discipline, strict moral accountability, and incessant, rigorous exercise" to its enervated visitors.

44. *Mitchell as Psychiatric Novelist* 20.

45. Kaledin 203.

46. Daniel J. Wilson, "Neurasthenia and Vocational Crisis in Post-Civil War America," *Psychohistory Review* 12.4 (1984): 31. Wilson continues, "men coming of age in the Civil War years and after and seeking professional careers were caught in the transition from the patterns of antebellum America to the newer professional and academic patterns that would be established by the 1880s. They sought careers which did not yet fully exist and the disjunction between their life-cycle and the world of work caused the problems so evident in this generation" (35).

47. Poirier repeats the oft-told story of Howells's daughter Winifred, who was labeled neurasthenic and endured Mitchell's treatment for ten years. Throughout, she complained of excruciating, unremitting physical pain. When Winifred died, an autopsy revealed an organic cause for her illness. "The Weir Mitchell Rest Cure" 30.

48. Mitchell, Letters to John K. Mitchell, November 29, 1873, SWM Papers.

49. F. G. Gosling, *Before Freud: Neurasthenia and the American Medical Community, 1870–1910* (Urbana: University of Illinois Press, 1987) 39. It seems clear that Mitchell was also countering the therapeutic value of Freud's "talking cure." In a speech in 1913 Mitchell mocks, if today's treatments were "aided by German perplexities, we would ask the victims a hundred and twenty-one questions, [and] consult their dreams and their subconscious minds." [The medical department in the Civil War], SWM Papers, 41.

50. *The Tragedy of Macbeth, The Complete Signet Shakespeare* 5.5.13 (San Diego: Harcourt Brace Jovanovich, 1972) 1259, 1258.

51. Quoted in Burr 98.

Chapter 2

1. C. F. Sprague, "What We Feel," *Atlantic Monthly* 20 (December 1867): 740–44. Subsequent references noted parenthetically as "We Feel."

2. Jean Baudrillard, *Simulacra and Simulation*, trans. Sheila Faria Glaser (1981; Ann Arbor: University of Michigan Press, 1994) 121.

3. Baudrillard 121, 123.

4. Elizabeth Stuart Phelps, Letters to S. Weir Mitchell, November 1887, ms. 2/0241–03, Box 9, SWM Papers. Phelps initially began their correspondence with a letter praising *In War Time*. She often mentions her many illnesses, which range from her "chief disease," insomnia, and its consequent nervousness, to more general "frailties," such as a sprained back and laryngitis. Mitchell apparently offered her a prescription for her insomnia that she politely declined by expressing her commitment to homeopathy (February 3, 1887). The letters end about a year after they began when Phelps and Mitchell disagree about the effi-

cacy of women doctors, the true character of female invalids, and the validity of her beloved homeopathic remedies.

5. Elizabeth Stuart Phelps, *The Gates Ajar* (Boston: Fields, Osgood & Co., 1868) 73. All subsequent references to the novel are taken from this edition and are cited parenthetically in the text as *Gates*.

6. Phelps's father, the eminent theologian Austin Phelps, had published his own influential notion of heaven, envisioning a place where we are freed from our bodies and rewarded with "an augmented intensity of mental powers." Quoted in Lori Duin Kelly, *The Life and Works of Elizabeth Stuart Phelps, Victorian Feminist Writer* (Troy, N.Y.: Whitson Publishing Co., 1983) 30.

7. The story was published posthumously in *Harper's New Monthly Magazine* 123 (August 1911) and in book form (New York: Harper's, 1911). Infirm, eighty-one-year-old Reuben Oaks had taken to calling his wife "Peter," for her given name, Patience, did not fit the "youth and vigor" of the woman (4). Peter's strength enables her husband to fulfill his Memorial Day duties at the cemetery.

8. Ann Douglas, *The Feminization of American Culture* (New York: Doubleday, 1977) 188. Phelps's quote is in her late-life autobiography, *Chapters from a Life* (Boston: Houghton, Mifflin and Company, 1896) 97–98. Subsequent quotes cited parenthetically as *Chapters*.

9. Jane E. Schultz, "The Inhospitable Hospital: Gender and Professionalism in Civil War Medicine," *Signs* 17.2 (1992): 365. Early influential work on Civil War literature, such as Lively's *Fiction Fights the Civil War* and Aaron's *The Unwritten War*, mention women writers only tangentially and largely unfavorably. Mary Boykin Chesnutt's diary is the most commonly cited work by a woman author; however, even she, Aaron contends, "tended to view the War on the home-front as a woman and to take women's side in a man-dominated world" (*Unwritten War* 253). The anthology *Civil War Women*, edited by Frank McSherry, Jr., Charles G. Waugh, and Martin Greenberg (New York: Simon & Schuster, 1988), reprints many significant war-related stories by women. However, the editors too circumscribe this group of writers, explaining that "someone packs the knapsacks of those warriors and bids them goodbye. Someone turns back to mundane labors, to the day-to-day responsibilities of a life that has suddenly, drastically changed. Someone runs the small farms and businesses that feed the hyperactive economics of war-time. Someone rears the next generation, and answers its questions about the killing of this one" (7). Recent work, notably Diffley's *Where My Heart Is Turning Ever*, begins to explore the ways in which matters of race, political section, and gender influenced individual authors' tellings of the Civil War. Shira Wolosky recontextualizes Emily Dickinson's war-era work in particular in *Emily Dickinson: A Voice of War* (New Haven, Conn.: Yale University Press, 1984). And finally, Young's *Disarming the Nation* rewrites a literary genealogy solidified in seminal treatments of Civil War literature. Young argues that we should look to mothers, daughters, and sisters, not to fathers, sons, and brothers, for compelling narratives of the Civil War. My own work has been inspired by these and similar arguments.

10. Kelly 12. For examples of scholarship that situate Phelps's work within the sentimental religion movement, see Ann Douglas and also Christine Stansell, "Elizabeth Stuart Phelps: A Study in Female Rebellion," *Massachusetts Review* 13 (1972): 239–56, and Barton Levi St. Armand's chapter on Phelps, "Dickinson, Phelps, and the Image of Heaven," *Emily Dickinson and Her Culture* (New York: Cambridge University Press, 1984). Nancy Schnog in "'The Comfort of My Fancying': Loss and Recuperation in *The Gates Ajar*," *Arizona Quarterly* 49.1 (1993):

21–24, sees Phelps's novel in terms of the nineteenth-century mourning rituals typically assigned to women. Gail K. Smith in "From the Seminary to the Parlor: The Popularization of Hermeneutics in *The Gates Ajar*," *Arizona Quarterly* 54.2 (1998): 99–133, argues that the novel is not as radical as critics like myself have made it out to be, in that it "attempts to reconcile the long history of Christian theology, new currents in biblical criticism, the needs of the contemporary believer, and the words of the Bible in a form accessible to the ordinary reader" (124).

11. In "The Heavenly Utopia of Elizabeth Stuart Phelps," *Women and Utopia: Critical Interpretations*, ed. Marleen Barr and Nicholas D. Smith (New York: University Press of America, 1983), Carol Farley Kessler places the novel squarely within a protofeminist tradition, labeling Phelps's *Gates* novels as "political actions" providing her mostly female readers with a feminist consciousness (94).

12. *Emily Dickinson* 118.

13. For example, Douglas 200. For psychobiography of Phelps also see Carol Farley Kessler, *Elizabeth Stuart Phelps* (Boston: Twayne Publishers, 1982), and Stansell.

14. See Douglas 205, and Gary Laderman, *The Sacred Remains: American Attitudes Toward Death, 1799–1883* (New Haven, Conn.: Yale University Press, 1996). Laderman explains that the Union dead were "buried unceremoniously near where they fell during an engagement, either in individual graves or mass trenches." The exigencies of war, he continues, "challenged the conventional and deeply rooted attitude about communal responsibilities, religious solemnities, and individual respect demanded in the disposal of corpses" during peacetime (104, 103).

15. Paludan, *"People's Contest"* 316, 325, 366.

16. Halttunen, *Confidence Men and Painted Women* 172, and Martha Pike, "In Memory Of: Artifacts Relating to Mourning in Nineteenth-Century America," *Rituals and Ceremonies in Popular Culture*, ed. Ray B. Browne (Bowling Green, Ohio: Bowling Green University Popular Press, 1980) 312–13. Pike also quotes from the most popular bereavement narrative of the midcentury, Nehemiah Adams's *Agnes and the Key to Her Little Coffin* (Boston: S. K. Whipple & Co., 1857), in which Adams reveals in loving detail the splendor of his dead daughter's casket.

17. In *Lincoln at Gettysburg* (New York: Touchstone, 1992), Wills sketches the horrendous conditions of the corpses found after the Battle of Gettysburg: "The debris was mainly a matter of rotting horseflesh and manflesh. . . . Even after most bodies were lightly blanketed, the scene was repellent. A nurse shuddered at the all-too-visible 'rise and swell of human bodies' in these furrows war had plowed. . . . Soon these uneasy graves were being rifled by relatives looking for their dead—reburying other bodies they turned up, even more hastily than had the first disposal crews" (20–21).

18. Daniel Aaron, "The Etiquette of Grief: A Literary Generation's Response to Death," *Prospects: An Annual of American Cultural Studies*, ed. Jack Salzman, vol. 4 (New York: Cambridge University Press, 1979) 206.

19. Alcott, *Hospital Sketches* 25.

20. The word *mausoleum* derives from the tomb his queen then built for Mausolas at Halicarnassus about 350 B.C. It is one of the seven wonders of the ancient world.

21. Phelps's vision of domestic felicity is also a far-flung yet recognizable permutation of Kathleen Diffley's "Old Homestead" narrative. As Diffley explains,

"Old Homestead stories relied in guaranteeing that no change would topple household gods. Instead, such stories answered the generic question 'Will we survive?' by promising continuity, safety, and ultimately restoration." *Where My Heart is Turning Ever* 5.

22. Gail K. Smith argues that Phelps's novel "was not alone in its defense of analogical heavenly rhetoric," engaging in historical and contemporaneous theological and pastoral conversations about the "materialist" vs. the "abstract" heaven (116–17).

23. Frothingham quoted in Paludan 363. From "A Sight in Camp in the Daybreak Gray and Dim" in *Portable Walt Whitman* 225. Timothy Sweet also explores the implications of Christian typology in *Traces of War* 24–27.

24. See *Inner Civil War*.

25. Although Susan Curtis sees Phelps's rebellion as responding directly to the oppressive influence of her distant and exacting father, I believe that Phelps also engages more probingly with the philosophical underpinnings of contemporaneous theological study. *A Consuming Faith: The Social Gospel and Modern American Culture* (Baltimore: Johns Hopkins University Press, 1991) 143.

26. "Albums of War: On Reading Civil War Photographs," *The New American Studies: Essays From* Representations, ed. Philip Fisher (Berkeley: University of California Press, 1991) 287. For further discussions of Civil War photography also see Sweet. Matthew Brady owned fashionable galleries in Washington and New York where he attracted large and enthusiastic crowds anxious to see battlefront photographs throughout the war. Brady arranged and published his images in 1862 as *Brady's Photographic Views of the War*. Alexander Gardner, the one-time manager of Brady's Washington gallery, published his own *Gardner's Photographic Sketch Book of the Civil War* in 1866.

27. Anne C. Rose, *Victorian America and the Civil War* (New York: Cambridge University Press, 1992) 17, and Sweet 55.

28. Ann Braude, *Radical Spirits: Spiritualism and Women's Rights in Nineteenth-Century America* (Boston: Beacon Press, 1989) 25, 34, 92, 165. Phelps also spends a great deal of time delineating the compelling nature of Winifred's physical presence (see *Gates* 41). Braude notes that Spiritualists often cited the overwhelming beauty and charisma of the young, female mediums as convincing new converts of the movement's validity.

Mitchell's description of his one meeting with a clairvoyant named Mrs. Piper, arranged by William James, is quite telling in this regard. He writes in his unpublished autobiography, "She was a good-looking woman of about 35 & as we sat down, she took my hand while Mr. James made notes at the table. She stretched herself out, began to quiver, face muscles twitched, & she appeared to have a mild hysterical spasm the reality of little doubt. . . . This interview lasted for two hours & absolutely not one thing came of it. It was a babble of utter nonsense." Mitchell's unpublished autobiography, SWM Papers, 59.

29. Braude 143. However, both doctors and clergy agreed that the inherently diseased souls and frail female reproductive organs of the daughters of Eve prevented them from venturing into public realms and required male supervision. Winifred's diseased breast does illustrate the physical frailty associated with "female organs" and in some measure mitigates her power.

30. Ironically, when Spiritualists began to enact the reembodiment, seances fell apart. In the 1870s, mediums began to perform "materializations," where they typically would withdraw into a cabinet or small room from which embodied spirits would then appear. Braude 145, 176.

31. Paludan 374, 342. In *American Apocalypse: Yankee Protestants and the Civil War, 1860–1869* (New Haven, Conn.: Yale University Press, 1978), James H. Moorhead argues that the millennial impulse that is an integral part of the American consciousness was foregrounded during the war period. However, the lofty expectations raised by such rhetoric left postbellum Americans bereft. Rose, too, addresses the spiritual renewal motivating a wartime fervor akin to antebellum revivalism (63).

32. In Paludan 349.

33. Gail Hamilton [Mary Abigail Dodge], "A Call to My Country-Women," *Atlantic Monthly* 11 (March 1863): 346. According to Kessler, Hamilton was the idol of Phelps's youthful devotion. *Elizabeth Stuart Phelps* 77.

34. In William G. McLoughlin, ed., *The American Evangelicals, 1800–1900: An Anthology* (Gloucester, Mass.: Peter Smith, 1976) 142–43.

35. Wills 37, and Laderman 125, 129. Lincoln does not mourn single soldiers; the cemetery he commemorates is the euphemistic "final resting place" of the uncounted "brave men" who fought there. "Our fathers" are the country's founders, not the soldiers' parents, whereas mothers are not mentioned. Rather Lincoln consecrates the continuation of total war on the graves of nameless, faceless corpses. Also see Sweet 14, and Kathy Newman, "Wound and Wounding in the American Civil War: A Visual History," *The Yale Journal of Criticism* 6.2 (1993): 63, 69. Newman shows us how the medical photographs taken by Civil War surgeon Reed B. Bontecou "contain the horror of war" in their gilt-edged frames through their "romantic softness," eroticization, and aestheticization of pain.

36. Halttunen shows how cultural anxiety about the sincerity of emotion eventually led to the rigidification and increasing complexity of mourning rituals by the middle of the nineteenth century. However, the war period, though brief, certainly disrupted Americans' ability to execute these rituals. Condolence calls, visitations, the laying out of the dead—all were traditionally conducted at a leisurely pace and often began even before the individual had died. Wartime shortages of fabrics and other goods made it difficult to obtain the outer signifiers of mourning. Deep mourning was an extended period, severely curtailing the activities of the bereaved, especially those of women, who were not allowed to leave home except to attend church for the first month of mourning.

37. Phelps's hyperbolic description is akin to the writings of Daniel Aaron's "veterans of grief"—Henry James and Henry Adams—whom Aaron describes as attaching their emotional battles to the martial project in which they did not participate. "Etiquette of Grief" 204.

38. Schnog 29.

39. Quoted in Kelly 60.

40. St. Armand 124.

41. Mary Louise Kete, *Sentimental Collaborations: Mourning and Middle-Class Identity in Nineteenth-Century America* (Durham, N.C.: Duke University Press, 1999) 62.

42. See Mark Twain, *Extract from Captain Stormfield's Visit to Heaven* (New York: Harper & Brothers, 1909). In *Chapters from a Life* Phelps laments that it was not women's lot to "offer life to the teeth of shot and shell, they 'gave their happiness instead'" (74).

43. Certainly Halttunen's observation that the "mourner had almost entirely upstaged the dearly departed for the lead role in the sentimental drama of death" holds true for this novel (127).

44. Eric T. Dean, Jr., "'We Will All Be Lost and Destroyed': Post-Traumatic Stress Disorder and the Civil War," *Civil War History* 37.2 (1991): 138–53. For another argument for Civil War combat fatigue, see Herbert Hendin and Ann Pollinger Haas, "Posttraumatic Stress Disorders in Veterans of Early American Wars," *Psychohistory Review* 12.4 (1984): 25–30.

45. Jay Martin has argued provocatively that Phelps responds to the disjunction between her age's growing materialism and fascination with spiritualism by providing readers with a concrete version of the unconscious in her heaven, a "spatial, a 'great good place'; that its activities were continuous, that its truths were superior to those of experience, its operations much more swift and intricate than those of the reasoning mind." "Ghostly Rentals, Ghostly Purchases: Haunted Imaginations in James, Twain, and Bellamy," *The Haunted Dusk: American Supernatural Fiction, 1820–1920*, ed. Howard Kerr, John W. Crowley, and Charles L. Crow (Athens: The University of Georgia Press, 1983). Martin also insists that writers of this period, including Phelps, were unable to write a fiction of the "self-haunted self," where the "spiritual, the uncanny, the mythical, the ghostlike, the haunted, and the hallucinatory" are allowed to "fracture the consciousness along innumerable planes" (126). I argue that Phelps's heaven, however, manufactures and responds to just such a haunted self.

46. *Beyond the Gates* (Boston: Houghton, Mifflin, and Company, 1883) 47. All quotes cited parenthetically as *Beyond.*

47. According to his biographers, Mitchell too began to associate his faith in the invisible knowledge of science with hopes for the invisible afterlife. Lovering writes that Mitchell was a theist, and he felt that "what was not clear to the mind here and now would be made clear elsewhere, just as the father's account to the child is often unclear" (159).

48. See Lears 33.

49. Mitchell, Letters to Elizabeth Kearsley Mitchell, SWM Papers.

50. Elizabeth Stuart Phelps, Letters to S. Weir Mitchell, November 25, 1887, SWM Papers.

Chapter 3

1. Quoted in William Quentin Maxwell's *Lincoln's Fifth Wheel: The Political History of the United States Sanitary Commission* (New York: Longmans, Green, 1956) 20. It is interesting to note that Olmsted's philosophy took form in many public parks and grounds throughout the country (notably Central Park).

For more information on the genesis and evolution of the USSC, also see Charles J. Stillé, *History of the United States Sanitary Commission, Being the General Report of Its Work During the War of the Rebellion* (Philadelphia, Penn.: Lippincott, 1866). George M. Frederickson devotes a substantial portion of *The Inner Civil War* to the Sanitary elite, as well. These books focus almost exclusively on powerful men's roles in shaping the USSC. In *Women and the Work of Benevolence: Morality, Politics, and Class in the Nineteenth-Century United States* (New Haven, Conn.: Yale University Press, 1990), and *Civil War Sisterhood: The U.S. Sanitary Commission and Women's Politics in Transition* (Boston: Northeastern University Press, 2000), Lori D. Ginzberg and Judith Ann Giesberg, respectively, counter those patriarchal narratives, examining the role of powerful, Northern women in shaping USSC policies.

2. Quoted in Maxwell 23.

3. *The Sanitary Commission of the United States Army: A Succinct Narrative of Its Works and Purposes* (1864; New York: Arno Press, 1972) 18. This document, subsequently cited within the text as *Succinct*, was compiled before the war ended, a collection of "outlines," "abstracts of current reports," and statistical records and tables intended to memorialize the "origin, purposes, progress, and present condition of the Commission's methods and departments of labor" (Intro.). Because the USSC was largely a charitable organization, a plethora of documents appeared before and after the war intended to raise funds for the commission, as well as to assure contributors that their money was being responsibly and well spent.

4. *The Incorporation of America: Culture & Society in the Gilded Age* (New York: Hill & Wang, 1982) 5. Trachtenberg defines the corporation literally in this era as the embodiment of a "legally sanctioned fiction . . . an association of people [that] constituted a single entity which might hold property, sue and be sued, enter contracts, and continue in existence beyond the lifetime or membership of any of its participants. The association itself was understood as strictly contractual, not necessarily comprised of people acquainted with each other or joined by any common motive other than profit seeking" (83). The resonance between corporate philosophy and army life is perhaps obvious: army life entailed the joining of unlike individuals in a narrowly common undertaking. One might argue that the prevalence of army experience for middle-aged Gilded Age men made the incorporation of America a comfortable inevitability.

5. *Where My Heart Is Turning Ever* 55. Diffley posits that romances "inherently based personal identity on choice twice over: once in embracing the lover, and then later in rejecting the decoy" that would entice the young protagonist to stay at home rather than renegotiate war-era loyalties (56).

Just one example of critics' common derision of Civil War romance plots is Michael Schaefer's disdain for De Forest's romance: "However much he desires to tell the whole truth as he saw it, [De Forest] could not break completely free from either the romantic literary conventions or the traditional conception of military professionalism prevailing in his era" (134). *Just What War Is: The Civil War Writings of De Forest and Bierce* (Knoxville: University of Tennessee Press, 1997) 134. Don Dingeldine, editor of Davis's *Waiting for the Verdict*, finds her romance less troubling, but notes nevertheless that one of the romance plots "dramatizes the clash between the romantic tradition deeply ingrained in American culture and the radical potential of a new literary realism" (xiii). Introduction, *Waiting for the Verdict* by Rebecca Harding Davis (1867; Albany, N.Y.: NCUP, Inc., 1995). Discussions of genre are at the heart of De Forest and Davis scholarship.

6. *Documents of the U.S. Sanitary Commission, vol. 1* (Numbers 1 to 60) (New York, 1866), and *Documents of the U.S. Sanitary Commission, vol. 2* (Numbers 61 to 95) (New York, 1866). Quote from No. 40. All citations extracted from these documents are cited by "No." in text. Because the books are not paginated continuously, I have noted the number of the document from which the citation is taken. The documents are comprised of letters, memos, declarations, and instructions, and that which appeared in various public forums throughout the war period. All ninety-five documents were gathered and bound in 1866, providing a coherent narrative of the organization's efforts.

7. Randall C. Jimerson, *The Private Civil War* (Baton Rouge: Louisiana State University Press, 1988) 227. In 1864, the author of *The Philanthropic Results of the War in America* (New York: Sheldon & Company, 1864), also alludes to the fact

that "the day laborer, the artisan, the mechanic, the operatives from the manu-factories, and the clerks from the stores sought employment, but in vain; there was not a full day's work for men in any department of labor except in tilling the soil" (11). This text will be cited parenthetically as *Philanthropic.* As Rebecca Harding Davis remembers, "With many laboring men the only choice was to enlist or starve." *Bits of Gossip* (Boston: Houghton, Mifflin, & Co., 1904) 124.

8. Robert E. Denney, *Civil War Medicine: Care & Comfort of the Wounded* (New York: Sterling Publishing Co., 1994) 8. Some USSC commissioners made the army sound as if it were comprised wholly of such misfits: "Feeble boys, toothless old men, consumptives, asthmatics, one-eyed, one-armed men, men with differ-ent length of legs, club-footed and ruptured, and, in short, men with every vari-ety of disability, and whose systems were replete with the elements of disease were accepted as recruits and started on the field." Quoted in Maxwell 32.

9. Mitchell, Letters to Elizabeth Kearsley Mitchell, August 1864, SWM Papers.

10. See James A. Hijiya, *J. W. De Forest and the Rise of American Gentility* (Han-over, N.H.: University Press of New England, 1988) 55–56.

11. *Philanthropic* 12. This little book, anonymously authored by "An American Citizen" but most likely written by Linus Pierpont Brockett, was prompted by the philanthropy of a "merchant of New York," eager to publicize the USSC's good works to eager citizens and, presumably, to encourage more charitable contributions.

12. De Forest scholarship in particular takes just such a position. See Robert Antoni, "*Miss Ravenel's Conversion:* A Neglected American Novel," *The Southern Quarterly* 24.3 (1986): 58–63, and Eric Solomon, "The Novelist As Soldier: Cooke and De Forest," *American Literary Realism* 19.3 (1987): 80–88. Antoni con-tends that "De Forest's work represents an important transition from romantic to realistic writing" (58). Solomon reads De Forest's generic mélange less chari-tably, noting "the mixture of sentiment and comedy with the brutal struggle for survival breaks down the aura of realism achieved by De Forest" at other points (83). Thomas Fick asserts that "'realism' and 'romance' are themselves among the novel's subjects." "Genre Wars and the Rhetoric of Manhood in *Miss Raven-el's Conversion from Secession to Loyalty,*" *Nineteenth Century Literature* 46.4 (1992): 474.

13. *Bodies and Machines* (New York: Routledge, 1992) 14. For an elaboration of Seltzer's notion of statistical persons see, for example, page 100.

14. References to De Forest's work come from *Miss Ravenel's Conversion from Secession to Loyalty* (1867; New York: Holt, Rinehart & Winston, 1955) 267, and are cited parenthetically as *Ravenel.*

James W. Gargano writes that *Miss Ravenel's Conversion* "was truly a *succes d'és-time,*" showered with critical recognition from reviews appearing in the *Atlantic, Harper's Monthly, Harper's Weekly, Peterson's,* and so on, as well as New York newspa-pers such as the *Times.* Introduction, *Critical Essays on John William De Forest,* ed. James W. Gargano (Boston: G. K. Hall & Co., 1981) 6, 10. The *Peterson's* reviewer pronounced it "one of the best novels that has appeared for years." Even less enthusiastic reviews, such as young Henry James's, praised the novel's realistic characterization. De Forest's success was mitigated, however, by *Harper's* unwill-ingness to print the gritty novel in their "family" magazine, thereby denying De Forest a large national audience for his work. And the excessive number of print-er's errors in the first edition discouraged many from buying the book. Though a critical success, *Miss Ravenel's Conversion* was an economic disappointment.

15. *Incorporation of America* 62. Trachtenberg draws on Melville's 1866 poetry to make his point but argues that Melville's observations are only a "premonition" of things to come. I argue that such a corporate ethos was full-blown during the war. USSC supporters deliberately deployed mechanistic language, one arguing for contributions to provide for the "maintenance," "restoration from sickness," and "the repairing of war's ravages" borne by men's bodies. *Philanthropic* 96. Such language clearly mechanizes soldiers' bodies.

16. After only two years USSC inspectors had logged more than 1,800 reports of camp visits. No. 69.

17. I'm using Seltzer's distinction between "deep embodiment and disembodiment" here (110). Reid Mitchell argues that the closeness of a soldier to his community could "undercut the traditional arrangements that armies make for discipline." He adds, however, that soldiers transferred domestic arrangements into their camp lives, making their companies an extension of their home communities. *The Vacant Chair: The Northern Soldier Leaves Home* (New York: Oxford University Press, 1993) 21. Mitchell does not explore the imperatives to abandon all such attachments.

18. Not surprisingly, when a USSC inspector comes upon an abandoned rebel outpost, he finds it the "dirtiest, nastiest (no other word will express it) place I have ever been in. I can scarcely imagine any kind of filth, or any combination of vile stench, which is not found here." *Succinct* 168.

19. The liberty of martial law produced an inordinately large number of executions. Carter praises a sentinel who shot a man dead for neglecting to halt when challenged. "'Good, by (this and that)' exclaimed the Colonel. 'Those fellows are redeeming themselves. . . . This is the second man the ninth fellows have shot within a week.'" *Ravenel* 220. Apparently, this passage mirrors an episode in De Forest's own life, for at the Battle of Fisher's Hill he ordered his men to shoot down a bluecoat who was fleeing the field. Hijiya 59. The USSC lauded strict punishment of even the most trifling of misdemeanors for, they claimed, "commiseration for what are erroneously considered technical offenders, and moderation or neglect in dealing with them, is costing the country more lives by far than the bullets of the enemy" (No. 40). Despite De Forest's lighthearted treatment of this summary execution and the USSC's tough talk, documents show that 276 men were executed during the Civil War, more than in all other United States conflicts combined. Robert Alotta's examination of government documents pertaining to the executions suggests that number falls far short of reality. See Robert Alotta, *Civil War Justice: Union Army Executions Under Lincoln* (Shippensburg, Penn.: White Mane Publications, 1989).

20. Hedges argues that such racial rhetoric was integral to the normalization of white bodies. "If Uncle Tom is White, Should We Call Him 'Auntie'? Race and Sexuality in Postbellum U.S. Fiction," *Whiteness: A Critical Reader*, ed. Mike Hill (New York: New York University Press, 1997) 226–47. Quote is located on page 229.

21. Giesberg xi. Giesberg's work counters arguments repeated in texts such as Maxwell's history of the USSC, where "the commission often found women difficult to direct. Their zeal sometimes outran good sense, demanding trifling attentions and wasting chatter. Unable to understand organizational precautions, some became impudent and caustic if crossed; others could never see problems in the whole, but rushed as though panic-stricken into a sea of details. Prima donnas of benevolence caused trouble in camps" (302).

22. Nina Silber and Elizabeth Young theorize the gendered implications of popular renderings of Confederate President Jefferson Davis eluding capture dressed in his wife's clothing. Silber contends that "northerners drew on the theme of depraved southern manliness, once again, as a way to establish their regional and political superiority in the postwar period." *Romance of Reunion* 33. Young argues that depictions of Davis in sexually vulnerable positions made him not only vulnerable to rape but also open to the possibilities of homosexuality. *Disarming the Nation* 183, 187.

23. Michael Barton has characterized the self-policing Northern soldier as "job-minded, mainly concerned with things and their production. But he produced not only things"; Barton argues that the truly arduous work of the martial worker was to produce a soldierly character in *Goodmen: The Character of Civil War Soldiers* (University Park: Pennsylvania State University Press, 1981) 16.

24. William Swinton, *Campaign of the Army of the Potomac* (New York: Charles R. Richardson, 1866) 614.

25. Ravenel's double professional identity seems particularly important as scholars note that the character was probably based on De Forest's father-in-law, Dr. Charles Upham Shepard (Hijiya 26–27). Dr. Shepard was a distinguished man of science with an "international reputation as a mineralogist." It seems likely that the addition of a medical degree to his honors was deliberate and somehow meaningful to De Forest in developing the science of the novel.

26. Swinton 634. James Russell Lowell, "A Great Public Character," *The Atlantic Monthly* 20 (1867): 632.

27. Quoted in Maxwell 316. Frederick Law Olmsted explicitly invoked sanitary rhetoric in his subsequent work as a designer of public spaces. Indeed, in the 1870s and 1880s the spread of cholera and yellow fever in urban areas was attributed in part to the "old-fashioned" arrangement of roads and neighborhoods. *Incorporation* 109.

28. All references to the text are cited internally and are taken from Don Dingeldine, ed., *Waiting For the Verdict* by Rebecca Harding Davis (1867; Albany, N.Y.: NCUP, 1995). As far as I can tell, Davis was not a member of any women's auxiliary organizations. However, in the novel she defends the efforts of such groups. An unsympathetic minor character, Mrs. Van Fitter, disparages the works of the "Sanitary Commission," finding any association with the carnage of the war "repulsive to a fine mind" (167). Yet none of Davis's admirable Northern war-supporting women are depicted attending a USSC meeting. Indeed, in writing of the future of "Women in Literature" in 1891 Davis exhorts new women to "leave something more permanent behind them than reports of Sanitary or Archeological clubs, and . . . paint as they only can do, for the next generation, the inner life and history of their times." "Women in Literature," *A Rebecca Harding Davis Reader*, ed. Jean Pfaelzer (Pittsburgh, Penn.: University of Pittsburgh Press, 1995) 404.

29. In *Bits of Gossip* (subsequent references to the text are cited internally as *Bits*) in a chapter entitled "The Civil War," Davis tells an anecdote about Abraham Lincoln and a young Springfield woman of his acquaintance, Mary. Meeting a young man whom he finds suitable for Mary, Lincoln contrives to bring the eligible P—— to Springfield, and the two young people fall in love. Wishing to provoke a proposal, Lincoln directs P—— to carry Mary home in a storm. "Carry her, P——," shouted Lincoln. "Drop that umbrella. Pick her up and carry her! Wade in, man!" (114). Although this story sounds apocryphal, it invokes Lincoln as a national father urging his children toward domestic stability.

30. Davis, however, denies the power of even the most careful breeding practices, arguing that they lead to degeneration rather than to purity. The "high-blooded," upper-class Strebling is "tainted an' cunnin, like thoroughbred horses full of nerves and tricks." Lower-class Joe Burley contends that "refinement of his'n is like the froth on that dirty pool outside the door" (*Waiting* 223). We also meet Mrs. Van Fitter, who is the product of familial inbreeding. Davis describes her as "a ponderous, yellow wooden tower" (*Waiting* 165). Though her careful attention to bloodlines would presumably make her "fitter" than others, Davis makes Mrs. Van Fitter's body as "yellow" as Sap/Dr. Broderip's "dirty" mulatto complexion.

31. Davis's most recent literary biographer, Sharon Harris, supposes that Davis was treated by Mitchell for nervous exhaustion in 1863. Though Davis never identified Mitchell as her doctor at that time, she later credited him with saving her life, and the Davises retained Mitchell as their family physician. More telling, Davis cryptically reveals at the time of her illness that "the doctor forbids the least reading or writing," which was a common and important component of Mitchell's extraordinary rest cure. In *Rebecca Harding Davis and American Realism* (Philadelphia: University of Pennsylvania Press, 1991) 107–8.

32. Toni Morrison, *Playing in the Dark: Whiteness and the Literary Imagination* (New York: Vintage Books, 1992). Morrison contends, "as a disabling virus within literary discourse, Africanism has become, in the Eurocentric tradition that American education favors, both a way of talking about and a way of policing matters of class, sexual license, and repression, formations and exercises of power, and meditations on ethics and accountability" (7). Particularly interesting is that Morrison phrases this phenomenon in the language of disease, suggesting the unstable bodies that found and disrupt this delicate system of meaning.

33. Hedges explains how white men in postbellum America were discouraged from acting "colorfully," a term that eventually connoted both blackness and effeminacy and allied black and effeminate men with homosexuality (228). Thus, reaction to Broderip's body could also be viewed as incipient homophobia.

Chapter 4

1. *Ravenel* 341.

2. Stephen J. Gould, *The Mismeasure of Man* (New York: W. W. Norton & Company, 1981) 71, and Sander L. Gilman, *Difference and Pathology: Stereotypes of Sexuality, Race, and Madness* (Ithaca, N.Y.: Cornell University Press, 1985) 138.

3. Benjamin Apthorp Gould, *Investigations in the Military and Anthropological Statistics of American Soldiers* (1869; New York: Arno Press, 1979). All quotes from this text are cited internally as *Investigations*.

4. Hedges, too, comments on the way the USSC studies set "statistical standards for a variety of racial types" (226). Hedges focuses especially on the andrometer, a measuring device that was used to define the boundaries of physical normality.

5. See John Higham, *Strangers in the Land: Patterns of American Nativism, 1860–1925* (New Brunswick, N.J.: Rutgers University Press, 1988). Higham argues that the war "completed the ruin of organized nativism by absorbing xenophones

and immigrants in a common cause" (13). However, this uneasy truce did not last long.

6. Quoted in S. Gould 33.

7. Mike Hawkins, *Social Darwinism in European and American Thought, 1860–1945* (Cambridge: Cambridge University Press, 1997) 105, and S. Gould 114. See E. D. Cope, *On the Hypothesis of Evolution: Physical and Metaphysical* (New Haven, Conn.: Chatfield and Co., 1870).

8. Such scientific racism, which gave full play to a confused logic about the physical differences allegedly attributable to genetics, bolstered negligent medical practices in the war. "As some race-conscious observers maintained, blacks did enjoy immunities to certain diseases . . . but along with special immunities, blacks also carried special susceptibilities," which went unrecognized by medical officers confident of the inhuman strength of African American bodies. Ira Berlin, ed. *Freedom: A Documentary History of Emancipation, 1861–1867,* ser. 2, *The Black Military Experience* (New York: Cambridge University Press, 1982) 635.

9. Benjamin Gould claims that researchers took anthropometric measurements of nearly 19,000 soldiers—3,000 of whom were "full-blooded Negroes" or "mulattos."

10. S. Gould 74, 31.

11. Brenda Stevenson, introduction, *The Journals of Charlotte Forten Grimké* (New York: Oxford University Press, 1988) 8, 15. All subsequent citations from Forten's journal are referenced internally as Forten.

12. Virginia Matzke Adams, introduction, *On the Altar of Freedom: A Black Soldier's Civil War Letters from the Front* (Amherst: University of Massachusetts Press, 1991) xxxiii. All citations from Gooding's newspaper articles and letters are referenced internally as *Altar.*

13. Wiegman 4.

14. As Wiegman explains, "the claim to sexual difference—to be a 'man' or a 'woman'—works to define and invoke a social subjectivity (and hence psychic interiority) previously denied the slave" (11).

15. Many have already theorized the ways in which domestic ideology transcended the private sphere to which it is so often delegated. Gillian Brown has persuasively argued that the "interiority" of domesticity—that is, its claim to privacy—is one and the same with the public, political economy in midcentury writings. She emphasizes that identity is fluid and that American selfhood is by definition "continually under construction, or at least renovation" at this time. *Domestic Individualism: Imagining Self in Nineteenth-Century America* (Berkeley: University of California Press, 1990) 1–2. Both Brown and Karen Sánchez-Eppler have argued that the mid-nineteenth-century house was the site of white domestic activity and the literal home of the racist slave economy. *Touching Liberty: Abolition, Feminism, and the Politics of the Body* (Berkeley: University of California Press, 1993). And Kathleen Diffley has elaborated on the crucial role of domestic ideology as recuperating and masking the real effects of war.

16. "A Call to My Country-Women," *Atlantic Monthly* 11 (March 1863): 349.

17. Young, *Disarming the Nation* 17.

18. Some Marxists still explicitly subordinate racism to classism, imagining African Americans as one class opposed to both the white ruling and working classes. For example, Stuart Blumin's book *The Emergence of the Middle-Class: Social Experience in the American City, 1760–1900* (New York: Cambridge University Press, 1989), considers the rise of the middle class in nineteenth-century America, yet race is never mentioned. One eventually realizes that "middle

class" really means white middle class. Gary Nash is one of a growing number of scholars who recognizes that by the second quarter of the nineteenth century "black society had become nearly as stratified as white society" in cities such as Forten's native Philadelphia. As is traditionally the case, however, Nash measures class in America by the "distribution of wealth, income, opportunity, work place task and authority, political power, [and] legal status." *Forging Freedom: The Formation of Philadelphia's Black Community, 1720–1840* (Boston: Harvard University Press, 1988).

19. Bettye Collier-Thomas and James Turner, "Race, Class and Color: The African American Discourse on Identity," *Journal of American Ethnic History* 14.1 (1994): 5–31. E. Franklin Frazier, *Black Bourgeoisie: The Rise of a New Middle Class in the United States* (New York: Free Press, 1957).

20. Jim Cullen, "'I's a Man Now': Gender and African American Men," *Divided Houses: Gender and the Civil War,* ed. Catherine Clinton and Nina Silber (New York: Oxford University Press, 1992) 82.

21. This poem is reprinted in Stevenson, Forten 583–86.

22. See *The Sable Arm: Negro Troops in the Union Army, 1861–1865* (New York: W. W. Norton & Company, 1966).

23. Quoted in James M. McPherson, *The Negro's Civil War: How American Blacks Felt and Acted during the War for the Union* (New York: Ballantine Books, 1991) 187.

24. *Altar* 9.

25. Martin E. Dann, *The Black Press, 1827–1890: The Quest for National Identity* (New York: G. P. Putnam's Sons, 1971) 22.

26. McPherson, *Negro's Civil War* xvi. Also see Cornish who writes, "From the middle of May on through the rest of 1862 the question of arming the Negro, slave or free, occupied column after column of newspaper space and stirred the expression of every kind of opinion, conviction, and reaction" (40).

27. Hondon Hargrove, *Black Union Soldiers in the Civil War* (Jefferson, N.C.: McFarland & Co., Inc., 1988) 125. Whereas Hargrove asserts that 80 percent of those executed were African American, Alotta contends that only 54.31 percent were foreign-born or African American. Alotta continues that the number of African American soldiers punished in such a manner was proportionately 133% higher than the army population of African Americans. *Civil War Justice* 187. Regardless of the precise number, it seems clear that the battlefield became the site of governmentally sanctioned racist violence. These statistics were not made available to the public until nineteen years after the war had ended.

28. H. Bruce Franklin, *Prison Literature: The Victim as Criminal and Artist* (New York: Oxford University Press, 1978) xxx.

29. Bonny Vaught, "Trying to Make Things Real," *Between Women: Biographers, Novelists, Critics, Teachers, and Artists Write about Their Work on Women,* ed. Carol Archer, Louise DeSalve, and Sara Ruddick (Boston: Beacon Press, 1984) 55. McPherson writes that by war's end, 900 teachers had provided 200,000 freedmen and women with a rudimentary education. Introduction, *Two Black Teachers during the Civil War* (New York: Arno Press, 1969) i, iii.

30. In *Hospital Sketches,* Alcott's thinly fictionalized account of her three-month stint in an army hospital, her energetic heroine laments, "I always owed fate a grudge because I wasn't a lord of creation instead of a lady (68).

31. In explaining his editorial strategy, Billington admits that he took "certain liberties with the text. Large sections in the period between 1854 and 1862 have been deleted. These describe the weather, family affairs, the landscape, and other matters of purely local interest" (40). Ray Allen Billington, introduction,

The Journal of Charlotte L. Forten (New York: Dryden, 1953) 1–40. Joanne Braxton labeled Billington's edition a "mutilated text." "Charlotte Forten Grimké and the Search for a Public Voice," *The Private Self: Theory and Practice of Women's Autobiographical Writings*, ed. Shari Benstock (Chapel Hill: University of North Carolina Press, 1988) 255. Gloria C. Oden has responded by reconstructing those family alliances Billington found extraneous, explaining "black history *is* genealogy." "*The Journal of Charlotte L. Forten*: The Salem-Philadelphia Years (1854–1862) Reexamined." *Essex Institute Historical Collections* 119 (1983): 120.

32. Billington 28.

33. See Emma Jones Lapsansky, "Feminism, Freedom, and Community: Charlotte Forten and Women Activists in Nineteenth-Century Philadelphia," *Pennsylvania Magazine of History and Biography* 113.1 (1989): 9–10, and Carla L. Peterson, *"Doers of the Word": African-American Women Speakers and Writers in the North, 1830–1880* (New York: Oxford University Press, 1995) 176.

34. Henry Louis Gates Jr., "The Master's Pieces: On Canon Formation and Afro-American Tradition," *The Bounds of Race: Perspectives on Hegemony and Resistance,*" ed. Dominick LaCapra (Ithaca, N.Y.: Cornell University Press, 1991) 122.

35. Braxton, "Charlotte Forten Grimké" 255.

36. Lapsansky 3.

37. Whittier quoted in Stevenson 32. Perhaps the greatest tribute to her lifelong commitment to dignity, education, and refinement was expressed in the loving epitaph written in 1914 by her husband, Francis Grimké: "Mrs. Grimké had a lovely disposition, was sweet and gentle, and yet she was a woman of great strength of character. She was a lady in the best sense of that term—a woman of great refinement. There was not the slightest trace of coarseness about her in any shape or form. She never grew old in spirit—she was always young, as young as the youngest. She had a fine mind, carefully trained and cultivated by hard study and contact [with] the best literature and with cultured people. She had the keenest appreciation for all that was best in literature and art. She loved books and pictures and flowers and everything that was beautiful and soul-uplifting. She had also charming manners—she was always thoughtful, always considerate for others, never allowing the thought of self to intrude or to interfere with the comfort and happiness of others. The plane upon which her life, inner and outer, moved was always high." Stevenson 55.

38. For further discussion see Dorothy Sterling, *We Are Your Sisters: Black Women in the Nineteenth Century* (New York: W. W. Norton & Co., 1984).

39. Frances Smith Foster, *Written by Herself: Literary Production by African American Women, 1746–1892* (Bloomington, Ind.: Indiana University Press, 1993) 17–18.

40. Quoted in Sterling 153. The character of speech is remarkably ephemeral—even when a written version remains. Though Truth was a prolific and powerful orator, she was illiterate, and thus the remaining transcriptions of her speeches are mediated—and perhaps corrupted—by the white women who made them. See Nell Irvin Painter's biography of Truth, *Sojourner Truth: A Life, A Symbol* (New York: Norton, 1996), for more on this episode. Painter argues that Truth's "speech act" was a "triumph of embodied rhetoric" (140).

41. See Deborah Gray White, *Ain't I a Woman: Female Slaves in the Plantation South* (New York: W. W. Norton & Co., 1985), and Patricia Morton, *Disfigured Images: The Historical Assault on Afro-American Woman* (New York: Praeger, 1991).

42. Forten mentions Stowe's *Sunny Memories of Foreign Lands* specifically among the many travel books she devoured (Forten 90). Just a few of the many

other Italian texts she mentions are: Stevens's "Travels in the East" (Forten 100); Ferguson's "History of Rome" (Forten 132); Macaulay's poem "Lays of Ancient Rome" (Forten 133); "Massacre of St. Bartholomew's," published in *Harper's* (Forten 197); "Diary of an Ennuyee" (Forten 230); and "Rienzi—the last of the Tribunes," an "exciting account of the ancient history of Rome" (Forten 233). In addition, she attended lectures on Italy; at one she learned about a saintly Italian cardinal's "untiring self-sacrificing devotion" to his missionary work (Forten 148). Roman Catholicism, too, comes to have meaning in her life as an admirable model of service and the possibilities of the sublime.

43. Leonardo Buonomo, *Backward Glances: Exploring Italy, Reinterpreting America, 1831–1866* (London: Associated University Press, 1996) 11, 14, 29. Peterson also notices Forten's passion for travel (186).

44. Her living conditions on the Sea Islands were much less restricted than those in New England. Whether living in Philadelphia or Salem, Forten was always under the watchful eye of an aunt, uncle, or benevolent family friend. On the Sea Islands she lived in a house with two other single women: Laura Towne and Ellen Murray.

45. Sterling 277.

46. Sterling 227.

47. Sterling 282.

48. There is no intimation that Dr. R. would ever leave his wife for Forten. Though he sends her expensive gifts and lavishes attention upon her, he also intermittently shares letters from his wife with Forten. For her part, Forten seems to take up a wifely role for the doctor, darning his stockings in the camp while he is preparing for rebel attack (Forten 475). Yet she claims she is not looking for marriage: "After all a marriage is a solemn thing. . . . I think *I* sh'ld dread a funeral much less" (Forten 483).

49. Robert B. Stepto, *From Behind the Veil: A Study of Afro-American Narrative* (Chicago: University of Illinois Press, 1979) 167.

50. Stevenson 281.

51. Foster, *Written by Herself* 81.

52. Peterson 183.

53. Towne was a committed abolitionist who stayed on in the South after the war to continue her school for the freedmen and freedwomen. However, her diary reveals that she was unable to extricate herself from the prevalent racist beliefs of her time, for she describes the Sea Island inhabitants as "savage," "uncouth and wild," and "very picteresque." Laura M. Towne, *Letters and Diary of Laura M. Towne, 1862–1884* (Cambridge, Mass.: Riverside, 1912) 20, 22, 70.

54. Both Towne and Higginson are quoted in Sterling 282.

55. Cited in Bert James Lowenberg and Ruth Bogin, eds., *Black Women in Nineteenth-Century American Life: Their Words, Their Thoughts, Their Feelings* (University Park: Pennsylvania State University Press, 1976) 284.

56. Peterson 179–80, and McKay, "The Journals of Charlotte L. Forten Grimké: *Les Lieux de Mémoire* in African-American Women's Autobiography," *History and Memory in African-American Culture*, ed. Genevieve Fabre and Robert O'Meally (New York: Oxford University Press, 1994): 261–71.

57. W. E. B. DuBois, *The Souls of Black Folk* (1903; New York: Bantam, 1989) 5–6.

58. Frazier 61.

59. Willie Lee Rose, *Rehearsal for Reconstruction: The Port Royal Experiment* (New York: Bobbs-Merrill Company, Inc., 1964) 88.

60. Booker T. Washington, *Up from Slavery* (1901; New York: Bantam, 1967) 122, 39–40.

61. Anna Julia Cooper, *A Voice from the South,* ed. Mary Helen Washington (1892; New York: Oxford University Press, 1988) 207.

62. Sterling 269.

63. The former enslaved of the Sea Islands were not left to fend for themselves. In addition to missionary schoolteachers such as Forten, superintendents were immediately sent down to "oversee" the plantations and keep cotton production high. The island was also crawling with Union soldiers, as a number of regiments were stationed there after it was captured. Forten comments briefly on the inadequacies of both groups. Her first experience on the Sea Island is with "several military gentleman [*sic*], *not* very creditable specimens, I sh'ld say. The little Commissary himself, Capt. T. is a perfect little popinjay, and he and a Col somebody who didn't look any too sensible, talked in a very smart manner, evidently for our special benefit. The word 'nigger' was plentifully used" (Forten 389). She writes that "some of the superintendents seem to be strongly prejudiced against [the former enslaved] and they have a contemptuous way of speaking of them that I do not like."

64. Lisa M. Koch comments briefly on Forten's illnesses, arguing that "portraying sickliness" was a "performative" act aimed at engaging "taboos against female bodily displays." "Bodies As Stage Props: Enacting Hysteria in the Diaries of Charlotte Forten Grimké and Alice James," *Legacy* 15 (1998): 59–64.

65. Forten is not the only African American woman who expressed her enthusiasm about the opportunities of the Civil War in the metaphors of health. Harriet Jacobs, whose *Incidents in the Life of a Slave Girl* (1861) anticipates Forten's own struggles with gender, sexuality, and single autonomy, worked with Southern refugees in Washington, D.C., during the war. "My health is better than it has been for years," she wrote to Amy Post. "The good God has spared me for this work. The last six months have been the happiest of all my life." Sterling 247.

66. See Diane Price Herndl, "The Invisible (Invalid) Woman: African-American Women, Illness, and Nineteenth-Century Narrative," *Women's Studies* 24 (1995): 553–72, 558, and Ann Folwell Stanford, "Mechanisms of Disease: African-American Women Writers, Social Pathologies, and the Limits of Medicine," *NWSA Journal* 6.1 (Spring 1994): 28–47.

67. Cited in Sterling 283.

68. Stanford 29.

69. *National Anti-Slavery Standard,* November 13, 1869, in Foner, *Reconstruction* 49.

70. The comment is by Henry McNeal Turner, chaplain of a black regiment who published this observation in the *Christian Recorder* in May 1865. Quoted in David W. Blight, *Frederick Douglass's Civil War: Keeping Faith in Jubilee* (Baton Rouge: Louisiana State University Press, 1989) 147.

Chapter 5

1. "Follow-up Studies of Patients with Nerve Injuries," ms. 2/024–93, Box 11, SWM Papers. The information cited in this first paragraph was garnered from the questionnaires and letters contained in Box 11. The letter from L. S. Benton is dated October 1892.

2. Letter to S. Weir Mitchell, February 10, 1906, ms. 2/0241, Box 11, SWM Papers.

3. Gosling, *Before Freud* xiii. Gosling offers a systematic analysis of the published case reports of neurasthenia during the four decades covered by his study. Of the 217 patients whose occupations were given, "seventy-nine were of the professional class" including bankers, lawyers, politicians, physicians, etc. Fifty-six patients belonged to the skilled and semiskilled laboring classes that made up a large part of the nineteenth-century work force; among them were "book-keepers, bank tellers, butchers, carpenters, clerks, storekeepers, tailors," etc. Finally, twenty-one were of the "unskilled laboring class, including waiters, waitresses, servants and housekeepers, a 'car cleaner,' [and] a stevedore" (31–32).

4. Lutz, *American Nervousness* 39, and Lears, *No Place of Grace* 117.

5. Ambrose Bierce, "An Occurrence at Owl Creek Bridge," *The Civil War Short Stories of Ambrose Bierce*, ed. Ernest J. Hopkins (Lincoln: University of Nebraska Press, 1988) 45–53. Citations noted internally as "An Occurrence."

6. *Devil's Dictionary* (1911; New York: Dover, 1993) 51.

7. Gail Bederman, *Manliness and Civilization: A Cultural History of Gender and Race in the United States, 1880–1917* (Chicago: University of Chicago Press, 1995) 5, 10.

8. "'The Right to Be Sick': American Physicians and Nervous Patients, 1885–1910," *Journal of Social History* 20.2 (1986): 251–67. This information is based on their examination of the 167 case records of neurasthenic patients published in American medical journals at the turn of the century. In *Before Freud,* Gosling's sample expands to 306, of which 154 were men and 152 were women. Such statistics do not erase the fact that neurasthenia was a distinct diagnosis for men and women.

9. The Red Badge of Courage *and Selected Prose and Poetry,* ed. William A. Gibson (1895; New York: Holt, Rinehart, and Winston, Inc., 1968) 538. Subsequent references are cited internally as *Red Badge.*

10. *The Double Life of Stephen Crane* (London: Andre Deutsch, 1992) 119. Benfey's reading of the novel largely confirms my own, for he sees that "Crane orchestrates Fleming's progress in and out of battle as an education in wounds and corpses. Accounts of the novel, in their attention to its 'psychological truth,' tend to overlook how physical the novel is in its focus, how minutely concerned with details of the fate of the body in war" (112).

11. Linderman, *Embattled Courage* 267–68; also see Aaron, *Unwritten War.*

12. Preface, *Battles and Leaders of the Civil War: Being for the Most Part Contributions by Union and Confederate Officers,* 4 vols., ed. Robert Underwood Johnson and Clarence Clough Buel (New York: The Century Company, 1894). Subsequent references cited internally as *Battles and Leaders.*

13. In *Race and Reunion* Blight points out that not all postwar publications were so harmonious. For example, the *Annals of the War* (1879) "illuminated many of the bitterest memories of modern warfare" (165). However, he does argue that *The Century* editors "quite purposefully intended to shape a culture of reunion" (175). See 173–81 for a more complete explanation of the series' development.

14. Wilson, *Patriotic Gore* 132.

15. Ulysses S. Grant, *Personal Memoirs of U. S. Grant* (1885; New York: Grosset & Dunlap, 1962) 584. Subsequent references cited internally as *Memoirs.*

16. "Wasted Magnanimity," *The New National Era,* August 10, 1871. In *The Life and Writings of Frederick Douglass,* ed. Philip S. Foner, vol. 4, *Reconstruction and After* (New York: International Publishers, 1955) 257.

17. Peter Novick, *That Noble Dream* 73.

18. James Ford Rhodes, *History of the United States from the Compromise of 1850 to the Final Restoration of Home Rule at the South in 1877*, 2 vols. (New York: Harper and Brothers, 1895). Though the book cost five dollars (per set of two volumes) at a time when a suit of men's clothing cost ten, and though it was released in the midst of an economic depression, the first edition sold so well that a second edition was issued almost immediately. See Robert Cruden, *James Ford Rhodes: The Man, the Historian, and His Work* (Westport, Conn.: Greenwood Press Publishers, 1961) 49.

19. Rhodes, vol. 2, 210 and vol. 1, 359.

20. *Political Science Quarterly* 8 (1893): 342–46. Quoted in Cruden, *James Ford Rhodes* 51.

21. Silber, *Romance of Reunion* 3.

22. Quoted in Lutz 63.

23. Benfey 230.

24. "Copy of Letter Written by General Smith," ms. 2/0241–93, Box 11, SWM Papers, 3, 7. There is no date on this later, but its placement among Mitchell's papers suggests that it was written right around the turn of the century. More critically, Mitchell does not identify which "General Smith" had written this essay. Yet it was apparently of such interest to him that Mitchell retyped it on his own letterhead and threw away the original document. My educated guess is that Mitchell was corresponding with Major-General William F. "Baldy" Smith. Two pieces of evidence lead me to this conclusion. First, this General Smith published a short article in *The North American Review* in February 1888 entitled "The Genius of Battle." Because Mitchell considered himself one of the literati, and because he had just published his Civil War novels *In War Time* and *Roland Blake*, one can surmise that Mitchell and Smith's paths may have crossed. Second, Smith died in Philadelphia in 1903, suggesting that he had been residing there at the turn of the century; Mitchell lived there nearly all of his life and was a prominent citizen. For information on William F. "Baldy" Smith, see Charles Royster, *The Destructive War: William Techumseh Sherman, Stonewall Jackson, and the Americans* (New York: Alfred A. Knopf, 1991) 337.

25. Anonymous, "A Green Private under Fire," *New York Times*, October 19, 1895, 3.

26. George Wyndham, "A Remarkable Book," *New Review* 14 (January 1896): 30–40.

27. Alexander McClurg, "The Red Badge of Hysteria," *Dial* 20 (April 1896): 228.

28. As Alfred Habegger writes, "Unrestrained speech brings a risk of combat and self-ostracism." "Fighting Words: The Talk of Men at War in *The Red Badge of Courage*," *Critical Essays on Stephen Crane's* The Red Badge of Courage, ed. Donald Pizer (Boston: G. K. Hall & Co., 1990) 233.

29. Donald Pease, "Fear, Rage, and the Mistrials of Representation in *The Red Badge of Courage*," *American Realism: New Essays*, ed. Eric Sundquist (Baltimore: Johns Hopkins University Press, 1982): 157.

30. McClurg 227.

31. Pease 162, and Robert M. Rechnitz, "Depersonalization and the Dream in *The Red Badge of Courage*," in *Critical Essays on Stephen Crane's* 152–63.

32. "Fighting Words" 236.

33. Andrew Delbanco, "The American Stephen Crane: The Context of *The*

Red Badge of Courage," New Essays on The Red Badge of Courage, ed. Lee Clark Mitchell (New York: Cambridge University Press, 1986): 65.

34. The Fanatics, ed. Lisa A. Long (1901; Acton, Mass.: Copley Publishing Group, 2001). Subsequent references are cited internally as Fanatics.

35. Indeed, Dunbar was keenly aware of the white co-optation of so-called plantation material. He did not condone the racist politics of such writers and advocated the "preserving by Afro-American—I don't like the word—writers these quaint old tales and songs of our fathers which have made the fame of Joel Chandler Harris, Thomas Nelson Page, Ruth McEnery Stuart and others!" Quoted in Joanne Braxton, introduction, The Collected Poetry of Paul Laurence Dunbar (Charlottesville: University Press of Virginia, 1993) xiv.

36. Paul Laurence Dunbar Papers, April 6, 1901, Roll 4, Box 18, Frame 350, Ohio Historical Society (Microfilm edition). All subsequent book reviews, references to contractual materials, and nonfiction essays are cited internally by the location of the materials in the microfilm.

37. Ralph Story, "Paul Laurence Dunbar: Master Player in a Fixed Game," College Language Association Journal 27.1 (1983): 43. Story goes on to dismiss all of Dunbar's novels as "attempts to cater to an audience desirous of (and only willing to accept) the black stereotypes by now entrenched in the national psyche" (40). Benjamin Brawley adds, "The novel is hardly more satisfying than [a shorter story that was equally disappointing], and the reception it received was a great disappointment to the author, who had labored earnestly upon it." Paul Laurence Dunbar, Poet of His People (Chapel Hill: University of North Carolina Press, 1936) 93. Finally, Addison Gayle states bluntly, "The Fanatics is a bad novel . . . [and] of all the failures of the book, Nigger Ed fails the most." Oak and Ivey: A Biography of Paul Laurence Dunbar (Garden City, N.Y.: Doubleday & Co., Inc., 1971) 140, 139.

38. Mia Bay, The White Image in the Black Mind: African-American Ideas about White People, 1830–1925 (New York: Oxford University Press, 2000) 75–76.

39. In his correspondence Dunbar expresses similarly classist sentiments; a letter to his lifetime benefactor, Dr. Tobey, expresses the hope that Dunbar would be able to go to "Washington, New York, Boston and Philadelphia, where [he] might see our Northern Negro at his best, before seeing his brother in the South." Quoted in Brawley 37.

40. Dunbar's papers contain a typewritten manuscript of the novel-in-progress, entitled "Copperheads," as well as the manuscript and proof version of The Fanatics.

41. Reviewers again and again remarked on Dunbar's amazing ability to see inside the tortured souls of Confederates and copperheads, suggesting that his meticulous narrative strategies gained him a rare hearing among many white readers. Words such as "tolerant," "sympathetic," "noble," and "unprejudiced" pepper reviews from the midwest to the southeast to New England. The New York Times says, "Above all, Mr. Dunbar is to be commended for his sobriety and for his broad liberality" in his sympathetic portrayal of Confederates as honorable gentlemen (April 6, 1901, Roll 5, Box 18, Frame 350). "One looks in vain for any bitterness of tone or morbid emphasis," the Des Moines, Iowa Leader testifies (April 14, 1901, Roll 5, Box 18, Frame 380).

42. Hazel Carby, "The Multicultural Wars," The Radical History Review 54 (Fall 1992): 7–18.

43. Act Like You Know: African-American Autobiography and White Identity (Chicago: University of Chicago Press, 1998) 9.

44. Gayle, *Oak and Ivey* 138.

45. Later in April Alice assured Dunbar that the *Kansas City Star* and the *New York Times* "are both almost eulogistic. . . . They make my heart warm." On April 15, she explains that the *Outlook* reviewer raises a point of fact about Dunbar's anachronistic use of Clement Vallandigham, "apologizing for doing so and calling it a very minor one." In *The Letters of Paul and Alice Dunbar: A Private History, Part 2*, ed. E. Metcalf (Ann Arbor, Mich.: University Microfilms International, 1981). Dunbar kept a scrapbook of his reviews, including appraisals of *The Fanatics* from all over the country. Not all reviews were eulogistic. Several reviewers criticized the plotting and characterization of the novel. However, most chalked up such infelicities to the inexperience of the young author and viewed the book a promising portent of better fiction to come.

46. Braxton, *Collected Poetry* 9–11. Subsequent poem references are cited internally as *Collected Poetry*.

47. See Allen Flint, "Black Response to Colonel Shaw," *Phylon* 45.3 (1984): 211–12. Flint singles out Dunbar's poem, for it is the first that hinted that Shaw's sacrifice had been in vain. As such, the poem may be read as a precursor of *The Fanatics*, where Dunbar makes a clear connection between the activities of wartime America and their disappointing consequences.

48. "Racial Fire in the Poetry of Paul Laurence Dunbar," *A Singer in the Dawn: Reinterpretations of Paul Laurence Dunbar*, ed. Jay Martin (New York: Dodd, Mead & Co., 1975) 83.

49. "Recession Never" appeared in the *Cincinnati Rostrum* on December 17, 1898 (Roll 19, Frames 799–800). According to Kenny G. Williams, the article received widespread circulation, appearing not only in many of the papers in Ohio and New York but also in many Chicago newspapers. "The Masking of the Novelist," *A Singer in the Dawn* 181. Jay Martin adds that the article was written originally for *McClure's*. However, this article proved "too strong" for the supposedly radical publication. "Paul Laurence Dunbar: Biography through Letters," *A Singer in the Dawn* 28. Addison Gayle was the first Dunbar critic to see that the "American Civil War, the product of national strife, might have served as the metaphor for a different kind of war—that between the races, which raged as intently in its own way as that between North and South during the 1860s." "Literature As Catharsis: The Novels of Paul Laurence Dunbar," *A Singer in the Dawn* 139–51.

50. Related in Virginia Cunningham, *Paul Laurence Dunbar and His Song* (New York: Dodd, Mead & Co., 1947) 207–11.

51. "Recession Never" 25.

52. K. Williams 169.

53. Morrison 5.

54. Morrison 19. K. Williams traces an interesting parallel between Dunbar's Nigger Ed and Twain's Nigger Jim in *Huckleberry Finn*. Ed, like Jim, "is the one Negro who is well known and with whom the entire race is identified" (186). Morrison continues that there is no way for Huck to obtain moral maturity without Jim's perpetual bondage.

55. "Recession Never" 26.

56. Lutz xii.

57. For a discussion of nervous bankruptcy, see Gosling, *Before Freud* 85.

58. Bederman 59, and Wiegman, *American Anatomies*.

59. Young, *Disarming the Nation* 198–200

60. G. Frank Lydston, M.D., *The Diseases of Society and Degeneracy: The Vice and*

Crime Problem (Philadelphia: J. B. Lippincott Co., 1904) 267. All subsequent references to this text are taken from this edition and are cited in the text as *Diseases*.

61. Lutz 5.

62. Lydston uses the recent Haymarket massacre, the Spanish-American war, and the assassination of President McKinley to generate his theories. Eugene S. Talbot refers to ancient history and the fall of the Roman Empire. *Degeneracy: Its Causes, Signs, and Results* (1898; New York: Garland Publishing Inc., 1984) 8. All subsequent references appear internally as *Degeneracy*. Still others discuss nineteenth-century European wars, such as the Napoleonic wars and the Thirty Years War. But the significance of the American Civil War in turn-of-the-century theories of race degeneracy seems absolutely taboo. Talbot is concerned solely with the institutional legacy of the Civil War, noting that it is a "natural" source of the "degradation" of American charitable and correctional institutions from 1861 to 1881 (21). Lydston goes a bit further, implying that those who began the Civil War were paranoid, for "the literal interpretation of State's rights on the part of the South precipitated the great Civil War" (242). However, he never admonishes Southerners directly. Lydston's only other reference to the Civil War is a seemingly offhand remark that "the unavoidable demoralization of the men of this country by the Civil War is well-nigh forgotten" (*Diseases* 264).

63. George Beard, *American Nervousness: Its Causes and Consequences* (1881; New York: Arno Press, 1972) vi.

64. Lydston also identifies the relationship between American nervousness, violence, and speech acts, which occupies all three historical novelists. He believes that "the flamboyant speech of the anarchist, like some of the more violent outward manifestations of hysteria, often serves to relieve nerve-tension" (*Diseases* 243). Thus, speech is directly related to neurasthenia. However, Lydston objects to efforts to control speech, for he finds the results of the "first serious attempt to 'bottle' anarchy in America," disastrous (*Diseases* 243). Read within this context, the "romance of reunion" dominating popular versions of the Civil War was detrimental to any efforts to heal the wounds of war.

65. Ambrose Bierce, "Chickamauga," *The Civil War Short Stories of Ambrose Bierce* 53–58. First published in the *San Francisco Examiner* on January 20, 1889, this story was subsequently reprinted in *Tales of Soldiers and Civilians* (1892).

66. Tubercular diseases such as those from which Crane and Dunbar suffered were among those contributing to the degeneracy of the race. Talbot explains that chronic disease "constitutes an element of degeneracy, since the victim of the chronic disease is able to leave more offspring than would be possible were the disorder acute. . . . The germ of the disease may be inherited, or general nutrition of the foetus may be so checked in development that the child inherits a predisposition to disease" (*Degeneracy* 121).

67. David Starr Jordan, *War and the Breed: The Relation of War to the Downfall of Nations* (1915; Washington, D.C.: The Cliveden Press, 1981) and Havelock Ellis, *Essays in War-Time: Further Studies in the Task of Social Hygiene* (Boston: Houghton, Mifflin and Company, 1917). All subsequent references to these texts are cited internally as *War* and *Essays* respectively.

68. Mitchell, *In War Time* 180.

Chapter 6

1. My reading of these nursing bodies has been influenced by Elizabeth Grosz's work in *Volatile Bodies: Toward a Corporeal Feminism* (Bloomington: Indi-

ana University Press, 1994). "Can it be that in the West, in our time," she asks, "the female body has been constructed not only as a lack or absence but with more complexity, as a leaking, uncontrollable, seeping liquid; as formless flow; as viscosity, entrapping, secreting; as lacking not so much or simply the phallus but self-containment—not a cracked or porous vessel, like a leaking ship, but a formlessness that engulfs all form, a disorder that threatens all order? I am not suggesting that this is how women *are*, that it is their ontological status. Instead, my hypothesis is that women's corporeality is inscribed as a mode of seepage" (203). Although I am intrigued by Grosz's view of the fluid permeability of women's bodies, I find that Civil War nurses do not ooze contaminating fluids but, rather, produce needed balm for injured Americans.

2. "Our Women and the War," *Harper's Weekly* 23 (August 1862): 568–70.

3. Jane E. Schultz has begun this sort of analysis on female hospital workers in "'Are We Not All Soldiers?' Northern Women in the Civil War Hospital Service," *Prospects: An Annual of American Cultural Studies*, ed. Jack Salzman, vol. 20 (New York: Cambridge University Press, 1996) 39–56. The nurses reclaimed by most feminist historians have been a homogeneous group. See Nina Bennett Smith, "The Women Who Went to War: The Union Army Nurse in the Civil War," diss., Northwestern University, 1981, 111; Ann Douglas Wood, "The War Within a War: Women Nurses in the Union Army," *Civil War History* 18 (September 1972): 197–212; Schultz, "Inhospitable Hospital"; and Ginzberg, *Women and Benevolence.* They recount the experiences of relatively powerful white women, i.e., Jane Stuart Woolsey, Mother Bickerdyke, and Georgeanna Woolsey.

4. "Woman," *Frank Leslie's Illustrated Newspaper* 27 (September 1862): 25.

5. See particularly Young's chapter entitled "A Wound of One's Own: Louisa May Alcott's Body Politic" in *Disarming the Nation,* where she explains Alcott's attraction to the "freeing dislocations caused by Civil War," which allowed Alcott to rebel against normative femininity (79). Both Young and Mary Capello in "'Looking about Me with All My Eyes': Censored Viewing, Carnival, and Louisa May Alcott's *Hospital Sketches,*" *Arizona Quarterly* 50.3 (Autumn 1994): 59–88, have written on the "topsy-turvy" and "carnivalesque" nature of the hospital zone, respectively. Young reads Alcott's disorder as enabling Trib's gender inversions, wheras Capello notes that Alcott's carnivalesque rendering of the nation's capitol makes gender and racial difference disturbingly indistinguishable. See also Jane E. Schultz, "Embattled Care: Narrative Authority in Louisa May Alcott's *Hospital Sketches,*" *Legacy* 9.2 (1992): 104–18.

6. See N. Smith, "Women Who Went to War" 111.

7. Schultz, "Inhospitable Hospital" 365.

8. Alcott, *Hospital Sketches.* All subsequent references taken from Showalter's *Alternative Alcott* and are cited internally as Alcott.

9. Young contends that Trib's delirious illness replicates the phantom limb pain accompanying the soldiers' amputations: "Even as she metaphorically feminizes the male soldier, Alcott also offers a metonymic displacement of war injury from bodies to minds and from men to women" (446).

10. See Jane Marcus, "Corpus/Corpse/Corps: Writing the Body in/at War," *Arms and the Woman: War, Gender and Literary Representation,* ed. Helen M. Cooper, Adrienne Auslander Munich and Susan Merrill Squier (Chapel Hill: University Press of North Carolina, 1989) 124–67, Young 75, and Schultz, "Embattled Care."

11. Cited in Sylvia G. L. Dannett, *Noble Women of the North* (New York: Thomas Yoseloff, 1959) 60.

12. Alcott's imagery suggests the nun-like aspects of Nurse Periwinkle's secular commitment, but Schultz's work explains the larger implications of that social paradigm. She writes, "Surgeons were especially fond of appointing Catholic sisters because the nuns did not require pay and asked for little in the way of accommodations" ("Inhospitable Hospital" 367). Some doctors even lobbied to have their more demanding, secular nurses removed and replaced with nuns. See Ellen Ryan Jolly, *Nuns of the Battlefield* (Providence: Providence Visitor Press, 1927), and Mary Denis Maher, *To Bind up the Wounds: Catholic Sister Nurses in the U.S. Civil War* (New York: Greenwood Press, 1989).

13. *The Journals of Louisa May Alcott*, ed. Joel Myerson and Daniel Shealy (Boston: Little, Brown & Company, 1989) 115.

14. *Louisa May Alcott: Her Life, Letters, and Journals*, ed. Ednah D. Cheney (Boston: Roberts Brothers, 1891) 150.

15. Elaine Showalter, introduction, *Alternative Alcott* by Louisa May Alcott (New Brunswick, N.J.: Rutgers University Press, 1988) xxvi.

16. "As *Hospital Sketches* crafts a new home, Hurly-burly House, for Alcott's domestic unrest, so too does the text translate her antebellum war fervor into actual war fever. In this translation, her illness gains new value, masculinized as battle service rather than essentialized as female hysteria" (Young 452). Capello interprets Alcott's illness as authorizing her to critique society: "Alcott further manipulates, in fact, re-appropriates the disempowered positions of seamstress and sick person to carve out a vantage point (in that middle section of the book titled 'Off Duty') from which to say that which was denied her" (68).

17. Reprinted as Mary Livermore, *My Story of the War: The Civil War Memoirs of the Famous Nurse, Relief Organizer and Suffragette*, ed. Nina Silber (1890; New York: Da Capo Press, 1995) 110. All subsequent references to this text will be cited parenthetically as *My Story*.

18. Nina Silber, introduction, *My Story* xi, vii.

19. Mary A. Gardner Holland, *Our Army Nurses: Interesting Sketches, Addresses, and Photographs of Nearly One Hundred of the Noble Women Who Served in Hospitals and on Battlefields during Our Civil War* (Boston: Press of Lousbery, Nichols & Worth, 1895). Subsequent references from this text cited internally as *Army Nurses*.

20. See Margaret Davis Burton, *The Women Who Battled for the Boys in Blue, Mother Bickerdyke: Her Life and Labor for the Relief of Our Soldiers* (San Francisco: A. T. Dewey, 1886); Julia A. Houghton Chase, *Mary A. Bickerdyke, "Mother": The Life Story of One Who, As Wife, Mother, Army Nurse, Pension Agent and City Missionary, Has Touched the Heights and Depths of Human Life* (Lawrence, Kans.: Journal Publishing House, 1896); Florence Shaw Kellogg, *Mother Bickerdyke, As I Knew Her* (Chicago: Unity Publishing Co., 1907).

21. S. Weir Mitchell, *Roland Blake* (New York: Century Company, 1886). Subsequent references from this text are cited internally as *Roland*.

22. S. Weir Mitchell, "Address before the Fiftieth Annual Meeting of the American Medico-Psychological Association, Held in Philadelphia, May 16th, 1894." Reprinted in *American Journal of Psychiatry, Sesquicentennial Supplement* 151.6 (June 1994): 32, 36.

23. S. Weir Mitchell, *Fat and Blood* (Philadelphia: J. B. Lippincott and Co., 1877) 6. Subsequent references from this text are cited internally as *Fat and Blood*.

24. *New York World*, May 11, 1866. Cited in Israel Kugler, *From Ladies to Women: The Organized Struggle for Woman's Rights in the Reconstruction Era* (New York: Greenwood Press, 1987).

25. Nicole Hahn Rafter, *White Trash: The Eugenic Family Studies* (Boston: Northeastern University Press, 1988).

26. The initial quote comes from Schultz, "Are We Not All Soldiers?" 43; Wood 199; and Schultz, "Inhospitable Hospital" 386.

27. Dale M. Bauer, *Edith Wharton's Brave New Politics* (Madison: The University of Wisconsin Press, 1995) 29, 51.

28. Hamilton 346.

29. Bauer 34.

30. According to Carroll Smith-Rosenberg, "In rejecting conventional female roles and asserting their right to a career, to a public voice, to visible power," New Women "laid claim to the rights and privileges customarily accorded bourgeois men." Carroll Smith-Rosenberg, *Disorderly Conduct: Visions of Gender in Victorian America* (New York: Oxford University Press, 1985) 176.

31. Gilman, *Difference and Pathology* 40.

32. Gilman, *Difference and Pathology* 24.

33. Claudia Tate contends that many African American writers believed that the "acquisition of their full citizenship would result as much or more from demonstrating their adoption of the 'genteel standard of Victorian sexual conduct' as from protesting racial injustice." *Domestic Allegories of Political Desire: The Black Heroine's Text at the Turn of the Century* (New York: Oxford University Press, 1992) 4.

34. African American Civil War nursing was not unprecedented in American literature. In the third incarnation of William Wells Brown's *Clotel, or the Colored Heroine: A Tale of the Southern States* (1867), the beautiful and pious octoroon, Clotel, returns from Europe to nurse Civil War soldiers. In her seminal treatment of *Iola Leroy*, Barbara Christian, too, recognizes Iola's affinity with Clotel, writing, "Like Clotel, the Angel of Mercy, Iola Leroy, when freed, nurses wounded soldiers. But Harper emphasized even more than Brown her heroine's commitment to the race." *Black Women Novelists: The Development of a Tradition, 1892–1976* (Westport, Conn.: Greenwood Press, 1980) 29. Nursing by enslaved women was also prominent. In *Incidents in the Life of a Slave Girl*, ed. Jean Fagan Yellin (1861; Cambridge, Mass.: Harvard University Press, 1987), Harriet Jacobs writes that her mother was weaned at three months so that the white daughter of the slave-owning family could be "nourished at [Jacobs's] grandmother's breast" (7).

35. Recall that she had removed her top at an antislavery meeting, claiming "that her breasts had suckled many a white babe, to the exclusion of her own offspring" and asking the audience "if they, too wished to suck!" Quoted in Sterling 153.

36. *Iola Leroy; or, Shadows Uplifted*, ed. Hazel Carby (1892; Boston: Beacon Press, 1987) 31. All subsequent references to Harper's text are cited internally as Harper.

37. Fannie Barrier Williams, "The Colored Woman and Her Part in Race Regeneration," *A New Negro for a New Century*, ed. Booker T. Washington (Chicago: American Publishing House, 1900) 424, 428.

38. Darlene Clark Hine, *Black Women in White: Racial Conflict and Cooperation in the Nursing Profession* (Bloomington: Indiana University Press, 1989) xxii. "From the very outset nurses were expected to deal with the patient as part of a broader social system." Hine adds later that one prominent African American founder of nursing schools, Daniel Hale Williams, extolled black women as "natural nurturers" who would teach the people "cleanliness, thrift, habits of indus-

try, sanitary housekeeping, the proper care of themselves and of their children" (13).

39. See Tate 132, and Young 278.

40. Reprinted in Melba Joyce Boyd, *Discarded Legacy: Politics and Poetics in the Life of Frances E. W. Harper, 1825–1911* (Detroit: Wayne State University Press, 1994) 116. From *Proceedings of the Eleventh National Woman's Rights Convention,* New York, May 10, 1866, Frances Harper Collection, the Historical Society of Pennsylvania, Philadelphia, Penn.

41. *Reminiscences of My Life in Camp with the 33rd U.S. Colored Troops, Late 1st South Carolina Volunteers,* reprinted as *A Black Woman's Civil War Memoirs,* ed. Patricia W. Romero and Willie Lee Rose (1902; New York: Markus Wiener Publishing, 1988) 62. All subsequent references to Taylor's text are cited internally as Taylor.

42. In exploring suffragist Elizabeth Cady Stanton's 1892 invocation of "hands"—a reference that is exactly contemporaneous to Harper's work in *Iola Leroy*—Gillian Brown explains the multiple connotations of "hands" as "grasping, producing, possessing, controlling, and authorizing." *Domestic Individualism* 4.

43. Washington quote cited in Hine 13.

44. Deborah McDowell, "'The Changing Same': Generational Connections and Black Women Novelists," *New Literary History* 18.2 (1987): 298.

45. Hazel Carby points out that Iola's fate subverts conventional plotting, in which heroines secure stability only through marriage. In Harper's novel, "Iola had not found a protector to lift her into a life of security; security had been achieved in other ways throughout the course of the novel." *Reconstructing Womanhood: The Emergence of the Afro-American Woman Novelist* (New York: Oxford University Press, 1987) 80.

46. It has often been argued that Harper, and I would add, Taylor, were attempting to counter the "Jezebel" image of African American women prevalent in nineteenth-century literature. See Patricia Morton, who observes that much of the hatred of the exotic mulatto was fueled by white men's frustration at the new sexual inaccessibility of black women. *Disfigured Images* 5, 30.

47. She might also invoke the simple dress of the Quakers here, for Harper maintained a political relationship with that group throughout her life. Boyd 132. Jacqueline Jones cogently explains the significance of postbellum African American dress. "Self indulgence" in clothes represented the "insolent, disrespectful" manner of newly outspoken freedwomen. Instead, "plain, neat dress" such as that worn by other "working classes" was commensurate with African Americans' eternal status as laborers. In *Freed Women?: Black Women, Work, and the Family During the Civil War and Reconstruction* (Wellesley, Mass.: Center for Research on Women, 1980) 47–48.

48. Young 189. Whereas African American mothers often take a central, heroic role in African American narratives, Civil War works are characterized by maternal absence.

49. M. Elizabeth Carnegie, *The Path We Tread: Blacks in Nursing, 1854–1984* (Philadelphia: Lippincott, 1985) 1.

50. See Barbara Melosh, *"The Physician's Hand": Work, Culture and Conflict in American Nursing* (Philadelphia: Temple University Press, 1982) 21. However, African American women were extremely active following the Civil War in their own separate project of education and professionalization. As Hine cogently has documented, the African American community created a network of about a dozen black hospitals and nurse training schools during the 1890s (188, x).

51. Schultz, "'Are We Not All Soldiers?'" 41.

52. Historian Benjamin Quarles confirms that Taylor often accompanied Barton on her rounds during Barton's eight months on the Sea Islands. *The Negro in the Civil War* (Boston: Little, Brown & Co., 1953) 228.

53. Reprinted in Boyd 222–225. Apparently, this speech inspired the publication of the journal *The Women's Era.*

54. *Black Women Writing Autobiography: A Tradition within a Tradition* (Philadelphia: Temple University Press, 1989) 66.

55. Jocelyn K. Moody contends that Taylor "supplants a community of black military men and women in place of the author as its focal point." "Twice Other, Once Shy: Nineteenth-Century Black Women Autobiographers and the American Literary Tradition of Self-Effacement" *a/b: Auto/Biography Studies* 7.1 (1992): 53.

56. Hine xvii.

57. In an 1878 essay, "Coloured Women of America," Harper notes how many African American women "have gone into medicine and have been practicing in different States of the Union. In the Woman's Medical College of Pennsylvania, two coloured women were last year pursuing their studies as Matriculants, while a young woman, the daughter of a former fugitive slave, has held the position of an assistant physician in one of the hospitals. Miss Cole, of Philadelphia, held for some time the position of physician in the State Orphan Asylum in South Carolina." She adds that "coloured women have been able to help each other in sickness" as well, setting up homes for the aged. Reprinted in Boyd 213.

58. Jane Campbell, *Mythic Black Fiction: The Transformation of History* (Knoxville: University of Tennessee Press, 1986) 28.

Chapter 7

1. Booker T. Washington, *A New Negro for a New Century* (Chicago: American Publishing House, 1900) 3.

2. "Black History's Antebellum Origins," *Black Mosaic: Essays in Afro-American History and Historiography* (Amherst: The University of Massachussets Press, 1988) 109–34, 109.

3. Quarles, *Black Mosaic* 107.

4. See *Order of Things*, for example, 367–69.

5. *A New Negro* 164.

6. *Reminiscences* 135.

7. *Conjugal Bonds: The Body, The House, and the Black American* (New York: Oxford University Press, 1999) 5.

8. Quarles, *Black Mosaic* 114, 119. Famous enthologist Samuel G. Morton asserted as early as 1839 that he could tell the difference between the Caucasian and Negro races in the skull remains of ancient Egypt.

9. Quoted in Quarles, *Black Mosaic* 110.

10. Quoted in Quarles, *Black Mosaic* 117.

11. George Washington Williams, *A History of the Negro Troops in the War of the Rebellion, 1861–1865* (1888; New York: Negro Universities Press, 1969) 332. All subsequent references to this text cited internally as Williams.

12. Williams's biographer, John Hope Franklin, has gathered all of Williams's reviews in *George Washington Williams: A Biography* (Chicago: University of Chi-

cago Press, 1985) 130–31. It is interesting to note that Williams's publisher, Harper and Brothers, revitalized more positive war-era imagery of African Americans in their presentation of his book. The cover "bore the impression of a Negro sergeant, dressed in the uniform of the Union Army and shouldering a rifle," as well as a "steel engraving of Williams dressed in full militia uniform and wearing a medal" (130).

13. Earl Thorpe, *Negro Historians in the United States* (Baton Rouge, La.: Fraternal Press, 1958) 29, and J. H. Franklin 131. Priscilla Wald explains how Du Bois's subsequent work, *The Souls of Black Folk* (1903), "makes scant claim to 'objectivity'; it is, rather about objectivity, and his generic hybridity depicts the struggle, against preconceptions as well as expedient sociohistorical narratives, to re-present a history of the United States that acknowledges and depicts the centrality of African Americans to that story." *Constituting Americans: Cultural Anxiety and Narrative Form* (Durham, N.C.: Duke University Press, 1995) 174.

14. Information on the popular reception to Wilson's work is taken from Thorpe, *Negro Historians* 39.

15. Norwood P. Hallowell, *The Negro As a Soldier in the War of the Rebellion* (Boston: Little, Brown & Co, 1897). Subsequent references appear internally as Hallowell. Whereas Williams, Wilson, and Fleetwood were African American veterans, Hallowell was white. Although an ardent abolitionist and leader of the 55th Massachusetts, Hallowell's racial privilege surely influenced his version of the Negro soldiers' accomplishments; his investment in this project of historical reclamation is not the same as that of his African American colleagues. However, he seems similarly committed to praising the Negro troops' heroism. For more information on Hallowell, see Luis F. Emilio, *History of the Fifty-Fourth Regiment of Massachusetts Volunteer Infantry, 1863–1865* (Boston: Boston Book Company, 1894). Williams, Wilson, and Fleetwood were all veterans who had marked themselves as leaders within their regiments and had gone on to work as journalists, academics, and politicians during Reconstruction.

16. "'What Will Peace among the Whites Bring?' Reunion and Race in the Struggle over the Memory of the Civil War in American Culture," *Massachusetts Review* 34.3 (Fall 1993): 397.

17. In Joseph T. Wilson, *The Black Phalanx* (1890; New York: Arno Press, 1968) 200. All subsequent references to this text cited internally as Wilson. For more information on the "ambivalence, ambiguity, and disillusionment that the military experience held" for African American men and women, see Cullen, "I's a Man Now" 84. And for a broader history of African American participation in the war, see Quarles, *Negro in the Civil War*; Cornish, *Sable Arm*; William A. Gladstone, *Men of Color* (Gettysburg, Penn.: Thomas Publications, 1993); Hargrove, *Black Union Soldiers*; Joseph T. Glatthaar, *Forged in Battle: The Civil War Alliance of Black Soldiers and White Officers* (New York: Free Press, 1990).

18. Eric Foner begins his towering study, *Reconstruction*, with emancipation. He comments that war is the "midwife of revolution" (3).

19. From a letter to the editor in the *Christian Recorder*, July 16, 1864; cited in McPherson, *Negro's Civil War.*

20. Sidney Kaplan, "The Black Soldier of the Civil War in Literature and Art," *American Studies in Black and White: Selected Essays, 1949–1989*, ed. Allan D. Austin (Amherst: University of Massachusetts Press, 1991) 108. He adds, "During the conflict, the newspapers and magazines of the day printed regular reports of the recruitment and battlefield activity of the black regiments, as well as articles and interviews dealing with the individual exploits of black infantrymen, artillerymen, scouts, and guerrillas, illustrated copiously" (103).

21. Kaplan 108.

22. "The Battleground of Historical Memory: Creating Alternative Culture Heroes in Post-bellum America," *Journal of Popular Culture* 20.1 (1986): 58. David Blight adds that the African American community was equally as anxious in many cases to forget the "origins and consequences as well as the sacrifices" of the Civil War. Blight reminds us of Frederick Douglass's postbellum diatribes against such "social forgetting." "'What Will Peace Among the Whites Bring?'" 98.

23. Christian A. Fleetwood, *The Negro as a Soldier* (Washington, D.C.: Howard University Print, 1895). This text is cited internally as Fleetwood. Fleetwood prepared this speech and the subsequent pamphlet for presentation to the "Cotton State and International Exposition" held in Atlanta, Georgia in November 1895. Fleetwood himself was one of the few commissioned Negro officers, obtaining the rank of Sergeant-Major in the 4th U.S. Colored Troops. He is cited in George Washington Williams's "Roll of Honor" for receiving a special medal for gallant conduct.

24. Earl Thorpe, *The Central Theme of Black History* (Durham, N.C.: Seeman Printery, 1969) 3.

25. Wiegman, *American Anatomies* 82.

26. Henry Louis Gates Jr., "The Trope of the New Negro and the Reconstruction of the Image of the Black," *The New American Studies*, ed. Philip Fisher (Berkeley: University of California Press, 1991) 319. For simplicity's sake, I will borrow Peter Novick's language in *That Noble Dream* to broadly outline the commonly held definition of *Objectivist or Scientific history*. Objectivist history garners its values/practices from scientific method: "Science must be rigidly factual and empirical, shunning hypothesis; the scientific venture was scrupulously neutral on larger questions of end and meaning; and, if systematically pursued, it might ultimately produce a comprehensive, 'definitive' history" (37). Additionally, Objectivism rests upon a "commitment to the reality of the past . . . and a sharp separation between knower and known" (2).

27. J. H. Franklin 100.

28. Thorpe, *Negro Historians* 25.

29. Novick 61. For example, prominent genteel historian James Ford Rhodes marshaled the war as evidence of Anglo-Saxon superiority (different aspects being illustrated by each side), and evidence that the Negro is "one of the most inferior races of mankind." Robert Cruden argues for the "awesome confidence of the American public in Rhodes' fairness, objectivity and integrity" in "James Ford Rhodes and the Negro: A Study in the Problem of Objectivity," *Understanding Negro History*, ed. Dwight D. Hoover (Chicago: Quadrangle Books, 1968) 97, 96.

30. Silber, *Romance of Reunion* 2, 124.

31. Novick 78, and J. H. Franklin 133. Also see John Higham's *History: The Development of Historical Studies in the United States* (Englewood Cliffs, N.J.: Prentice-Hall, 1965), and W. Stull Holt's *Historical Scholarship in the United States* (Seattle: University of Washington Press, 1967).

32. Stepto, *Behind the Veil* 3. Although Stepto goes to great lengths to distinguish among nineteenth-century male-authored slave narratives, for my purpose I use his analysis piecemeal.

33. Michael O'Malley, "Specie and Species: Race and the Money Question in Nineteenth-Century America" *American Historical Review* 99.2 (1994): 370, 372. O'Malley also traces the root of turn-of-the-century racial economics to the

greenbacks that African American troops were initially given as pay. "'The greenback was the first thing they ever earned that they could call their own, the first thing, save the flag, that stood before them, a symbol of their freedom.' Greenbacks symbolized the power of government to overturn the natural law arguments that justified slavery. . . . Greenbacks made it possible for slaves to own property and establish families, the two bulwarks of republican citizenship. . . . But could citizens created with the help of valueless currency ever acquire any genuine value of their own?" Also see Nell Irvin Painter's article in the same issue of *AHR*, "Thinking about the Languages of Money and Race: A Response to Michael O'Malley, 'Specie and Species,'" *American Historical Review* 99.2 (1994): 396–404. Painter nuances O'Malley's argument, insisting, "Before 1865, the vast majority of African Americans were, literally, property, and they served simultaneously as an embodied currency and a labor force" (398).

34. J. H. Franklin 104.

35. Charles Victor Langlois and Charles Segnobos, *Introduction to the Study of History* (New York: Henry Holt & Co, 1898).

36. Novick 2.

37. Thorpe asserts that fully one-half of Wilson's history consists of direct quotations. *Negro Historians* 30. He also emphasizes the wide variety of resources consulted: libraries in Boston, New York, Cincinnati and New Bedford, private libraries, records from the War Department, letters, and newspapers. Additionally, Thorpe claims that Williams consulted more than twelve thousand volumes in researching his *History of the Negro Race* (32).

38. J. H. Franklin 127.

39. Novick 38.

40. Donald J. Mrozek, "The Habit of Victory: The American Military and the Cult of Manliness," *Manliness and Morality: Middle-Class Masculinity in Britain and America, 1800–1940*, ed. J. A. Mangan and James Walvin (New York: St. Martin's Press, 1987) 221.

41. Higham 95. Also see Dickson D. Bruce Jr., "The Ironic Conception of American History: The Early Black Historians, 1883–1915," *Journal of Negro History* 69.2 (1984): 53–62. Bruce points out that Williams argues "black civilizations, and what they had created, provided the foundations for all of western civilization" in his general history of the race (57).

42. *American Anatomies* 87.

43. Hart quoted in James M. McPherson, *The Abolitionist Legacy: From Reconstruction to the NAACP* (Princeton, N.J.: Princeton University Press, 1975) 337–38.

44. Wiegman 82.

45. Jacquelyn Dowd Hall, "'The Mind that Burns in Each Body': Women, Rape, and Racial Violence," *Powers of Desire: The Politics of Sexuality*, ed. Ann Snitow, Christine Stansell, and Sharon Thompson (New York: Monthly Review Press, 1983) 328–49.

46. Although strength and bravery are most often associated with military life, Mrozek explains that "military courage and manliness inspired a rhetoric of 'softening' as much as 'toughening'" in the nineteenth century (224). Because class standing and wealth were traditional requirements for an officer's commission, and because much of the manpower of the military came from outside the upper and middle classes, Mrozek argues that the development of "grace under pressure" was just as important as brute strength.

47. Chaplain Henry M. Turner, *Christian Recorder*, May 17, 1865.

48. Michael Hatt, "'Making a Man of Him': Masculinity and the Black Body in Mid-Nineteenth-Century American Sculpture," *Oxford Art Journal* 15.1 (1992): 21–35.

49. For a brief look at the treatment of Negro soldiers by Confederate troops, see Richard M. Reid, "Black Experience in the Union Army: The Other Civil War," *Canadian Review of American Studies* 21 (1990): 145–55. In 1905 James Elbert Cutler defined lynching as "an illegal and summary execution at the hands of a mob, or a number of persons, who have in some degree the public opinion of the community behind them." *Lynch-Law: An Investigation into the History of Lynching in the United States* (1905; New York: Negro University Press, 1969) 276. For more detailed discussions of lynching, see Sandra Gunning, *Race, Rape, and Lynching: The Red Record of American Literature, 1890–1912* (New York: Oxford University Press, 1996); W. Fitzhugh Brundage, *Lynching in the New South: Georgia and Virginia, 1880–1930* (Urbana: University of Illinois Press, 1993). Lynching still remains ill-defined.

50. Cullen, "I's a Man Now" 91.

51. William J. Moses, "Dark Forests and Barbarian Vigor: Paradox, Conflict, and Africanity in Black Writing Before 1914," *American Literary History* 1.3 (Fall 1989): 641.

52. Reviews taken from J. H. Franklin 130, 131.

53. J. H. Franklin 106.

54. Bruce 56.

Epilogue

1. James Marten, *The Children's Civil War* (Chapel Hill: The University of North Carolina Press, 1998) 189.

2. Jane Addams, *Twenty Years at Hull-House* (1910; New York: Penguin Books, 1981) 36–37. All subsequent references to this edition are cited parenthetically as Addams.

3. Tony Horwitz, *Confederates in the Attic: Dispatches from the Unfinished Civil War* (New York: Vintage Books, 1998) 1. All subsequent references to this edition are cited parenthetically as Horwitz.

4. For example, when Horwitz interviews popular Civil War historian Shelby Foote, Foote explains, "If you look at American history as the life span of a man, the Civil War represents the great trauma of our adolescence" (146).

5. Louisa May Alcott's well-loved and enduring novel of white girls and the Civil War, *Little Women* (1868), was reissued in the 1880s after Alcott's death; however, as far as I have been able to tell, few writers followed in Alcott's wake. Alice Fahs details the way that girls were provisionally included in war-era Civil War fiction. *Dora Darling, the Daughter of the Regiment* (1864) by Jane Goodwin Austin, makes her way through war-era battlefields. However, Fahs emphasizes that "the sexually-charged instability of her identity as girl heroine was explicitly acknowledged in the text," as two grown men wrangle over postwar custodianship of the "coquettish" twelve-year-old. *The Imagined Civil War* 278.

6. Cullen, *Civil War in Popular Culture* 182. Cullen reveals that several of these events were held in New Jersey during the late 1870s and 1880s.

7. Randal Allred also notes that many Civil War buffs "search for a more meaningful paradigm of conviction and purpose in our time of fragmented self-absorption" (2). "Catharsis, Revision, and Re-enactment: Negotiating the Mean-

ing of the American Civil War," *Journal of American Culture* 19.4 (Winter 1996): 1–13. Allred goes on to argue that reenacting may be an "effort to re-contruct a deconstructing universe" (7). However, I contend that it is the war's ability to express the "deconstruction" at play throughout time in different forms that constitutes its lasting power. Dennis Hall, too, notes that reenactors seek to conjure a time seemingly "free from the complexities and ambiguities of the post-1960s era" (8). "Civil War Reenactors and the Postmodern Sense of History," *Journal of American Culture* 17.3 (Fall 1994): 7–12.

8. Jim Murphy, *The Journal of James Edmond Pease: A Civil War Union Soldier* (New York: Scholastic Inc., 1998). All subsequent references to this text will be cited internally as Murphy. *When Will This Cruel War Be Over?: The Civil War Diary of Emma Simpson* by Barry Dennenberg (New York: Scholastic Inc., 1996), a book in the "Dear America" series, takes place on a Virginia plantation. The protagonist's family has been ravaged by war, and she traditionally represents her family's grief. Indeed, the first scene of the novel mirror's that of Phelps's *The Gates Ajar*, as Emma's brother's coffin is brought home.

9. According to most scholars, including Ruth Elson, "apart from the Bible, the books most widely read in the nineteenth century were not those written by intellectuals, but schoolbooks written by printers, journalists, teachers, ministers, and future lawyers earning their way through college" (vii). This claim holds true into the middle of the twentieth century. The ambitions of some authors and publishers, as well as the budgetary requirements of many school districts, were instrumental in shaping turn-of-the-century and early twentieth-century versions of the Civil War. Few teachers who taught outside the large cities had much education beyond that of the schools in which they taught. Thus rote memorization became the pedagogical tool of choice. Publishers and historians responded to classroom needs, leaving their histories unedited for decades, for school boards would continue to order their books if they ensured textual uniformity. Teachers could conduct mass recitations if the page numbers and text remained unchanged over the years. Consequently, when new material was added to the books it was simply appended to the end of older editions and the copyright date remained unchanged. See *Guardians of Tradition: American Schoolbooks of the Nineteenth Century* (Lincoln: University of Nebraska Press, 1964).

10. Joel Dorman Steele and Esther Baker Steele, *Barnes's School History of the United States* (New York: American Book Company, 1903) 277. Though Joel Steele is awarded most of the credit for the series' success, his wife apparently wrote most of the books. First published in 1871, their text was widely used as late as the 1930s. See John A. Nietz, *Old Textbooks* (Pittsburgh: University of Pittsburgh Press, 1961) 267–68.

11. As one educational historian wonders, "It is somewhat difficult to understand how [such books], each one of which was scarcely more than a syllabus in style . . . could have been as successful as they were. Charles Carpenter, *History of American Schoolbooks* (Philadelphia: University of Pennsylvania Press, 1963) 10.

12. D. H. Montgomery, *The Leading Facts of American History* (Boston: Ginn & Company Publishers, 1893) 302. For background information on this history see Carpenter 206.

13. *Disarming the Nation* 289.

14. See Stuart McConnell, *Glorious Contentment: The Grand Army of the Republic, 1865–1900* (Chapel Hill: University of North Carolina Press, 1992).

15. *Camp Chase Gazette*, "Publisher's Note" (September 1990): 30. This publication is sponsored by the National Regiment, a national reenactors organiza-

tion, and considers itself "The Voice of Civil War Reenacting." Quoted in Cullen, *Civil War in Popular Culture* 181.

16. R. Lee Hadden, *Reliving the Civil War: A Reenactor's Handbook* (Mechanicsburg, Penn.: Stackpole Books, 1999) 36. Cited internally as Hadden.

17. Neil Johnson, *The Battle of Gettysburg* (New York: Four Wings Press, 1989). Cited internally as Johnson.

18. Margaret Whitman Blair, *Brothers at War* (Shippensburg, Penn.: White Mane Publising Co., Inc., 1997). All subsequent quotes cited internally as Blair. Another popular juvenile novel, *The Root Cellar* by Janet Lunn (New York: Puffin Books, 1981), tells of the time travels of a young orphan girl, who finds adventure and enduring friendship in Civil War-era America.

19. Judith Butler, "Imitation and Gender Insubordination," *The Lesbian and Gay Studies Reader*, ed. Henry Abelove, Michèle Aina Barale, and David M. Halperin (New York: Routledge, 1993): 314. The connection between Butler and Civil War renactments might seem a specious one; Butler would emphasize the way that gender is stabilized by such performances. However, I do believe that Butler's larger claim about the truth the body supposedly speaks is useful here.

20. See Young's "Afterword," in which she analyzes the plight of Lauren Cook Burgess, a female reenactor who sued the National Park Service when she was told she could not participate in battles as a male soldier because such a performance would not be authentic.

21. Hall 10.

Bibliography

Aaron, Daniel. "The Etiquette of Grief: A Literary Generation's Response to Death." *Prospects: An Annual of American Cultural Studies.* Ed. Jack Salzman. Vol. 4. New York: Cambridge University Press, 1979. 197–213.

———. *The Unwritten War: American Writers and the Civil War.* New York: Oxford University Press, 1973.

Adams, Nehemiah. *Agnes and the Key to Her Little Coffin.* Boston: S. K. Whipple & Co., 1857.

Adams, Virginia Matzke. Introduction. *On the Altar of Freedom: A Black Soldier's Civil War Letters from the Front.* By James Henry Gooding. Amherst: University of Massachusetts Press, 1991. xv–xxxvii.

Addams, Jane. *Twenty Years at Hull-House.* 1910. New York: Penguin Books, 1981.

Alcott, Louisa May. *Hospital Sketches, Alternative*   ine Showalter. New Brunswick, N.J.: Rutgers University Press, 19

———. *The Journals of Louisa May Alcott.* Ed. Joel Myerson and Daniel Shealy. Boston: Little, Brown & Co., 1989.

———. *Little Women.* Boston: Roberts Brothers, 1868.

———. *Louisa May Alcott: Her Life, Letters, and Journals.* Ed. Ednah D. Cheney. Boston: Roberts Brothers, 1891.

Allred, Randal. "Catharsis, Revision, and Re-enactment: Negotiating the Meaning of the American Civil War." *Journal of American Culture* 19 (Winter 1996): 1–13.

Alotta, Robert. *Civil War Justice: Union Army Executions under Lincoln.* Shippensburg, Penn.: White Mane Publications, 1989.

Antoni, Robert. "*Miss Ravenel's Conversion*: A Neglected American Novel." *The Southern Quarterly* 24.3 (1986): 58–63.

Barton, Michael. *Goodmen: The Character of Civil War Soldiers.* University Park: Pennsylvania State University Press, 1981.

Baudrillard, Jean. *Simulacra and Simulation.* 1981. Trans. by Sheila Faria Glaser. Ann Arbor: University of Michigan Press, 1994.

Bauer, Dale M. *Edith Wharton's Brave New Politics.* Madison: University of Wisconsin Press, 1995.

Bay, Mia. *The White Image in the Black Mind: African-American Ideas about White People, 1830–1925.* New York: Oxford University Press, 2000.

Beard, George. *American Nervousness: Its Causes and Consequences.* 1881. New York: Arno Press, 1972.

Bederman, Gail. *Manliness and Civilization: A Cultural History of Gender and Race in the United States, 1880–1917.* Chicago: University of Chicago Press, 1995.

Benfey, Christopher. *The Double Life of Stephen Crane.* London: Andre Deutsch, 1992.

Berlin, Ira, ed. *Freedom: A Documentary History of Emancipation, 1861–1867.* The

Black Military Experience. Ser. II. New York: Cambridge University Press, 1982.

Bierce, Ambrose. *The Civil War Short Stories of Ambrose Bierce.* Ed. Ernest J. Hopkins. Lincoln: University of Nebraska Press, 1988.

———. *Devil's Dictionary.* 1911. New York: Dover, 1993.

Billington, Ray Allen. Introduction. *The Journal of Charlotte L. Forten.* By Charlotte L. Forten. New York: Dryden, 1953. 1–40.

Blair, Margaret Whitman. *Brothers at War.* Shippensburg, Penn.: White Mane Publising Co., 1997.

Blight, David W. *Frederick Douglass's Civil War: Keeping Faith in Jubilee.* Baton Rouge: Louisiana State University Press, 1989.

———. *Race and Reunion: The Civil War in American Memory.* Cambridge, Mass.: Harvard University Press, 2001.

———. " 'What Will Peace among the Whites Bring?' Reunion and Race in the Struggle over the Memory of the Civil War in American Culture." *Massachusetts Review* 34.3 (Fall 1993): 393–410.

Blumin, Stuart. *The Emergence of the Middle-Class: Social Experience in the American City, 1760–1900.* New York: Cambridge University Press, 1989.

Boyd, Melba Joyce. *Discarded Legacy: Politics and Poetics in the Life of Frances E. W. Harper, 1825–1911.* Detroit, Mich.: Wayne State University Press, 1994.

Braude, Anne. *Radical Spirits: Spiritualism and Women's Rights in Nineteenth-Century America.* Boston: Beacon Press, 1989.

Brawley, Benjamin. *Paul Laurence Dunbar, Poet of His People.* Chapel Hill: University of North Carolina Press, 1936.

Braxton, Joanne. *Black Women Writing Autobiography: A Tradition within a Tradition.* Philadelphia: Temple University Press, 1989.

———. "Charlotte Forten Grimké and the Search for a Public Voice." *The Private Self: Theory and Practice of Women's Autobiographical Writings.* Ed. Shari Benstock. Chapel Hill: University of North Carolina Press, 1988. 254–71.

———. Introduction. *The Collected Poetry of Paul Laurence Dunbar.* Charlottesville: University Press of Virginia, 1993. ix–xxxvi.

Brody, Howard. *Stories of Sickness.* New Haven, Conn.: Yale University Press, 1987.

Brooks, Stewart. *Civil War Medicine.* Springfield, Ill.: Charles C. Thomas, 1966.

Brown, Gillian. *Domestic Individualism: Imagining Self in Nineteenth-Century America.* Berkeley: University of California Press, 1990.

Bruce, Dickson D., Jr. "The Ironic Conception of American History: The Early Black Historians, 1883–1915." *Journal of Negro History* 69.2 (1984): 53–62.

Brundage, W. Fitzhugh. *Lynching in the New South: Georgia and Virginia, 1880–1930.* Urbana: University of Illinois Press, 1993.

Buonomo, Leonardo. *Backward Glances: Exploring Italy, Reinterpreting America, 1831–1866.* London: Associated University Press, 1996.

Burbick, Joan. *Healing the Republic: The Language of Health and the Culture of Nationalism in Nineteenth-Century America.* New York: Cambridge University Press, 1994.

Burr, Anna Robeson Brown. *Weir Mitchell: His Life and Letters.* New York: Duffield & Co., 1929.

Burton, Margaret Davis. *The Women Who Battled for the Boys in Blue, Mother Bickerdyke: Her Life and Labor for the Relief of Our Soldiers.* San Francisco: A. T. Dewey, 1886.

Butler, Judith. *Bodies That Matter: On the Discursive Limits of "Sex."* New York: Routledge, 1993.

————. "Imitation and Gender Insubordination." *The Lesbian and Gay Studies Reader.* Ed. Henry Abelove, Michèle Aina Barale, and David M. Halperin. New York: Routledge, 1993. 307–20.

Campbell, Jane. *Mythic Black Fiction: The Transformation of History.* Knoxville: University of Tennessee Press, 1986.

Capello, Mary. "'Looking about Me with All My Eyes': Censored Viewing, Carnival, and Louisa May Alcott's *Hospital Sketches*." *Arizona Quarterly* 50.3 (Autumn 1994): 59–88.

Carby, Hazel. "The Multicultural Wars." *The Radical History Review* 54 (Fall 1992): 7–18.

————. *Reconstructing Womanhood: The Emergence of the Afro-American Woman Novelist.* New York: Oxford University Press, 1987.

Carnegie, M. Elizabeth. *The Path We Tread: Blacks in Nursing, 1854–1984.* Philadelphia: J. B. Lippincott, 1985.

Carpenter, Charles. *History of American Schoolbooks.* Philadelphia: University of Pennsylvania Press, 1963.

Carpenter, F. B. *Six Months at the White House with Abraham Lincoln.* New York, 1866.

Chase, Julia A. Houghton. *Mary A. Bickerdyke, "Mother": The Life Story of One Who, As Wife, Mother, Army Nurse, Pension Agent and City Missionary, Has Touched the Heights and Depths of Human Life.* Lawrence, Kans.: Journal Publishing House, 1896.

Christian, Barbara. *Black Women Novelists: The Development of a Tradition, 1892–1976.* Westport, Conn.: Greenwood Press, 1980.

Clinton, Catherine, and Nina Silber, eds. *Divided Houses: Gender and the Civil War.* New York: Oxford University Press, 1992.

Collier-Thomas, Bettye, and James Turner. "Race, Class and Color: The African American Discourse on Identity." *Journal of American Ethnic History* 14.1 (1994): 5–31.

Cooper, Anna Julia. *A Voice from the South.* 1892. Ed. Mary Helen Washington. New York: Oxford University Press, 1988.

Cope, E. D. *On the Hypothesis of Evolution: Physical and Metaphysical.* New Haven, Conn.: Chatfield & Co., 1870.

Cornish, Dudley. *The Sable Arm: Negro Troops in the Union Army, 1861–1865.* New York: W. W. Norton & Company, 1966.

Crane, Stephen. *The Red Badge of Courage and Selected Prose and Poetry.* 1895. Ed. William A. Gibson. New York: Holt, Rinehart, and Winston, Inc., 1968.

Cruden, Robert. *James Ford Rhodes: The Man, the Historian, and His Work.* Westport, Conn.: Greenwood Press, 1961.

————. "James Ford Rhodes and the Negro: A Study in the Problem of Objectivity." *Understanding Negro History.* Ed. Dwight W. Hoover. Chicago: Quadrangle Books, 1968. 95–105.

Cullen, Jim. *The Civil War in Popular Culture: A Reusable Past.* Washington, D.C.: Smithsonian Institution Press, 1995.

————. "'I's a Man Now': Gender and African American Men." *Divided Houses: Gender and the Civil War.* Ed. Catherine Clinton and Nina Silber. New York: Oxford University Press, 1992. 76–96.

Cullen, Thomas Frankford. "Observations on the Influence of the Present War upon American Medicine and Surgery." Speech read before the Medical Society of New Jersey, 1864. Library of the College of Physicians of Philadelphia.

Cunningham, Virginia. *Paul Laurence Dunbar and His Song.* New York: Dodd, Mead & Co., 1947.

Curtis, Susan. *A Consuming Faith: The Social Gospel and Modern American Culture.* Baltimore: Johns Hopkins University Press, 1991.

Cutler, James Elbert. *Lynch-Law: An Investigation into the History of Lynching in the United States.* 1905. New York: Negro University Press, 1969.

Daniel, Stephen L. "The Patient As Text: A Model of Clinical Hermeneutics." *Theoretical Medicine* 7 (1986): 195–210.

Dann, Martin E. *The Black Press, 1827–1890: The Quest for National Identity.* New York: G. P. Putnam's Sons, 1971.

Dannett, Sylvia G. L. *Noble Women of the North.* New York: Thomas Yoseloff, 1959.

Davis, Rebecca Harding. *Bits of Gossip.* Boston: Houghton, Mifflin & Co., 1904.

———. *A Rebecca Harding Davis Reader.* Ed. Jean Pfaelzer. Pittsburgh: University of Pittsburgh Press, 1995.

———. *Waiting For the Verdict.* 1867. Ed. Don Dingeldine. Albany, N.Y.: NCUP, 1995.

Davis, Robert Leigh. *Whitman and the Romance of Medicine.* Berkeley: University of California Press, 1997.

Dean, Eric T., Jr. "'We Will All Be Lost and Destroyed': Post-Traumatic Stress Disorder and the Civil War." *Civil War History* 37.2 (1991): 138–53.

Dearing, Mary K. *Veterans in Politics: The Story of the G.A.R.* Baton Rouge: Louisiana State University Press, 1952.

De Forest, John William. *Miss Ravenel's Conversion from Secession to Loyalty.* 1867. New York: Holt, Rinehart & Winston, 1955.

Delbanco, Andrew. "The American Stephen Crane: The Context of *The Red Badge of Courage.*" *New Essays on* The Red Badge of Courage. Ed. Lee Clark Mitchell. New York: Cambridge University Press, 1986. 49–76.

Denney, Robert E. *Civil War Medicine: Care & Comfort of the Wounded.* New York: Sterling Publishing Co., 1994.

Diffley, Kathleen. *Where My Heart Is Turning Ever: Civil War Stories and Constitutional Reform, 1861–1876.* Athens: University of Georgia Press, 1992.

Dingeldine, Don. Introduction. *Waiting for the Verdict.* By Rebecca Harding Davis. Albany, N.Y.: NCUP, Inc., 1995. iii–xxxix.

Documents of the U.S. Sanitary Commission. Vol. 1 (Numbers 1 to 60). New York, 1866.

Documents of the U.S. Sanitary Commission. Vol. 2 (Numbers 61 to 95). New York, 1866.

Douglas, Ann. *The Feminization of American Culture.* New York: Doubleday, 1977.

Douglass, Frederick. *The Life and Writings of Frederick Douglass.* Ed. Philip S. Foner. Vol. 4, *Reconstruction and After.* New York: International Publishers, 1955.

Du Bois, W. F. B. *The Souls of Black Folk.* 1903. New York: Bantam, 1989.

Dunbar, Paul Laurence. *The Collected Poetry of Paul Laurence Dunbar.* Ed. Joanne Braxton. Charlottesville: University Press of Virginia, 1993.

———. *The Fanatics.* 1901. Ed. Lisa A. Long. Acton, Mass.: Copley Publishing Group, 2001.

———. *Lyrics of Love and Laughter.* 1900. New York: Dodd, Mead & Co., 1903.

———. The Paul Laurence Dunbar Papers, Ohio Historical Society. Dayton, Ohio. Microfilm edition.

Dunbar, Paul Laurence, and Alice Dunbar Nelson. *The Letters of Paul and Alice Dunbar: A Private History, Part 2.* Ed. E. Metcalf. Ann Arbor, Mich.: University Microfilms International, 1981.

Earnest, Ernest. *S. Weir Mitchell, Novelist and Physician.* Philadelphia: University of Pennsylvania Press, 1950.

Eiselein, Gregory. *Literature and Humanitarian Reform in the Civil War Era.* Bloomington: Indiana University Press, 1996.

Eisenberg, Leon. "The Physician As Interpreter." *Comprehensive Psychiatry* 22.3 (May/June 1981): 239–48.

Ellis, Havelock. *Essays in War-Time: Further Studies in the Task of Social Hygiene.* Boston: Houghton, Mifflin & Co., 1917.

Elson, Ruth. *Guardians of Tradition: American Schoolbooks of the Nineteenth Century.* Lincoln: University of Nebraska Press, 1964.

Emanuel, James. E. "Racial Fire in the Poetry of Paul Laurence Dunbar." *A Singer in the Dawn: Reinterpretations of Paul Laurence Dunbar.* Ed. Jay Martin. New York: Dodd, Mead & Co., 1975. 79–93.

Emilio, Luis F. *History of the Fifty-Fourth Regiment of Massachusetts Volunteer Infantry, 1863–1865.* Boston: Boston Book Company, 1894.

Evans, Robert J. *In Defense of History.* New York: W. W. Norton & Company, 1999.

Fahs, Alice. *The Imagined Civil War: Popular Literature of the North and South, 1861–1865.* Chapel Hill: University of North Carolina Press, 2001.

Fick, Thomas. "Genre Wars and the Rhetoric of Manhood in *Miss Ravenel's Conversion from Secession to Loyalty.*" *Nineteenth Century Literature* 46.4 (1992): 473–94.

Fleetwood, Christian A. *The Negro As a Soldier.* Washington, D.C.: Howard University Print, 1895.

Flint, Allen. "Black Response to Colonel Shaw." *Phylon* 45.3 (1984): 210–19.

Foner, Eric. *Reconstruction: America's Unfinished Revolution, 1863–1877.* New York: Harper & Row Publishers, 1988.

Foster, Frances Smith. *Written by Herself: Literary Production by African American Women, 1746–1892.* Bloomington: Indiana University Press, 1993.

Foster, Susan Leigh. "Choreographing History." *Choreographing History.* Ed. Susan Leigh Foster. Bloomington: Indiana University Press, 1995. 3–24.

Foucault, Michel. *The Order of Things: An Archaeology of the Human Sciences.* New York: Vintage Books, 1970.

Fox, William F. *Regimental Losses in the American Civil War, 1861–65.* Albany, N.Y.: Albany Publishing Co., 1889.

Franklin, H. Bruce. *Prison Literature: The Victim As Criminal and Artist.* New York: Oxford University Press, 1978.

Franklin, John Hope. *George Washington Williams: A Biography.* Chicago: University of Chicago Press, 1985.

Frazier, E. Franklin. *Black Bourgeoisie: The Rise of a New Middle Class in the United States.* New York: Free Press, 1957.

Frederic Edwin Church: An Exhibition Organized by the National Collection of Fine Arts. Washington, D.C.: Smithsonian Publications, 1966.

Frederickson, George. *The Inner Civil War: Northern Intellectuals and the Crisis of the Union.* New York: Harper & Row Publishers, 1965.

———. "Nineteenth-Century American History," *Imagined Histories: American Historians Interpret the Past.* Ed. Anthony Molho and Gordon S. Wood. Princeton, N.J.: Princeton University Press, 1998. 164–84.

Gallman, J. Matthew. *The North Fights the Civil War: The Home Front.* Chicago: Ivan R. Dee, 1994.

Gargano, James W., ed. *Critical Essays on John William De Forest.* Boston: G. K. Hall & Co., 1981.

Gates, Henry Louis, Jr. "The Master's Pieces: On Canon Formation and Afro-American Tradition." *The Bounds of Race: Perspectives on Hegemony and Resistance.* Ed. Dominick LaCapra. Ithaca, N.Y.: Cornell University Press, 1991. 17–38.

————. "The Trope of the New Negro and the Reconstruction of the Image of the Black." *The New American Studies.* Ed. Philip Fisher. Berkeley: University of California Press, 1991. 379–45.

Gayle, Addison. "Literature As Catharsis: The Novels of Paul Laurence Dunbar." *A Singer in the Dawn: Reinterpretations of Paul Laurence Dunbar.* Ed. Jay Martin. New York: Dodd, Mead & Co., 1975. 139–51.

————. *Oak and Ivey: A Biography of Paul Laurence Dunbar.* Garden City, N.Y.: Doubleday & Co., Inc., 1971.

Giesberg, Judith Ann. *Civil War Sisterhood: The U.S. Sanitary Commission and Women's Politics in Transition.* Boston: Northeastern University Press, 2000.

Gilman, Charlotte Perkins. *The Living of Charlotte Perkins Gilman.* 1935. Madison: University of Wisconsin Press, 1988.

Gilman, Sander L. *Difference and Pathology: Stereotypes of Sexuality, Race, and Madness.* Ithaca, N.Y.: Cornell University Press, 1985.

Ginzberg, Lori D. *Women and the Work of Benevolence: Morality, Politics, and Class in the Nineteenth-Century United States.* New Haven, Conn.: Yale University Press, 1990.

Gladstone, William A. *Men of Color.* Gettysburg, Penn.: Thomas Publications, 1993.

Glatthaar, Joseph T. *Forged in Battle: The Civil War Alliance of Black Soldiers and White Officers.* New York: Free Press, 1990.

Gooding, James Henry. *On the Altar of Freedom: A Black Soldier's Civil War Letters from the Front.* Ed. Virginia Matzke Adams. Amherst: University of Massachusetts Press, 1991.

Gosling, F. G. *Before Freud: Neurasthenia and the American Medical Community, 1870–1910.* Urbana: University of Illinois Press, 1987.

Gosling, F. G., and Joyce Ray. "'The Right to Be Sick': American Physicians and Nervous Patients, 1885–1910." *Journal of Social History* 20.2 (1986): 251–67.

Gould, Benjamin Apthorp. *Investigations in the Military and Anthropological Statistics of American Soldiers.* 1869. New York: Arno Press, 1979.

Gould, Stephen J. *The Mismeasure of Man.* New York: W. W. Norton & Company, 1981.

Grant, Ulysses S. *Personal Memoirs of U. S. Grant.* 1885. New York: Grosset & Dunlap, 1962.

"A Green Private Under Fire." *New York Times,* October 19, 1895: 3.

Grimké, Charlotte Forten. *The Journals of Charlotte Forten Grimké.* Ed. Brenda Stevenson. New York: Oxford University Press, 1988.

Grosz, Elizabeth. *Volatile Bodies: Toward a Corporeal Feminism.* Bloomington: Indiana University Press, 1994.

Gunning, Sandra. *Race, Rape, and Lynching: The Red Record of American Literature, 1890–1912.* New York: Oxford University Press, 1996.

Habegger, Alfred. "Fighting Words: The Talk of Men at War in *The Red Badge of Courage.*" *Critical Essays on Stephen Crane's* The Red Badge of Courage. Ed. Donald Pizer. Boston: G. K. Hall & Co., 1990. 185–203.

Hadden, R. Lee. *Reliving the Civil War: A Reenactor's Handbook.* Mechanicsburg, Penn.: Stackpole Books, 1999.

Hall, Dennis. "Civil War Reenactors and the Postmodern Sense of History." *Journal of American Culture* 17.3 (Fall 1994): 7–12.

Hall, Jacquelyn Dowd. "'The Mind that Burns in Each Body': Women, Rape, and Racial Violence." *Powers of Desire: The Politics of Sexuality.* Ed. Ann Snitow, Christine Stansell, and Sharon Thompson. New York: Monthly Review Press, 1983. 328–49.

Hallowell, Norwood P. *The Negro As a Soldier in the War of the Rebellion.* Boston: Little, Brown & Co, 1897.

Hallwas, John E. "Civil War Accounts As Literature: Illinois Letters, Diaries, and Personal Narratives." *Western Illinois Regional Studies* 13.1 (1990): 46–59.

Halttunen, Karen. *Confidence Men and Painted Women: A Study of Middle-Class Culture in America, 1830–1870.* New Haven, Conn.: Yale University Press, 1982.

Hamilton, Gail [Mary Abigail Dodge]. "A Call to My Country-Women." *Atlantic Monthly* 11 (March 1863): 345–49.

Hargrove, Hondon. *Black Union Soldiers in the Civil War.* Jefferson, N.C.: McFarland & Co., 1988.

Harper, Frances Ellen Watkins. *Iola Leroy; or, Shadows Uplifted.* 1892. Ed. Hazel Carby. Boston: Beacon Press, 1987.

Harris, Sharon. *Rebecca Harding Davis and American Realism.* Philadelphia: University of Pennsylvania Press, 1991.

Hatt, Michael. "'Making a Man of Him': Masculinity and the Black Body in Mid-Nineteenth-Century American Sculpture." *Oxford Art Journal* 15.1 (1992): 21–35.

Hawkins, Mike. *Social Darwinism in European and American Thought, 1860–1945.* Cambridge: Cambridge University Press, 1997.

Hedges, Warren. "If Uncle Tom Is White, Should We Call Him 'Auntie'? Race and Sexuality in Postbellum U.S. Fiction." *Whiteness: A Critical Reader.* Ed. Mike Hill. New York: New York University Press, 1997. 226–47.

Hendin, Herbert, and Ann Pollinger Haas. "Posttraumatic Stress Disorders in Veterans of Early American Wars." *Psychohistory Review* 12.4 (1984): 25–30.

Herndl, Diane Price. "The Invisible (Invalid) Woman: African-American Women, Illness, and Nineteenth-Century Narrative." *Women's Studies* 24 (1995): 553–72

Higham, John. *History: The Development of Historical Studies in the United States.* Englewood Cliffs, N.J.: Prentice-Hall, 1965.

———. *Strangers in the Land: Patterns of American Nativism, 1860–1925.* New Brunswick, N.J.: Rutgers University Press, 1988.

Hijiya, James A. *J. W. De Forest and the Rise of American Gentility.* Hanover, N.H.: University Press of New England, 1988.

Hine, Darlene Clark. *Black Women in White: Racial Conflict and Cooperation in the Nursing Profession.* Bloomington: Indiana University Press, 1989.

Holland, Mary A. Gardner. *Our Army Nurses: Interesting Sketches, Addresses, and Photographs of Nearly One Hundred of the Noble Women Who Served in Hospitals and on Battlefields During Our Civil War.* Boston: Press of Lounsbery, Nichols & Worth, 1895.

Holt, W. Stull. *Historical Scholarship in the United States.* Seattle: University of Washington Press, 1967.

Horwitz, Tony. *Confederates in the Attic: Dispatches from the Unfinished Civil War.* New York, Vintage Books, 1998.

Jacobs, Harriet. *Incidents in the Life of a Slave Girl.* 1861. Ed. Jean Fagan Yellin. Cambridge, Mass.: Harvard University Press, 1987.

Jimerson, Randall C. *The Private Civil War.* Baton Rouge: Louisiana State University Press, 1988.

Johnson, Neil. *The Battle of Gettysburg.* New York: Four Winds Press, 1989.

Johnson, Robert Underwood, and Clarence Clough Buel, eds. *Battles and Leaders of the Civil War: Being for the Most Part Contributions by Union and Confederate Officers.* 4 Vols. New York: Century Company, 1894.

Jolly, Ellen Ryan. *Nuns of the Battlefield.* Providence, R.I.: Providence Visitor Press, 1927.

Jones, Jacqueline. *Freed Women? Black Women, Work, and the Family during the Civil War and Reconstruction.* Wellesley, Mass.: Center for Research on Women, 1980.

Jordan, David Starr. *War and the Breed: The Relation of War to the Downfall of Nations.* 1915. Washington, D.C.: The Cliveden Press, 1981.

Journet, Deborah. "Phantom Limbs and 'Body-Ego': S. Weir Mitchell's 'George Dedlow.'" *Mosaic* 23.1 (Winter 1990): 87–99.

Kaledin, Eugenia. "Dr. Manners: S. Weir Mitchell's Novelistic Prescription for an Upset Society." *Prospects* 11 (1986): 199–216.

Kaplan, Sidney. "The Black Soldier of the Civil War in Literature and Art." *American Studies in Black and White: Selected Essays, 1949–1989.* Ed. Allan D. Austin. Amherst: The University of Massachusetts Press, 1991. 101–26.

Katz, Leslie. "Flesh of His Flesh: Amputation in *Moby Dick* and S. W. Mitchell's Medical Papers." *Genders* 4 (Spring 1989): 1–10.

Keen, William W., M.D., S. Weir Mitchell, M.D., and George R. Morehouse, M.D. "On Malingering, Especially in Regard to Simulation of Diseases of the Nervous System." *Philadelphia Medical Journal* (October 1864): 367–94.

Kellogg, Florence Shaw. *Mother Bickerdyke, As I Knew Her.* Chicago: Unity Publishing Co., 1907.

Kelly, Lori Duin. *The Life and Works of Elizabeth Stuart Phelps, Victorian Feminist Writer.* Troy, N.Y.: Whitson Publishing Co., 1983.

Kessler, Carol Farley. *Elizabeth Stuart Phelps.* Boston: Twayne Publishers, 1982.

———. "The Heavenly Utopia of Elizabeth Stuart Phelps." *Women and Utopia: Critical Interpretations.* Ed. Marleen Barr and Nicholas D. Smith. New York: University Press of America, 1983. 85–95.

Kete, Mary Louise. *Sentimental Collaborations: Mourning and Middle-Class Identity in Nineteenth-Century America.* Durham, N.C.: Duke University Press, 1999.

Koch, Lisa. "Bodies As Stage Props: Enacting Hysteria in the Diaries of Charlotte Forten Grimké and Alice James." *Legacy* 15 (1998): 59–64.

Kugler, Israel. *From Ladies to Women: The Organized Struggle for Woman's Rights in the Reconstruction Era.* New York: Greenwood Press, 1987.

Laderman, Gary. *The Sacred Remains: American Attitudes toward Death, 1799–1883.* New Haven, Conn.: Yale University Press, 1996.

Langlois, Charles Victor, and Charles Segnobos. *Introduction to the Study of History.* New York: Henry Holt & Co, 1898.

Lapsansky, Emma Jones. "Feminism, Freedom, and Community: Charlotte Forten and Women Activists in Nineteenth-Century Philadelphia." *Pennsylvania Magazine of History and Biography* 113.1 (1989): 3–19.

Lears, T. J. Jackson. *No Place of Grace: Antimodernism and the Transformation of American Culture, 1880–1920.* Chicago: University of Chicago Press, 1981.

Leonard, Elizabeth. *Yankee Women: Gender Battles in the Civil War.* New York: W. W. Norton, 1994.

Linderman, Gerald. *Embattled Courage: The Experience of Combat in the American Civil War.* New York: Free Press, 1987.

Lively, Robert A. *Fiction Fights the Civil War: An Unfinished Chapter in the Literary History of the American People.* Chapel Hill: University of North Carolina Press, 1957.

Livermore, Mary. *My Story of the War: The Civil War Memoirs of the Famous Nurse, Relief Organizer and Suffragette.* Ed. Nina Silber. 1890. New York: Da Capo Press, 1995.

"The Lounger." Editorial. *Harper's Weekly*, August 10, 1861: 499.

Lovering, Joseph P. *S. Weir Mitchell.* New York: Twayne Publishers, 1971.

Lowell, James Russell. "A Great Public Character." *The Atlantic Monthly* 20 (1867): 618–32.

Lowenberg, Bert James, and Ruth Bogin, eds. *Black Women in Nineteenth-Century American Life: Their Words, Their Thoughts, Their Feelings.* University Park: Pennsylvania State University Press, 1976.

Lunn, Janet. *The Root Cellar.* New York: Puffin Books, 1981.

Lutz, Tom. *American Nervousness, 1903: An Anecdotal History.* Ithaca, N.Y.: Cornell University Press, 1991.

Lydston, G. Frank, M.D. *The Diseases of Society and Degeneracy: The Vice and Crime Problem.* Philadelphia: J. B. Lippincott Co., 1904.

Maher, Mary Denis. *To Bind up the Wounds: Catholic Sister Nurses in the U.S. Civil War.* New York: Greenwood Press, 1989.

Malmsheimer, Richard. *"Doctors Only": The Evolving Image of the American Physician.* New York: Greenwood Press, 1988.

Manthorne, Katherine. *Creation and Renewal: Views of Cotopaxi by Frederic Edwin Church.* Washington, D.C.: National Museum of American Art and Smithsonian Institution Press, 1985.

Marcus, Jane. "Corpus/Corpse/Corps: Writing the Body in/at War." *Arms and the Woman: War, Gender and Literary Representation.* Ed. Helen M. Cooper, Adrienne Auslander Munich, and Susan Merrill Squier. Chapel Hill: University of North Carolina Press, 1989. 124–67.

Marten, James. *The Children's Civil War.* Chapel Hill: University of North Carolina Press, 1998.

Martin, Jay. "Ghostly Rentals, Ghostly Purchases: Haunted Imaginations in James, Twain, and Bellamy." *The Haunted Dusk: American Supernatural Fiction, 1820–1920.* Ed. Howard Kerr, John W. Crowley, and Charles L. Crow. Athens: University of Georgia Press, 1983. 123–31.

———. "Paul Laurence Dunbar: Biography Through Letters." *A Singer in the Dawn: Reinterpretations of Paul Laurence Dunbar.* Ed. Jay Martin. New York: Dodd, Mead & Co., 1975. 13–35.

Maxwell, William Quentin. *Lincoln's Fifth Wheel: The Political History of the United States Sanitary Commission.* New York: Longmans, Green, 1956.

May, William F. "Dealing With Catastrophe." *Dax's Case: Essays in Medical Ethics and Human Meaning.* Ed. Lonnie D. Kliever. Dallas: Southern Methodist University Press, 1989. 131–50.

McClurg, Alexander. "The Red Badge of Hysteria." *Dial* 20 (April 1896): 228.

McConnell, Stuart. *Glorious Contentment: The Grand Army of the Republic, 1865–1900.* Chapel Hill: University of North Carolina Press, 1992.

McDowell, Deborah. "'The Changing Same': Generational Connections and Black Women Novelists." *New Literary History* 18.2 (1987): 281–302.

McKay, Nellie Y. "The Journals of Charlotte L. Forten Grimké: *Les Lieux de Mémoire* in African-American Women's Autobiography." *History and Memory in African-American Culture.* Ed. Genevieve Fabre and Robert O'Meally. New York: Oxford University Press, 1994. 261–71.

McLoughlin, William G., ed. *The American Evangelicals, 1800–1900: An Anthology.* Gloucester, Mass.: Peter Smith, 1976.

McPherson, James M. *The Abolitionist Legacy: From Reconstruction to the NAACP.* Princeton, N.J.: Princeton University Press, 1975.

———. *The Negro's Civil War: How American Blacks Felt and Acted During the War for the Union.* New York: Ballantine Books, 1991.

———. Introduction. *Two Black Teachers during the Civil War.* Ed. James M. McPherson. New York: Arno Press, 1969. i–vi.

———. "The War That Never Goes Away." *Drawn with the Sword: Reflections on the American Civil War.* New York: Oxford University Press, 1996. 55–65.

McPherson, James M., and William J. Cooper Jr., eds. *Writing the Civil War: The Quest to Understand.* Columbia: University of South Carolina Press, 1998.

McSherry, Frank, Jr., Charles G. Waugh, and Martin Greenberg, eds. *Civil War Women.* New York: Simon & Schuster, 1988.

Melosh, Barbara. *"The Physician's Hand": Work, Culture and Conflict in American Nursing.* Philadelphia: Temple University Press, 1982.

Mitchell, Reid. *The Vacant Chair: The Northern Soldier Leaves Home.* New York: Oxford University Press, 1993.

Mitchell, S. Weir. "Address before the Fiftieth Annual Meeting of the American Medico-Psychological Association, Held in Philadelphia, May 16th, 1894." Reprinted in *American Journal of Psychiatry, Sesquicentennial Supplement* 151.6 (June 1994): 29–36.

———. "The Case of George Dedlow." *Atlantic Monthly* 18 (July 1866): 1–11.

———. *Fat and Blood.* Philadelphia: J. B. Lippincott and Co., 1877.

———. *In War Time.* 1884. New York: Century Company, 1912.

———. *Roland Blake.* New York: Century Company, 1886.

———. The S. Weir Mitchell Papers, The Francis Clark Wood Institute for the History of Medicine, The Library of the College of Physicians of Philadelphia.

Mitchell, S. Weir, M.D., George R. Morehouse, M.D., and William W. Keen, M.D. *Gunshot Wounds and Other Injuries of Nerves.* Philadelphia: J. B. Lippincott & Co., 1864.

Montgomery, D. H. *The Leading Facts of American History.* Boston: Ginn & Company Publishers, 1893.

Moody, Jocelyn K. "Twice Other, Once Shy: Nineteenth-Century Black Women Autobiographers and the American Literary Tradition of Self-Effacement." *a/b: Auto/Biography Studies* 7.1 (1992): 46–61.

Moorhead, James H. *American Apocalypse: Yankee Protestants and the Civil War, 1860–1869.* New Haven, Conn.: Yale University Press, 1978.

Morris, David B. *The Culture of Pain.* Berkeley: University of California Press, 1991.

Morrison, Toni. *Playing in the Dark: Whiteness and the Literary Imagination.* New York: Vintage Books, 1992.

Morton, Patricia. *Disfigured Images: The Historical Assault on Afro-American Women.* New York: Praeger, 1991.

Moses, William J. "Dark Forests and Barbarian Vigor: Paradox, Conflict, and Africanity in Black Writing Before 1914." *American Literary History* 1.3 (Fall 1989): 637–55.

Mrozek, Donald J. "The Habit of Victory: The American Military and the Cult of Manliness." *Manliness and Morality: Middle-Class Masculinity in Britain and America, 1800–1940.* Ed. J. A. Mangan and James Walvin. New York: St. Martin's Press, 1987. 220–41.

Murphy, Jim. *The Journal of James Edmond Pease: A Civil War Union Soldier.* New York: Scholastic Inc., 1998.

Nash, Gary. *Forging Freedom: The Formation of Philadelphia's Black Community, 1720–1840.* Cambridge, Mass.: Harvard University Press, 1988.

Newman, Kathy. "Wound and Wounding in the American Civil War: A Visual History." *The Yale Journal of Criticism* 6.2 (1993): 63–86.

Nietz, John A. *Old Textbooks.* Pittsburgh: University of Pittsburgh Press, 1961.

Novick, Peter. *That Noble Dream: The "Objectivity Question" and the American Histori-cal Profession.* New York: Cambridge University Press, 1988.

O'Connor, Erin. "'Fractions of Men': Engendering Amputation in Victorian Culture." *Comparative Studies in Society and History* 39.4 (October 1997): 742–78.

Oden, Gloria C. "*The Journal of Charlotte L. Forten*: The Salem-Philadelphia Years (1854–1862) Reexamined." *Essex Institute Historical Collections* 119 (1983): 119–36.

O'Malley, Michael. "Specie and Species: Race and the Money Question in Nine-teenth-Century America." *American Historical Review* 99.2 (1994): 369–95.

"Our Women and the War." *Harper's Weekly* 23 (August 1862): 568–70.

Painter, Nell Irvin. *Sojourner Truth: A Life, A Symbol.* New York: Norton, 1996.

———. "Thinking about the Languages of Money and Race: A Response to Michael O'Malley, 'Specie and Species.'" *American Historical Review* 99.2 (1994): 396–404.

Paludan, Phillip Shaw. "*A People's Contest": The Union and the Civil War.* New York: Harper & Row Publishers, 1988.

Pease, Donald. "Fear, Rage, and the Mistrials of Representation in *The Red Badge of Courage.*" *American Realism: New Essays.* Ed. Eric Sundquist. Baltimore: Johns Hopkins University Press, 1982. 155–175.

Peterson, Carla L. *"Doers of the Word": African-American Women Speakers and Writers in the North, 1830–1880.* New York: Oxford University Press, 1995.

Pfister, Joel. "On Conceptualizing the Cultural History of Emotional and Psy-chological Life in America." *Inventing the Psychological: Toward a Cultural His-tory of Emotional Life in America.* Ed. Joel Pfister and Nancy Schnog. New Haven, Conn.: Yale University Press, 1997. 17–62.

Phelps, Elizabeth Stuart. *Beyond the Gates.* Boston: Houghton, Mifflin & Co., 1883.

———. *Chapters from a Life.* Boston: Houghton, Mifflin & Co., 1896.

———. *Comrades.* New York: Harper's, 1911.

———. *The Gates Ajar.* Boston: Fields, Osgood & Co., 1868.

The Philanthropic Results of the War in America. New York: Sheldon & Company, 1864.

Pike, Martha. "In Memory Of: Artifacts Relating to Mourning in Nineteenth-Century America." *Rituals and Ceremonies in Popular Culture.* Ed. Ray B. Browne. Bowling Green, Ohio: Bowling Green University Popular Press, 1980. 296–316.

Poirier, Suzanne. "The Physician and Authority: Portraits by Four Physician-Writers." *Literature and Medicine* 2 (1983): 21–40.

———. "The Weir Mitchell Rest Cure: Doctor and Patients." *Women's Studies* 10 (1983): 15–40.

Quarles, Benjamin. *Black Mosaic: Essays in Afro-American History and Historiogra-phy.* Amherst: University of Massachusetts Press, 1988.

———. *The Negro in the Civil War.* Boston: Little, Brown and Co., 1953.

Rafter, Nicole Hahn. *White Trash: The Eugenic Family Studies.* Boston: Northeast-ern University Press, 1988.

Raymond, Henry J. Editorial. *Harper's Weekly,* August 10, 1861: 491.

Rechnitz, Robert M. "Depersonalization and the Dream in *The Red Badge of Cour-age.*" *Critical Essays on Stephen Crane's* The Red Badge of Courage. Ed. Donald Pizer. Boston: G. K. Hall & Co., 1990. 152–63.

Reid, Richard M. "Black Experience in the Union Army: The Other Civil War." *Canadian Review of American Studies* 21 (1990): 145–55.

Reid-Pharr, Robert. *Conjugal Bonds: The Body, The House, and the Black American.* New York: Oxford University Press, 1999.

Rhodes, James Ford. *History of the United States from the Compromise of 1850 to the Final Restoration of Home Rule at the South in 1877.* 2 Vols. New York: Harper and Brothers, 1895.

Rien, David. *S. Weir Mitchell As a Psychiatric Novelist.* New York: International University Press, 1952.

Rose, Anne C. *Victorian America and the Civil War.* New York: Cambridge University Press, 1992.

Rose, Willie Lee. *Rehearsal for Reconstruction: The Port Royal Experiment.* New York: Bobbs-Merrill Company, Inc., 1964.

Royster, Charles. *The Destructive War: William Techumseh Sherman, Stonewall Jackson, and the Americans.* New York: Alfred A. Knopf, 1991.

Sánchez-Eppler, Karen. *Touching Liberty: Abolition, Feminism, and the Politics of the Body.* Berkeley: University of California Press, 1993.

The Sanitary Commission of the United States Army: A Succinct Narrative of Its Works and Purposes. 1864. New York: Arno Press, 1972.

Sartwell, Crispin. *Act Like You Know: African-American Autobiography and White Identity.* Chicago: University of Chicago Press, 1998.

Scarry, Elaine. *The Body in Pain: The Making and Unmaking of the World.* New York: Oxford University Press, 1985.

———. Introduction. *Literature and the Body: Essays on Populations and Persons.* Ed. Elaine Scarry. Baltimore: Johns Hopkins University Press, 1988. vii–xxvii.

Schaefer, Michael. *Just What War Is: The Civil War Writings of De Forest and Bierce.* Knoxville: University of Tennessee Press, 1997.

Schnog, Nancy. "'The Comfort of My Fancying': Loss and Recuperation in *The Gates Ajar.*" *Arizona Quarterly* 49.1 (1993): 21–47.

Schultz, Jane E. "'Are We Not All Soldiers?' Northern Women in the Civil War Hospital Service." *Prospects: An Annual of American Cultural Studies.* Ed. Jack Salzman. Vol. 20. New York: Cambridge University Press, 1996. 39–56.

———. "Embattled Care: Narrative Authority in Louisa May Alcott's *Hospital Sketches.*" *Legacy* 9.2 (1992): 104–18.

———. "The Inhospitable Hospital: Gender and Professionalism in Civil War Medicine." *Signs* 17.2 (1992): 353–92.

Seltzer, Mark. *Bodies and Machines.* New York: Routledge, 1992.

Shakespeare, William. *The Tragedy of Macbeth. The Complete Signet Shakespeare.* Ed. Sylvan Barnet. San Diego: Harcourt Brace Jovanovich, 1972. 1227–63.

Showalter, Elaine. Introduction. *Alternative Alcott.* By Louisa May Alcott. New Brunswick, N.J.: Rutgers University Press, 1988. ix–xlvii.

Silber, Nina. Introduction. *My Story of the War: The Civil War Memoirs of the Famous Nurse, Relief Organizer and Suffragette.* By Mary Livermore. New York: Da Capo Press, 1995. v–xii.

———. *The Romance of Reunion: Northerners and the South, 1865–1900.* Chapel Hill: University of North Carolina Press, 1993.

Smith, Bonnie G. *The Gender of History: Men, Women, and Historical Practice.* Cambridge, Mass.: Harvard University Press, 1998.

Smith, Gail K. "From the Seminary to the Parlor: The Popularization of Hermeneutics in *The Gates Ajar.*" *Arizona Quarterly* 54.2 (1998): 99–133.

Smith, Nina Bennett. "The Women Who Went to War: The Union Army Nurse in the Civil War." Diss. Northwestern University, 1981.

Smith-Rosenberg, Carroll. *Disorderly Conduct: Visions of Gender in Victorian America.* New York: Oxford University Press, 1985.

Solomon, Eric. "The Novelist As Soldier: Cooke and De Forest." *American Literary Realism* 19.3 (1987): 80–88.

Sprague, C. F. "What We Feel." *Atlantic Monthly* 20 (December 1867): 740–44.

St. Armand, Barton Levi. *Emily Dickinson and Her Culture.* New York: Cambridge University Press, 1984.

Stanford, Ann Folwell. "Mechanisms of Disease: African-American Women Writers, Social Pathologies, and the Limits of Medicine." *NWSA Journal* 6.1 (Spring 1994): 28–47.

Stansell, Christine. "Elizabeth Stuart Phelps: A Study in Female Rebellion." *Massachusetts Review* 13 (1972): 239–56.

Starr, Paul. *The Social Transformation of American Medicine.* New York: Basic Books, Inc., 1982.

Steele, Joel Dorman, and Esther Baker Steele. *Barnes's School History of the United States.* New York: American Book Company, 1903.

Stepto, Robert B. *From Behind the Veil: A Study of Afro-American Narrative.* Urbana: University of Illinois Press, 1979.

Sterling, Dorothy. *We Are Your Sisters: Black Women in the Nineteenth Century.* New York: W. W. Norton & Co., 1984.

Stevenson, Brenda. Introduction. *The Journals of Charlotte Forten Grimké.* By Charlotte Forten Grimké. New York: Oxford University Press, 1988. 3–55.

Stillé, Charles J. *History of the United States Sanitary Commission, Being the General Report of Its Work During the War of the Rebellion.* Philadelphia: J. B. Lippincott, 1866.

Story, Ralph. "Paul Laurence Dunbar: Master Player in a Fixed Game." *College Language Association Journal* 27.1 (1983): 30–55.

Stowe, Harriet Beecher. *Uncle Tom's Cabin or, Life among the Lowly.* 1852. Ed. Ann Douglas. New York: Penguin, 1981.

Sweet, Timothy. *Traces of War: Poetry, Photography, and the Crisis of the Union.* Baltimore: Johns Hopkins University Press, 1990.

Swinton, William. *Campaign of the Army of the Potomac.* New York: Charles R. Richardson, 1866.

Talbot, Eugene S. *Degeneracy: Its Causes, Signs, and Results.* 1898. New York: Garland Publishing Inc., 1984.

Tate, Claudia. *Domestic Allegories of Political Desire: The Black Heroine's Text at the Turn of the Century.* New York: Oxford University Press, 1992.

Taylor, Susie King. *A Black Woman's Civil War Memoirs.* Ed. Patricia W. Romero and Willie Lee Rose. New York: Markus Wiener Publishing, 1988. Rpt. of *Reminiscences of My Life in Camp with the 33rd U.S. Colored Troops, Late 1st South Carolina Volunteers.* 1902.

Thorpe, Earl. *The Central Theme of Black History.* Durham, N.C.: Seeman Printery, 1969.

———. *Negro Historians in the United States.* Baton Rouge, La.: Fraternal Press, 1958.

Tichi, Cecelia. "Pittsburgh at Yellowstone: Old Faithful and the Pulse of Industrial America." *American Literary History* 9.3 (Fall 1997): 522–41.

Towne, Laura M. *Letters and Diary of Laura M. Towne, 1862–1884.* Cambridge, Mass.: Riverside Press, 1912.

Trachtenberg, Alan. "Albums of War: On Reading Civil War Photographs." *The New American Studies: Essays from Representations.* Ed. Philip Fisher. Berkeley: University of California Press, 1991. 287–318.

————. *The Incorporation of America: Culture and Society in the Gilded Age.* New York: Hill & Wang, 1982.

Turner, Chaplain Henry M. Letter. *Christian Recorder,* May 17, 1865.

Twain, Mark. *Extract from Captain Stormfield's Visit to Heaven.* New York: Harper & Brothers, 1909.

Van De Berg, William. "The Battleground of Historical Memory: Creating Alternative Culture Heroes in Post-bellum America." *Journal of Popular Culture* 20.1 (1986): 49–62.

Vaught, Bonny. "Trying to Make Things Real." *Between Women: Biographers, Novelists, Critics, Teachers, and Artists Write about Their Work on Women.* Ed. Carol Archer, Louise DeSalve, and Sara Ruddick. Boston: Beacon Press, 1984. 55–70.

Wald, Priscilla. *Constituting Americans: Cultural Anxiety and Narrative Form.* Durham, N.C.: Duke University Press, 1995.

Walter, Richard D., M.D. *S. Weir Mitchell, M.D., Neurologist: A Medical Biography.* Springfield, Ill.: Charles C. Thomas, 1970.

Warner, John Harley. *The Therapeutic Perspective: Medical Practice, Knowledge, and Identity in America, 1820–1885.* Cambridge, Mass.: Harvard University Press, 1986.

Washington, Booker T. *A New Negro for a New Century.* Chicago: American Publishing House, 1900.

————. *Up from Slavery.* 1901. New York: Bantam, 1967.

White, Deborah Gray. *Ain't I a Woman: Female Slaves in the Plantation South.* New York: W. W. Norton & Co., 1985.

White, Hayden. "Bodies and Their Plots." *Choreographing History.* Ed. Susan Leigh Foster. Bloomington: Indiana University Press, 1995. 229–34.

————. *The Content of the Form: Narrative Discourse and Historical Representation.* Baltimore: Johns Hopkins University Press, 1987.

————. "Historical Emplotment and the Problem of Truth." *Probing the Limits of Representation: Nazism and the "Final Solution."* Ed. Saul Friedlander. Cambridge, Mass.: Harvard University Press, 1992. 37–53.

Whitman, Walt. *The Civil War Poems of Walt Whitman.* New York: Barnes & Noble Books, 1994.

————. *The Portable Walt Whitman.* Ed. Mark Van Doren. New York: Penguin, 1973.

Wiegman, Robyn. *American Anatomies: Theorizing Race and Gender.* Durham, N.C.: Duke University Press, 1995.

Williams, Fannie Barrier. "The Colored Woman and Her Part in Race Regeneration." *A New Negro for a New Century.* Ed. Booker T. Washington. Chicago: American Publishing House, 1900. 406–428.

Williams, George Washington. *A History of the Negro Troops in the War of the Rebellion, 1865–1888.* New York: Negro Universities Press, 1969.

Williams, Kenny G. "The Masking of the Novelist." *A Singer in the Dawn: Reinterpretations of Paul Laurence Dunbar.* Ed. Jay Martin. New York: Dodd, Mead & Co., 1975. 152–207.

Wills, Gary. *Lincoln at Gettysburg.* New York: Touchstone, 1992.

Wilson, Daniel J. "Neurasthenia and Vocational Crisis in Post-Civil War America." *Psychohistory Review* 12.4 (1984): 31–38.

Wilson, Edmund. *Patriotic Gore: Studies in the Literature of the American Civil War.* New York: Farrar, Straus and Giroux, 1962.

Wilson, Joseph T. *The Black Phalanx.* 1890. New York: Arno Press, 1968.

Winslade, William J. "Taken to the Limits: Pain, Identity and Self-Transformation." *Dax's Case: Essays in Medical Ethics and Human Meaning.* Ed. Lonnie D. Kliever. Dallas: Southern Methodist University Press, 1989. 115–130.

Wolosky, Shira. *Emily Dickinson: A Voice of War.* New Haven, Conn.: Yale University Press, 1984.

"Woman." *Frank Leslie's Illustrated Newspaper* 27 (September 1862): 25.

Wood, Ann Douglas. "The War within a War: Women Nurses in the Union Army." *Civil War History* 18 (September 1972): 197–212.

Woodward, C. Vann. Editor's Introduction. *Battle Cry of Freedom: The Civil War Era.* New York: Oxford University Press, 1988.

Wyndham, George. "A Remarkable Book." *New Review* 14 (January 1896): 30–40.

Young, Elizabeth. *Disarming the Nation: Women's Writing and the American Civil War.* Chicago: University of Chicago Press, 1999.

Index

Aaron, Daniel: and mourning, 68, 272n37; *Unwritten War, The*, 6, 16, 149, 259–60n7, 269n9

Adams, Virginia Matzke, 123

Addams, Jane, 30, 238–40, 257

adolescents: affinity for the Civil War, 238–41, 248, 251, 257; during the Civil War, 21, 177, 238–39; unstable bodies of, 240–41, 244, 246, 252. *See also* juvenile fiction

African American men, 25; defined through money, 127–28, 225–26; discipline of, 198–99, 221, 230–33; domestic role of, 120–21, 200, 229; evolution and, 231–32; exhumation of, 127, 211, 215–16, 228, 232, 237; fear of, 108, 122, 218, 220; feminization of, 107, 109–10, 174; in heaven, 112, illnesses of, 154, 166, 220; lynching and sexuality of, 221, 229–30, 232–34; strength of, 122, 126, 128, 168, 220, 232–33; as symbol of citizenship, 199–220; violent war work of, 218, 220–21, 228–29, 232–35. *See also* Negro regiments; white men

African Americans: biological theories of, 8–9, 114–16, 128, 144–45, 197–98, 210, 279n8; caricatures of, 149–51, 162; class among, 119–20, 123–24, 126, 130–33, 139–44, 279n18; clothing and, 25, 292n47; in consumer culture, 117–21, 125, 127, 129, 173, 225; criminalization of, 129; degeneracy and, 9, 26, 116, 118, 180, 198, 210, 212–13; education during enslavement, 202–4, 206; education during war, 132, 139, 143–44, 280n29; evolution and, 9, 114–16, 212, 231–32; experiments on, 99, 114–16, 124–25, 129–30; families of, 102–3, 106, 108–9, 111–12, 229, 280–81n31; gender roles of, 118–20, 142; insensibility of, 181, 197; prejudice against, incidents of,

102–3, 106–10, 123, 125–26, 140–41, 170, 283n63; racial impurity of, 88, 103, 112, 144; racial passing and, 102, 106, 108–9, 111–12; racial uplift and, 130, 142–43, 209; recapitulation theory and, 103, 110, 118, 231–32; reenactments and, 242; rebelliousness of, 127–28, 199, 221–22, 228–29, 232, 235; regional differences among, 140–42, 163, 172; rehabilitated through Civil War service, 24–25, 116–19, 121, 135, 137–39, 145, 210–11, 219; relation to Civil War disease, 1–5, 117, 279n8; skin color and, 103, 106, 130, 141, 202, 214; strikes and, 129, 218; textuality and, 212–16, 222–24, 235–37; turn-of-the-century economic plight of, 220; turn-of-the-century violence against, 25–26, 169–70, 208, 213–14, 218, 220, 229. *See also* African American men; African American women; Negro histories; Negro regiments

African American women: activism of, 133–35, 143, 198–99, 207–8, 283n65, 292n50; biological theories of, 8, 26, 144–45, 180–81, 197–98; class and, 130–32, 134–35, 140–41, 292n47; as doctors, 201, 293n57; economics and, 25, 120–21, 130–32, 206–8; enslavement of, 131, 198–99, 201, 247, 205–6, 291–92n34; gender performance of, 118–19; heroism of, 199–200; illnesses of, 130, 132, 137, 140, 144–45, 201–2, 283n65; mothering and, 198, 204–6, 247, 291n35; nursing tradition and, 26, 135, 182–83, 198–99, 205–7, 291–92n38; regenerative power of, 26, 181, 183, 198, 200–201, 204–6, 208; and relation to Civil War story, 9, 17, 130–31, 182–84, 262n31, 269n9; representative experience of, 130–31; romantic relationships of, 137–

Acknowledgments

I begin by gratefully recognizing the institutions that have supported my book. A University of Wisconsin fellowship helped to speed early work along. A Francis Clark Wood Fellowship from the College of Physicians of Philadelphia allowed me to examine S. Weir Mitchell's papers. Charles Grifenstein, a fellow Mitchell enthusiast, was particularly helpful in Philadelphia. And I thank North Central College for supporting the last stages of the project through summer research grants and a Junior Faculty Enhancement Fellowship. The North Central librarians, particularly June Johnson, have been a great help. I also acknowledge the following institutions for granting me permission to reproduce material from their collections and for the helpful and efficient staff members with whom I have corresponded at each: the Photographs and Prints Division of the Schomburg Center for Research on Black Culture, The New York Public Library, for the photograph of Susie King Taylor; the Ohio Historical Society for extracts from their Paul Laurence Dunbar Papers; the College of Physicians of Philadelphia for quotations and a photograph from their S. Weir Mitchell Papers; and the National Museum of Health and Medicine for the cover image.

The day-to-day work of writing is relieved mainly by the dinners, phone calls, and e-mails of colleagues and friends. My thanks go to the special people in my life during the many years that I have lived with this project. Some have generously read my work, others have given me a place to stay when I needed it, and all have provided emotional support and a sense of intellectual community at different points in my life: Richelle Munkhoff, William Kuskin, Denise Aulik, Christine Damrow, Theresa Strouth Gaul, and Melvina Young when we were all at Wisconsin; my lecturer compatriots during our stint at Michigan State University, Phoebe Jackson, Tersh Palmer, Greg Garvey, Carl Eby, Leon Jackson, Charles Hannon, and especially Lisa Rashley, who has since become a great friend and a valued editor; and my North Central colleagues, Sara Eaton, Richard Glejzer, Jennifer Jackson, and Anna Leahy.

I am also grateful to the Civil War scholars who have become my friends while I have been working on this project: Elizabeth Young, Jane Schultz, and especially Kathleen Diffley and Timothy Sweet, both of whom provided valuable, meticulous readings of the entire manuscript. Not only their fine scholarship but also their generosity and collegiality have inspired me. This book has benefited from the attentions of many colleagues, all of whom have brought their unique skills to bear on my work. I want to acknowledge Tom Lutz for his careful and encouraging review, Jeffrey Steele for his early and unwavering enthusiasm, Sargent Bush for his astute editorial eye, and Steven Kantrowitz for a valuable historical perspective. I owe my sincerest thanks to Dale Bauer. She has read endless versions of this book, patiently, efficiently, always insightfully, and with a sense of humor. I am lucky, indeed, to have had such a marvelous teacher and to now have such a wonderful friend.

Many others have offered advice and support at key moments: Sharon Harris, Jean Pfaelzer, Steven Arch, Cynthia Davis, Denise Knight, John Ernest, Philip Gould, Carol Farley Kessler, Don Dingeldine, Lucy Frank, Doug Noverr, and Gordon Hutner. Their keen insights have sharpened my work in important ways. Bob Brugger's enthusiasm for the project was instrumental in bringing it to print. Finally, I am fortunate to have had the opportunity to publish with the University of Pennsylvania Press. I owe Jerry Singerman a great debt for believing in the book and for deftly nudging me in all the right directions. I also thank Rebecca Rich, Erica Ginsburg, and the editorial staff at Penn for their cheerful aid.

Last but certainly not least, my heartfelt thanks go to my family. I am grateful to Joel Long, Kady Long, Andrew Long, and now Garet Long for providing joyful, laughter-filled breaks to the writing routine. Joe and Donna Long have offered constant encouragement. Glen and Barty Amundson, Laurie Keinberger, and Gwen and Dayton Carlson have welcomed me into their family with open arms. My mother, Lou Ann Long, and the memory of my grandmother, Stacy Estenson, continue to inspire my work, for they serve as examples of women's extraordinary endurance and grace. Their love and care are the foundation of all that I do. Finally, I owe my love and gratitude to James Amundson. I couldn't ask for a more generous and supportive partner. He makes it all possible.

The following material was previously published in different form: part of Chapter 2 appeared as " 'The Corporeity of Heaven': Rehabilitating the Civil War Body in *The Gates Ajar*" in *American Literature* 69.4 (December 1997); part of Chapter 4 appeared as "Charlotte Forten's Civil War Journals and the Quest for 'Genius, Beauty, and Deathless Fame'" in *Legacy* 16.1 (Spring 1999); and part of Chapter 5 appeared in the critical introduction to my edition of Paul Laurence Dunbar's *The Fanatics* (Acton, Mass.: Copley Publishing Group, 2001).